# Illustrated Pediatric Dentistry (Part 4)

Edited by

**Satyawan Damle**
*Former Professor of Pediatric Dentistry,
Dean Nair Hospital Dental College,
Mumbai, India*


*Former Vice Chancellor,
Maharishi Markandeshwar University,
Mullana, Ambala, India*

**Ritesh Kalaskar**
*Department of Pedodontic and Preventive Dentistry,
Government Dental College & Hospital, Nagpur,
India*


&


**Dhanashree Sakhare**
*Founder, Lavanika Dental Academy
Melbourne
Australia*

# Illustrated Pediatric Dentistry (Part 4)

Editors: Satyawan Damle, Ritesh Kalaskar and Dhanashree Sakhare

ISBN (Online): 978-981-5080-83-4

ISBN (Print): 978-981-5080-84-1

ISBN (Paperback): 978-981-5080-85-8

need for a court order if at any point you breach any terms of this License Agreement. In no event will any delay or failure by Bentham Science Publishers in enforcing your compliance with this License Agreement constitute a waiver of any of its rights.

3. You acknowledge that you have read this License Agreement, and agree to be bound by its terms and conditions. To the extent that any other terms and conditions presented on any website of Bentham Science Publishers conflict with, or are inconsistent with, the terms and conditions set out in this License Agreement, you acknowledge that the terms and conditions set out in this License Agreement shall prevail.

**Bentham Science Publishers Pte. Ltd.**
80 Robinson Road #02-00
Singapore 068898
Singapore
Email: subscriptions@benthamscience.net

**BENTHAM
SCIENCE**

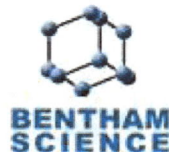

# CONTENTS

**CHAPTER 4 DRUGS USED IN PEDIATRIC DENTISTRY** .......... 116
*Abdulkadeer M. Jetpurwala, Shely P. Dedhia* and *Vidya Iyer*

*Sarita Fernandes* and *Esha Kodal*

# FOREWORD 1

It is my great pleasure to pen down a foreword for this tremendous book on Pediatric Dentistry for a legend and doyen of the subject, a mentor and guide to the brightest of minds in the field of dentistry.

Rising from the fundamentals, comprehensive in-built, contemporary and authoritative in construct and approach, and hands-on to the core, *Illustrated Pediatric Dentistry* is a wonderful work engineered by some of the best-known academics in this noble realm. The chief author, *Professor Satyawan Damle*, is a colossus among giants, having been a celebrated teacher, distinguished leader, and dynamic policymaker at several dental institutions and universities, including the most prized, the University of Mumbai.

Prof. Satyawan Damle is the rare blend of a gifted clinician and a carved-out academic guru whose intellect has emerged with decades of practice. It is no secret that the degree of acquisition of knowledge by students is one of the measures of the effectiveness of a medical curriculum; and with Pediatric Dentistry being one of the crucial epicentres of growth, it has the potential to make momentous advancements in the evolutionary trajectory of oral and general health.

His co-editors *Ritesh Kalaskar*, and *Dhanashree Sakhare* are examples excellence in their arena. The work reflects their collective understanding of where pediatric dentistry stands today, what have been the treasures and well-kept secrets of the past, and where this tree of knowledge finds fruition today pawing way for the future.

Embedding best care practices of all times, *Illustrated Pediatric Dentistry* is a comprehensive yet concise work, which fulfills the essentials of the pediatric dentistry curriculum both for graduates and postgraduates across all universities.

Walking you through the nitty-gritties of preventive, curative and restorative childhood dentistry, be it the behavioral challenges, cariology, endodontics, traumatology, para-surgical themes such as the use of conscious sedation and general anaesthesia at that age, and the management of medically compromised children, the work is a tree of knowledge, nurtured with experiential learning, and carries wonderful blossoms of practical wisdom.

Let us savour and celebrate the chef-d'oeuvre. Indeed, *Illustrated Pediatric Dentistry* is a must-read and must-assimilate work for each one of us. Students, practitioners and teachers of Pediatric dentistry will cherish it as a treasured possession on their shelves. I congratulate Prof. Damle and Bentham Science, Singapore, for publishing this irreplaceable tome.

**Prof. (Dr.) Mahesh Verma**
Vice Chancellor
Guru Gobind Singh
Indraprastha University,
New Delhi,
India

# FOREWORD 2

I am delighted to write this foreword for a Book of Illustrated Pediatric Dentistry authored by Professor Satyawan Damle and other academicians. Prof. Satyawan Damle is a well-known researcher and academician with over 44 years of clinical and teaching experience in Dentistry. Besides the several posts and hats he wore in the various roles he played for the profession, he is also a recipient of several awards and recognitions, including the Lifetime Achievement Awards, Outstanding Public Servant Awards, and Research Awards and Fellowships. He is an active member of the Indian Council of Medical Research. Despite his extraordinary achievements as a Pediatric dentist, researcher, and academician, Prof Satyawan Damle will always be known as the longest-serving chief editor of Indexed journals. For almost 35 years. He dedicated himself to overseeing the publication of the highest-quality peer-reviewed studies and opinion pieces on child dental health.

Prof. Damle is actively involved in writing several books on Pediatric Dentistry and Dentistry, which is the testimony of his in-depth knowledge of the subject. The Book of Illustrated Pediatric Dentistry is their new venture initiated by him. I am confident that this book will be accepted by students and faculty involved in teaching Pediatric Dentistry. His work as a teacher, researcher, innovator, visionary and extraordinary academician made him a legend. His role as a mentor and friend made him a role model to those of us who know him and worked with him. His legacy persists not only in academics but also as an able administrator, as he proved his mettle as the Dean of a dental school, Director of Medical Education, Joint Municipal.

Commissioner of Mumbai and, ultimately, the Vice Chancellor of a University. Prof. Damle has worked conscientiously and untiringly to present an unmatched educational endeavour. The topics in this book display a clear and succinct clinical expertise and the capability of imparting updated education and information to Oral Health Professionals. The entire volume of this book deals with ultramodern and current state-of-the-art techniques. I take this opportunity to congratulate Prof. Satyawan Damle and his team of contributors - Ritesh Kalaskar, and Dhanashree Sakhare for having published this Textbook for Bentham Sciences.

**Dr. Ashok Dhoble. Hon. Secretary**
General, Indian Dental Association H.O.
India

# PREFACE

It is imperative to have an established approach to handling Children's oral diseases. **'Illustrated Pediatric Dentistry'** is an unpretentious endeavour to integrate the latest developments and up-to-date reviews in the field of Pediatric dentistry by distinguished writers. The book intends to allow students to understand the conceptions of Pediatric dentistry and create a spur to discover the subject by advance reading. Several illustrations, descriptions and graphic drawings have been included to attract the students and make the subject simple to comprehend. A healthy mouth is a gateway to a healthy body and the best time to inculcate healthy habits is through childhood. Prevention of the initiation of oral diseases and training appropriate oral hygiene methods are commenced best throughout the formative years of the child. With a substantial percentage of the worldwide population being in the Pediatric age group, it is imperious to have a scientific approach to behaviour management, prevention and treatment modalities in the dental office, as Pediatric dentistry is a fast-growing division of dental disciplines that lays the basis for the impending dental health of the populace.

The book has been divided into several sections. The sections on child psychology and the emotional development of children are important to learn the basics of various behaviour management strategies. The section on dental caries sensitizes the reader towards the most common dental disorder that is seen in children, and preventive procedures aimed towards lessening dental caries are the necessity of the hour. While an endeavour has been made to include the growth and development of the facial structures and dentition and along with their disturbances and the interceptive and preventive procedures to monitor the erupting teeth.

Pediatric Operative techniques, including endodontics and management of teeth with immature apices affected due to Dental caries and traumatic injuries have been given prominence. Innovations in the field of Pediatric Dentistry are transpiring amazingly fast, and it is crucial to stay up to date with the latest materials, equipment and techniques to deliver the highest quality of care to our little patients.

The New Book cannot be successfully compiled without the collective contribution regarding meticulous reviews of the manuscript to keep pace with the latest innovative novelties. The credit for introducing a New Textbook goes to the contributors for their engrossment, devotion and dedication in presenting a manuscript after applying prudent and well-adjudged scrutiny and analytical approach and have excelled in exploring things to the ultimate.

Accumulation of information and its cogent management would not have been conceivable without the efforts of the contributors who have painstakingly submitted their manuscripts to shape this gargantuan task and introduce this book in the service of Pediatric dentistry.

**Satyawan Damle**
Former Professor of Pediatric Dentistry,
Dean Nair Hospital Dental College,
Mumbai, India

Former Vice-Chancellor,
Maharishi Markandeshwar University,
Mullana, Ambala, India

**Ritesh Kalaskar**
Department of Pedodontic and Preventive Dentistry
Government Dental College & Hospital, Nagpur
India

&

**Dhanashree Sakhare**
Founder,
Lavanika Dental Academy,
Melbourne
Australia

# ACKNOWLEDGEMENTS

We do not find such appropriate words to praise the unique nature of Dr. Mahesh Verma, Vice Chancellor of Guru Gobind Singh Indraprastha University, New Delhi, who himself being a great resolute and connoisseur of dentistry occupying an illustrious position with an eminent background in dentistry, has spared his valuable time from his busy schedule to inscribe the foreword for the Textbook of" Illustrated Pediatric Dentistry." We take it as inventiveness and encouragement rather than a morale-boosting for us to uphold and keep up our determination to satisfy our hunger for academics for the advantage of budding dental professionals.

We also do not find such befitting words to laud the unique nature of Dr. Ashok Dhoble Hon, General Secretary Indian, Dental Association Head Office, who himself is a great advocate and connoisseur of dentistry occupying a distinguished position with an illustrious background in dentistry has spared his precious time from his busy schedule to write the foreword for the Textbook of Illustrated Pediatric Dentistry. I take it as an inspiration and encouragement rather than a morale-boosting for us to uphold and keep up our determination to satisfy our hunger for academics for the advantage of budding dental professionals.

We are also indebted and beholden to the contributors for their altruistic and substantial contribution to make this Textbook of Illustrated Pediatric Dentistry, a great academic endeavour. The contributors are highly competent and knowledgeable clinicians known for their aptitude and capability, which have successfully recognized the most complex and convoluted details of each topic, duly integrating and blending the latest advancements and innovations in Pediatric Dentistry. They are a terrific hard worker and legendary luminaries known for their admirable accomplishments and remarkable involvement in dental education. They have made lots of efforts to lead things to excellence. Credit goes to these patrons and benefactors for the benevolent bequest of their vast knowledge and experience for the betterment of dental education.

We would also like to thank Dr. Priyanka Bhaje, Dr. Parag Kasar, Dr. Sharath Chandra, Dr. Prachi Goyal and Dr. Vidya Iyer for their painstaking efforts and intransigent toil during the editing of this book. They displayed exceptional patients, forbearance, and commitment during the preparation of the book Our dream has come true due to the support of our past and present students. Credit also goes to our family members for their tolerance, Love, and affection.

We would like to appreciate the efforts of Mrs. Humaira Hashmi & Mrs. Fariya Zulfiqar of Bentham Science for giving us an opportunity to pen down our ideas and academic work into reality. We also convey our kind and sincere appreciation to Pascali Pascalis.

Representative of Porter Instrument Business Unit of Parker Hannifin Matrx by Parker and Parker-Porter Product for permitting us to use the company products in our book.

Lastly, we would like to state that fortune favours those who defy complexities and overcome them on their own. We also passionately believe that Man is the architect of his own destiny, and God is on the side of those who toil and perspire to make their providence.

We place our sincerest admiration and gratitude to all those who have delightfully contributed to this cause and for their wishes and devotions made for understanding our dream.

**Satyawan Damle**
Former Professor of Pediatric Dentistry,
Dean Nair Hospital Dental College,
Mumbai, India

Former Vice-Chancellor,
Maharishi Markandeshwar University,
Mullana, Ambala, India

**Ritesh Kalaskar**
Department of Pedodontic and Preventive Dentistry
Government Dental College & Hospital, Nagpur
India

&

**Dhanashree Sakhare**
Founder,
Lavanika Dental Academy,
Melbourne
Australia

# List of Contributors

| | |
|---|---|
| **Abdulkadeer Jetpurwala** | Department of Pediatric Dentistry, Nair Hospital Dental College, Mumbai, India |
| **Abi M. Thomas** | Christian Dental College Ludhiana, Ludhiana, Punjab 141008, India |
| **Alka Halbe** | Breach Candy Hospital Trust, Mumbai, India |
| **Alireza Mirzaei** | RWTH Aachen University, 52062 Aachen, Germany |
| **Amit Jain** | Consultant Implantologist, Mumbai, India |
| **Anahita Bagheri** | RWTH Aachen University, 52062 Aachen, Germany |
| **Andi Setiawan Budihardja** | Department of Oral Maxillofacial Surgery, Faculty of Medicine, University of Pelita Harapan, Tangerang, Indonesia |
| **Armelia Sari Widyarman** | Department of Oral Biology, Faculty of Dentistry, Trisakti University, Jakarta, Indonesia |
| **Bahman Seraj** | Department of Pediatric Dentistry, Dental Faculty, Tehran University of Medical Science, Tehran, Iran |
| **Bhagyashree Shetty** | Junior Research Officer, Pune, India |
| **Bhavna H. Dave** | Department of Pediatric and Preventive Dentistry, K.M. Shah Dental College and Hospital, Sumandeep Vidyapeeth Deemed to Be University, Vadodara, Gujarat, India |
| **Deepashri Meshram** | Department of Oral and Maxillofacial Surgery, Nair Hospital Dental College, Mumbai, India |
| **Devendra Nagpal** | Department of Pediatric Dentistry, VSPM Dental College and Research Centre, Nagpur, India |
| **Dhanashree Sakhare** | Founder, Lavanika Dental Academy, Melbourne, Australia |
| **Esha Kodal** | Department of Anesthesiology, TNMC & BYL Nair Ch. Hospital, Mumbai, India |
| **Falguni Shah** | Lilavati hospital and Research Centre, Mumbai, India |
| **Gholam Hossein Ramezani** | Department of Pediatric Dentistry, Dental Faculty, Islamic Azad University of Medical Science, Tehran, Iran |
| **Harsimran Kaur** | Department of Pedodontics and Preventive Dentistry, Teerthanker Mahaveer Dental College and Research Centre, Moradabad, U.P, India |
| **Jeddy** | Department of Pediatric Dentistry, Faculty of Dentistry, Trisakti University, Jakarta, Indonesia |
| **Mona Sohrabi** | Department of Pediatric Dentistry, Qazvin University of Medical Sciences, Qazvin, Iran |
| **Madulika Kabra** | Division of Medical Genetics, Department of Pediatrics, AIIMS, New Delhi, India |
| **N. Venugopal Reddy** | Mamata Dental College & Hospital, Khammam, Telangana 507002, India |
| **Naveen Manuja** | Department of Pediatric and Preventive Dentistry, Kothiwal Dental College, Moradabad, India |

**Neeraj Gugnani** — Department of Pediatric and Preventive Dentistry, DAV (C) Dental College, Yamuna Nagar, Haryana, India

**Niraja Gupta** — Division of Medical Genetics, Department of Pediatrics, AIIMS, New Delhi, India

**Nilima Thosar** — Department,of Pediatric and Preventive Dentistry, Sharad Pawar Dental College and Hospital, Datta Meghe Institute of Medical Sciences (Deemed to be University), Wardha-442107, India

**Parag D. Kasar** — Deep Dental Clinic, Navi Mumbai, Maharashtra 400706, India

**Prachi Goyal** — Department of Pediatric and Preventive Dentistry, MMCDSR, Mullana, Ambala, India

**Pratik B. Kariya** — Department of Pediatric and Preventive Dentistry, K.M. Shah Dental College and Hospital, Sumandeep Vidyapeeth Deemed to Be University, Vadodara, Gujarat, India

**Ramakrishna Yeluri** — Department of Pedodontics and Preventive Dentistry, Teerthanker Mahaveer Dental College and Research Centre, Moradabad, U.P, India

**Razieh Jabbarian** — Department of Pediatric Dentistry, Qazvin University of Medical Sciences, Qazvin, Iran

**Rishika** — Department of Pedodontics and Preventive Dentistry, Teerthanker Mahaveer Dental College and Research Centre, Moradabad, U.P, India

**Sarita Fernandes** — Department of Anesthesiology, TNMC & BYL Nair Ch. Hospital, Mumbai, India

**Satyawan Damle** — Former Professor of Pediatric Dentistry, Dean Nair Hospital Dental College, Mumbai, India; Former Vice Chancellor, Maharishi Markandeshwar University, Mullana, Ambala, India

**Shely P. Dedhia** — Department of Pediatric and Preventive Dentistry, Nair Hospital Dental College, Madurai, Tamilnadu, India

**Vidya Iyer** — Ex Associate Professor, Department of Pediatric and Preventive Dentistry, CSI College of Dental Sciences, East Veli Street, Madurai, Tamilnadu, India

**Vishwas Chaugule** — Ex Professor, Department of Paediatric and Preventive Dentistry, Sinhgad Dental College and Hospital, Pune, India

**Vishwas Patil** — Ex Professor, Department of Paediatric and Preventive Dentistry, Dr. D.Y. Patil Dental College and Hospital, Pimpri, Pune, India

# CHAPTER 1

# Local Anesthesia in Pediatric Dentistry

**Devendra Nagpal**[1], **Deepashri Meshram**[2,*] and **Abdulkadeer Jetpurwala**[3]

[1] *Department of Pediatric Dentistry, VSPM Dental College and Research Centre. Nagpur, India*

[2] *Department of Oral and Maxillofacial Surgery, Nair Hospital Dental College, Mumbai, India*

[3] *Department of Pediatric Dentistry, Nair Hospital Dental College, Mumbai, India*

**Abstract:** Dental treatment has been associated with pain by adults and children alike. The fear associated with the perceived pain causes a lot of anxiety and is a common cause for patients to show avoidance towards basic dental care. A painless experience during dental treatment allows children to look forward to future dental appointments and allows the dentist to establish a good rapport with the child. Various agents are available for the administration of local anesthesia with lignocaine being the most common agent. As children have unique physiology and anatomic variations, the techniques for local anesthesia require minor modifications. Advances in local anesthesia materials and techniques have provided the dental surgeon to accomplish the goal of true painless dentistry.

**Keywords:** Dental Treatment, Lignocaine, Local Anesthesia, Pain.

## INTRODUCTION

Local anesthesia is the temporary or reversible loss of sensation including pain in a specific part of the body produced by a topically applied or injected agent without depressing the level of consciousness. Providing a pain-free experience to children is the most important aspect of pediatric dentistry which helps to alleviate anxiety and instill a positive attitude towards dental treatment. Considering the innate fear of pain and injections in children it is all the more vital to carry out this key step in a child-friendly manner.

As with any anesthetic medical, dental, or surgical procedure, a careful and thorough preoperative evaluation must be conducted before the selection of technique and agents. This should include a review of medical history with special emphasis on past anesthetic experiences, a focused physical examination, determination of physical risk, and the potential for adverse drug interactions. The

* **Corresponding author Deepashri Meshram:** Department of Oral and Maxillofacial Surgery, Nair Hospital Dental College, Mumbai, India; E-mail: 24deemes@gmail.com

**Satyawan Damle, Ritesh Kalaskar & Dhanashree Sakhare (Eds.)**

patient's weight and body mass index are also important considerations. The historical perspective of local anesthesia has been shown in Table **1**.

Table 1. History of local anesthesia.

| 1859-60 | Albert Niemann was the first to isolate cocaine and discover its anesthetic properties |
|---|---|
| 1884 | Karl Koller introduced cocaine into clinical practice of medicine, using it as topical anesthetic for opthalmological surgical procedures |
| 1892 | Alfred Einhorn initiated the search and in 1905 for injectable local anesthetics |
| 1905 | Procaine (novocaine), the first injectable local anesthetic |
| 1948 | Introduction of Lidocaine |

## Physiology of Nerve

**Nerve** – It is a cord-like bundle of fibers surrounded by a sheet that connects the nervous system with other parts of the body. The nerve conducts impulses towards and away from the central nervous system.

**Neuron** – It is a structural and functional unit of the nervous system.

Parts of Neurons

1. **The Cell body** – It contains the nucleus & other cell organelles.

2. **Dendrites** – It extends from the cell body & receives nerve impulses from the neurons.

3. **The Axon** – It is a long extension of the cell body that transmits nerve impulses to other cells.

The axon branches at the end, forming axon terminals. These are the points where neurons communicate with other cells.

Normal **depolarization** causes changes in the nerve membrane that allow for the passage of sodium ions through specific channels resulting in the propagation of action potential along the nerve.

An **action potential** is defined as a sudden, fast, transitory, and propagating change of the resting membrane potential. Only neurons and muscle cells are capable of generating an action potential and this property is called **excitability**.

There is a passage of an electrical impulse along the length of the axon. This flow of electricity is due to the movement of ions across the membrane of the axon. An action potential travels down an axon causing a change in polarity across the membrane of the axon. In response to a signal from another neuron, sodium ($Na^+$) and potassium ($K^+$) gated ion channels open and close as the membrane reaches its threshold potential. $Na^+$ channels open at the beginning of the action potential and $Na^+$ moves into the axon, causing depolarization. Repolarization occurs when the $K^+$ channels open and $K^+$ moves out of the axon, creating a change in polarity between the intra and extracellular fluid. The impulse travels down the axon unidirectional to the axon terminal where it signals other neurons [1].

Five Phases of action potential (Fig. **1**):

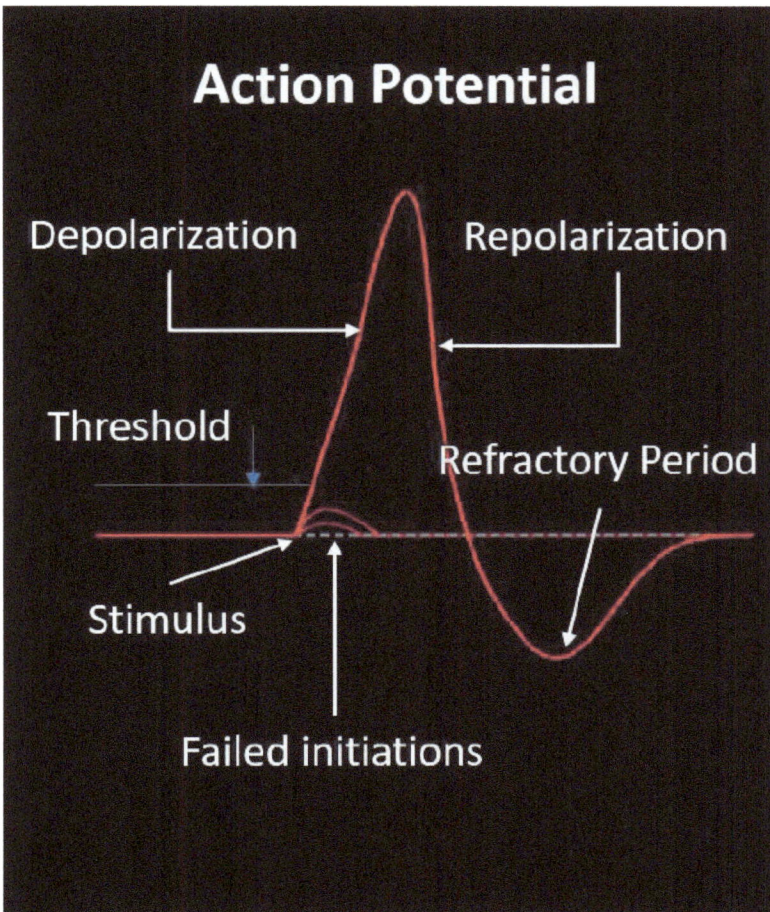

**Fig. (1).** Stages of nerve impulse.

1. **Rising Phase** – During this phase, the membrane potential depolarizes (becomes more positive).

2. **Peak Phase** – The point at which depolarization stops and the membrane potential reaches a maximum.

3. **Falling Phase** – During this phase, the membrane potential becomes negative returning towards resting potential.

4. **The Undershoot (after hyperpolarization) Phase** – It is the period during which the membrane potential temporarily becomes more negatively charged than when at rest (hyperpolarized).

5. **Refractory Period** – This is the phase during which subsequent action potential is impossible or difficult to fire and there will be no response to stimuli. It lasts for 1 millisecond.

6. **Saltatory Conduction** – It is the propagation of action potential along myelinated axons from one node of Ranvier to the next node.

**General Principles of Local anesthesia (LA)**

1. LA binds to specific sites within sodium channels and thus impairs conduction.

2. As more receptors bind to LA there is a progressive reduction in the rate and degree of depolarization until conduction fails.

3. Nerve conduction will get disrupted when a critical length of a nerve is exposed to a local anesthetic solution.

4. For halting saltatory conduction, a longer critical length of the nerve is required for exposure to local anesthetic for a block to occur.

5. There is a differential sensitivity to the effects of local anesthetic as influenced by the diameter of the nerve fiber and frequency of the impulses along nerve fibers.

6. Larger diameter myelinated fibers have a greater internodal distance than smaller myelinated fibers.

7. When local anesthetics are applied to a nerve trunk, pain fibers are blocked first, followed by temperature, touch, pressure, and motor functions.

8. Smaller nerve fibers, either myelinated or unmyelinated, typically transmit pain and proprioceptive impulses, whereas larger myelinated fibers carry motor impulses.

9. High-frequency impulses make more sodium channels available to exposure by LA and these fibers are blocked faster than slower frequency fibers.

10. During the diffusion of LA through the nerve bundle the outer or mantle axons are affected first and the core later.

11. In the case of the inferior alveolar nerve, proximal structures are innervated by the mantle fibers (outer) and distal structures are innervated by the core. The onset of an inferior alveolar nerve block is therefore proximal to the distal, molars to incisors, and lower lip. Recovery is also proximal to the distal, with the lip being the last to recover from the block.

## Action of LA

1. LA exists in the ionized (cation) and unionized (anion) form.

2. Action of LA depends upon both the ionized and unionized form of the drug.

3. The ionized form of the drug is water-soluble.

4. The nonionized form of the drug is lipid-soluble (soluble in the plasma membrane of a cell/axon).

5. The ionized form of LA is most active at the receptor site. It binds at the receptor site by inhibiting sodium influx.

6. Sodium channels are lipoproteins.

7. The nonionized form is the one that is important for membrane penetration.

8. The pH and pKa are important in determining the ionization of the drug.

9. When the LA is injected into the infected tissue the local tissue pH is low which leads to a more ionized form.

10. LA is not only specific for sensory neurons but also blocks motor fibers, hence the dropping mouth following a visit to a dentist occurs.

## LA Shares a Common Structure Comprising Three Elements

1. A lipophilic aromatic ring

2. An ester or amide link

3. A terminal amine group – The amine group may exist as a tertiary form *i.e.*, unionized and lipid-soluble, or as a quaternary form *i.e.*, ionized and water-

soluble. Lipid solubility enhances potency.

## Calcium and Magnesium Ions

1. The extracellular $Ca^{2+}$ helps to close the sodium channels.

2. An increase in Magnesium enhances the potency of lidocaine at high stimulation frequency [2].

## Ideal Properties of Local Anesthetic Agent [3]

1. Its action must be reversible.

2. It must be non-irritating to the tissues and produce no secondary local reaction.

3. It should have a low degree of systemic toxicity.

4. It should have a rapid onset and be of sufficient duration.

5. It should be able to anesthetize the tissue completely without any harm.

6. It should be effective as the topical anesthetic.

7. It should not produce any allergic reactions.

8. It should be stable in solution and undergo biotransformation readily within the body.

9. It should be sterile are capable of being sterilized without deterioration.

## Classification of LA

They are categorized into 2 different classes based on their structure: - (Table **2**)

1. Para-aminobenzoic acid (PABA) based known as **esters**.

2. Non-PABA-based anesthetics are termed as an **amide**.

**Table 2. Types of local anesthesia according to their structure.**

| Amides | Esters |
|---|---|
| Lidocaine (or lignocaine) | Cocaine |
| Prilocaine | Procaine |
| Mepivacaine | Chloroprocaine |
| Etidocaine | Tetracaine (Amethocaine) |

*(Table 2) cont.....*

| Amides | Esters |
|---|---|
| Bupivacaine | Benzocaine |
| Ropivacaine | - |
| Levobupivacaine | - |

## Classification of Local Anesthetic Agents Depending Upon Their Duration

Ultra-short acting anesthetics – (less than 30 minutes)

- Procaine without a vasoconstrictor
- 2-chloroprocaine without a vasoconstrictor
- 2% lidocaine without the vasoconstrictor
- 4% prilocaine without vasoconstrictor for infiltration
  Short-acting anesthetics– (45 to 75 minutes)
- 2% lidocaine with 1: 100000 epinephrine
- 2% mepivacaine with 1: 200000epinephrine
- 4% prilocaine when used for nerve block
- 2% procaine, 4% propoxycaine with a vasoconstrictor
  Medium acting anesthetics- (90 to 150 minutes)
- 4% prilocaine with 1:200000 epinephrine
- 2% lidocaine and 2% mepivacaine with the vasoconstrictor may produce pulpal anesthesia of this duration
  Long-acting anesthetics – (180 minutes or longer)
- 5% Bupivacaine with 1:200000 epinephrine
- 5% or 1.5% etidocaine with 1:20000 epinephrine

## Lidocaine (Lignocaine)

Chemically lignocaine is 2-diethylaminoaceto-2', 6'-xylidide ($C_{14}H_{22}N_2O$). It is a stable, crystalline, colorless solid whose hydrochloride salt is water-soluble. Solutions for injections are available with or without adrenaline added in the ratio of 1: 2000000 or 1: 80000. All lignocaine solutions should be protected from light and maintained at room temperature of approximately 25°C or 77°F. It has a pKa – 7.7. Inflamed tissue may have pH as low as 6.8 while normal tissue pH of extracellular fluid is 7.4. Lidocaine is sometimes given with bicarbonate to alkalinize the area and make the drug more lipid soluble and enhance the action of the drug. Lignocaine is absorbed rapidly into the blood from the site of injection. The duration of action is limited but can be prolonged if the blood flood is reduced. Its effect depends upon the dose given, the concentration used, type of nerve blocked, and status of the patient.

## Indications

1. Local neuraxial, regional, or peripheral anesthesia.

2. Infiltration, block, or topical application

3. Prophylaxis or treatment of life-threatening ventricular arrhythmias.

## Absorption

1. The speed of onset of LA is 1-5 minutes after local infiltration

2. 5-15 minutes after peripheral nerve block

3. Absorption is dependent upon the total dose administered, the route, by which it is delivered, and the blood supply at the site of the injection.

4. Peak serum level occurred 20-30 minutes following injection.

5. The addition of adrenaline (1:200000) to the local anesthetic solution reduces peak levels and delays the rate of absorption.

### Antiarrhythmic Effect

LA decreases action potential length and refractory period duration of Purkinje fibers.

### Anti-nociceptive Effects

LA blocks the neuronal sodium channels and potassium currents and the blockage of presynaptic muscarinic and class 1B dopamine receptors [4].

### Anti-inflammatory Effects

Lignocaine has been documented to block the release of interleukin 1(IL-1), an inflammatory mediator acting on polymorphonuclear granulocytes, which in turn activates phagocytosis, respiratory burst, degranulation, and chemotaxis. This reduction in the release of interleukins may contribute to the lignocaine anti-inflammatory effect.

### Antibacterial Activity

Both amide and ester-type local anesthetics can inhibit bacteria in high enough concentration, for example, gram-positive Staphylococcus aureus and Staphylocoocus pneumonia, gram-negative Haemophilus influenza, and Pseudomonas aeruginosa [4].

## Protein Binding

- The plasma binding of lignocaine is inversely proportional to the drug concentration. Plasma binding also depends on the plasma level of the acute phase reactant α-1-glycoproteins.
- Lignocaine has been shown to cross the placenta and blood-brain barrier by simple passive diffusion.
- Maternal protein binding is greater than fetal protein.
- Lignocaine crosses the placenta in the unionized form in fetal acidosis.

## Metabolism [3]

- Lignocaine is dealkylated in the liver by the cytochrome p-40 system
- Metabolism takes place in the liver.
- Monoethyl glycine xylidide and glycine xylidide are the key active metabolites.
- The rate of metabolism is slower in patients with congestive cardiac failure, chronic liver disease, and hepatic insufficiency and after acute myocardial infarction
- Lignocaine and its metabolites are predominantly excreted by kidneys while less than 10% of lignocaine is excreted without being metabolized.
- Its metabolite para-aminobenzoic acid (PABA) is responsible for allergic reactions in patients who have this enzyme in abnormal or inadequate form.

**Elimination Half-life** is defined as the rate at which the amount of the drug in the blood is reduced by half. The elimination half-life of lidocaine is biphasic and around 90 minutes to 120 minutes in most patients. This may be prolonged in congestive heart failure and hepatic impairment.

## Contraindications

1. Known hypersensitivity

2. Sinoatrial disorders

3. All grades of atrioventricular block

4. Severe myocardial depression

5. Porphyria

6. Complete heart block

7. Hypovolemia

## Instructions for Use/ Handling

- Adequate precautions should be taken to avoid prolonged contact between local anesthetic solutions containing adrenaline (epinephrine) (low PH) and metal surfaces. *e.g.*, needle or metal part of syringe since dissolved metal ions particularly copper ions may cause severe local irritation (swelling, edema) at the injection site and accelerate the degradation of adrenaline.
- Surface sterilization should be done using undiluted isopropyl alcohol 91% or 70% ethyl alcohol on the skin and dry mucosa.
- In the oral cavity, surface disinfection may be done by a betadine soaked cotton swab (Fig. **2**)
- The solutions which are free from preservatives should be used immediately after opening the vial.
- Aspiration before the injection is recommended to reduce the possibility of intravascular injection.
- Atraumatic techniques should be used to avoid nerve injury.

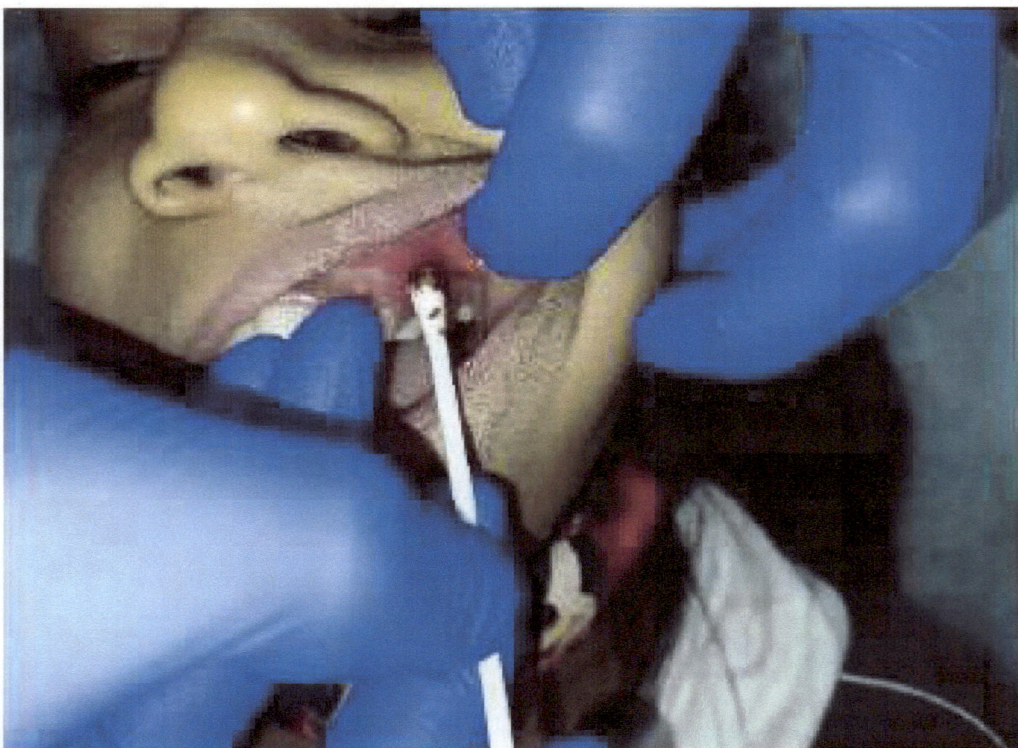

**Fig. (2).** Application of betadine at the injection site.

## Composition of LA (Fig. 3)

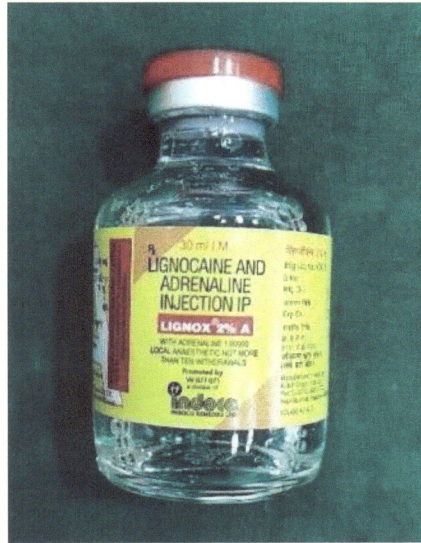

**Fig. (3).** Local anesthesia.

1. Lignocaine hydrochloride monohydrate is the active ingredient 2% (20mg/ml)

Lidocaine 1% means 1:100 dilution

Therefore 2 ml of the solution will contain,

2 x10 mg = 20 mg of lidocaine

Lidocaine is generally available as a 2% solution

A standard vial of lignocaine contains 1.8 ml of solution = 20 X 1.8 = 36 mg of LA

2. Reducing agent/ antioxidant/ antibacterial- Sodium Metabisulfite (0.5 mg)

3. Preservative- Methyl paraben 0.1% (1mg)

4. Diluting agent- distilled water

5. Fungicide- Thymol

6. Isotonic solution- Sodium chloride or Ringer's solution (6mg)

7. Vasoconstrictor- adrenaline (1:80,000 or 1:2,00,000)

8. Sodium Hydroxide: - to adjust pH

9. Nitrogen bubble - 1-2 mm in diameter to prevent oxygen from being trapped in the cartridge and potentially destroying the vasopressor.

The most used local anesthetics for pediatric dentistry are **amide-type agents**. Lidocaine hydrochloride (2% with 1:100000 epinephrine) is preferred because of its low allergenic characteristics and its greater potency at a lower concentration. Local anesthetics without vasoconstrictors should be used with caution due to rapid systemic absorption which may result in overdose.

A long-acting local anesthetic (*i.e.* Bupivacaine) is not recommended for a child or the physically or mentally disabled patient due to its prolonged effect, which increases the risk of post-operative soft tissue self-self-injury.

## Patient Management While Administering Local Anesthetic Injections

The most common fear in children is that of a needle. When a child has to undergo an injection, in the oral cavity it increases the level of difficulty for the operator as obtaining the profound effect of the drug, it has to be done with the right technique and the site of injection should be as close to the nerve trunk as possible. This may be difficult to achieve if the child is moving and resisting during the administration of the anesthetic solution.

The fear of needles and pins is also called 'belonephobia.' It is a common condition seen in many children and adults as well. The fear gets deep-rooted as the child grows older if the resolution of the fears does not take place at a younger age. During adolescence, a phobic child can be extremely difficult to manage without adjuvant use of inhalational sedation.

A relaxed and calm child during the administration of local anesthesia is important for the success of the clinical process as well. The tell-show-do technique, animism, and desensitization of an apprehensive child are important tools of behavior management. Introducing the child to the procedure by using euphemisms and also informing them about how they will feel during and after the injection also allay their fears. Anxiety-provoking words like injection, pain should be avoided when taking with the child. Few key procedures are common to all techniques.

1. Control of child's head

2. The dental assistant should be prepared to restrain the child's hand, gently but firmly.

3. Topical anesthesia- the topical anesthetic agent must be applied on mucosa and left in place for at least one minute to achieve maximum effect and to minimize the painful sensation of needle penetration into the soft tissue.

4. The topical anesthetic agent benzocaine 20% or lidocaine as a solution or ointment-5% and spray-10% should be used.

5. Topical lidocaine has low incidences of allergic reactions, but it is absorbed systematically and can combine with an injected amide.

6. Localized allergic reactions may occur after prolonged or repeated use.

## Syringes Used for Local Anesthesia (Fig. 4)

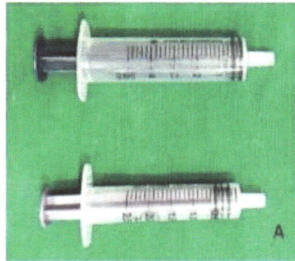

**Fig. (4A).** Syringe of 2 ml and 5 ml.

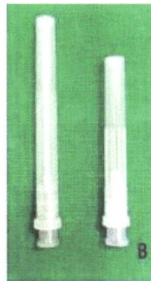

**Fig. (4b).** Short and long needle.

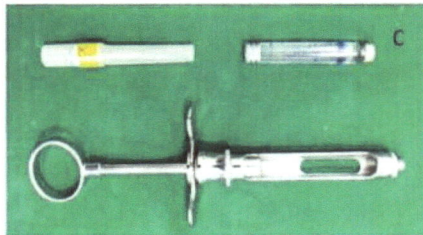

**Fig. (4C).** Cartridge and special syringe for anesthesia.

Disposable syringes are commonly used for administrating local anesthesia. They are available in various sizes according to their volume. 2cc and 5cc syringes are most commonly preferred. Depending on the mechanism by which the needle hub is attached to the syringe, they can be of friction lock or Luer lock types. When the anesthetic solution is expected to be delivered under pressure like intra-pulpal, intra-ligamentary, or intra-osseous techniques the Luer lock types are preferred. The desired amount of local anesthetic solution is loaded from vials before injection.

There are specially autoclavable and reusable syringes, which hold specially designed prefilled cartridges that were commonly used earlier but are getting less popular due to the easy availability of disposable syringes.

**Needle Size and Length (Fig. 4)**

1. A short (20 mm) or long (32 mm) 27- 30-gauge needle may be used for most intraoral injections in children.

2. An extra shot (10 mm) 30-gauge needle has been suggested for maxillary anterior injections and infiltration techniques in children.

3. Long needles are frequently recommended for inferior alveolar nerve blocks (pterygomandibular block).

**Duration of Injection**

Injection of local anesthetics should always be made slowly preceded by aspirations to avoid intra-vascular injections and systemic reactions to LA and vasoconstrictor as well.

**Post-operative Soft Tissue Injury**

1. Self-induced soft tissue trauma is an unfortunate clinical complication of local anesthetics used in the oral cavity for children and patients with special health care needs.

2. Most lip and cheek biting legions of this nature are self-limiting and heal without complications and require only palliative care.

3. Bleeding and infection from the injection site may be seen.

4. Parents should be given a realistic time, depending on the agent used for the duration of numbness, and be informed of the possibility of soft tissue trauma.

## Failure of Local Anesthesia

Several factors contribute to the failure of local anesthesia as below-

- Choice of a LA agent
- Improper technique
- Anatomical variations
- Local infection, causing an acidic environment
- Severe anxiety

When local anesthetic fails, generally, it is best to repeat the injection keeping in mind the permissible dose of the anesthetic agent.

## Conventional Methods of Obtaining Local Anesthesia

- Maxillary teeth – infiltration technique is the choice of anesthesia.
- The needle should penetrate the mucobuccal fold and be inserted to the depth of the apices of buccal roots of the teeth.
- The solution is deposited supra-periosteally and infiltrates through the alveolar bone to reach root apices
- A little local anesthetic may be sufficient to produce anesthesia as the alveolar bone in children is more permeable than it is in adults.

## Infiltration Technique

- The buccal mucosa is stretched, and a small amount of solution is deposited with shallow penetration of the needle.
- Position the needle as close to the periosteum as possible.
- After a few seconds, the needle can be slowly advanced 1-2 mm followed by aspiration, another small amount of solution can be deposited then.

## Anesthesia of Mandibular Primary Molars

- Usually achieved by infiltration in children up to the age of 5 years
- Mandibular block - inferior alveolar nerve block or pterygomandibular block is advisable for mandibular permanent and primary molar and while treating multiple mandibular teeth in one appointment.

## Inferior Alveolar Nerve Block (Pterygomandibular Block) (Fig. 5):

## Anatomic Considerations

Boundaries of pterygomandibular space:

- Anterior: - Pterygomandibular raphe
- Posterior: - Deep part of the parotid gland
- Medial: - Lateral aspect of medial pterygoid muscle
- Lateral: - Medial surface of the mandible
- Superior: - Lateral pterygoid muscle and the infratemporal surface of the greater wing of the sphenoid bone.

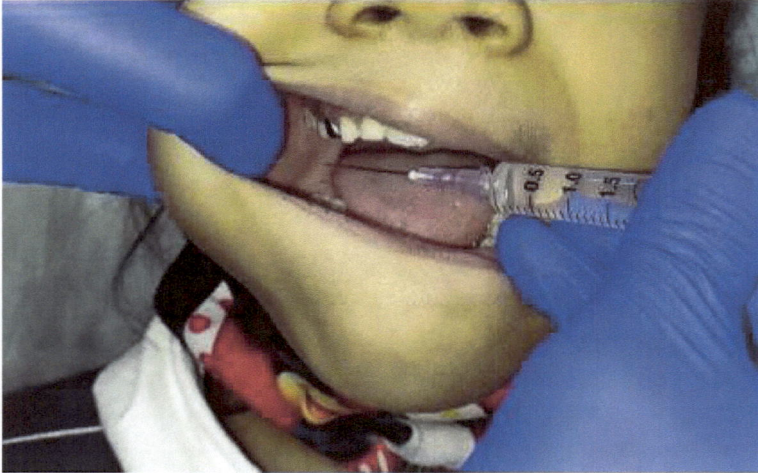

**Fig. (5).** Inferior alveolar nerve block.

## Technique

1. The child is asked to open his mouth wide.

2. The thumb/index finger is positioned in the buccal vestibule and gently moved backward to identify the deepest portion of the anterior border of the ramus *i.e.* Coronoid notch.

3. The needle is inserted between the internal oblique ridge and ptery-gomandibular raphe by positioning the barrel of the syringe over the two primary molars on the opposite side, parallel to the occlusal plane.

4. A small amount of solution is deposited and after negative aspiration, the needle is very gently and slowly advanced to contact bone.

5. The final position of the needle is in the pterygomandibular space.

6. Long buccal anesthesia may also require which is achieved by infiltrating a few drops of solution in buccal vestibule posterior primary mandibular molars or below permanent first molar if erupted.

7. A major consideration for inferior alveolar nerve block in the pediatric patient is that the position of the mandibular foramen may show variation according to the age of the child. (Table **3**).

Table 3. Position of mandibular foramen according to the age of the child.

| Age of Child | Position of Mandibular Foramen |
|---|---|
| < 6 years | Below the occlusal plane |
| 6 – 12 years | At the level of the occlusal plane |
| >12 years | Above the occlusal plane |

## Complications

1. Hematoma formation.

2. Trismus either because of multiple needle insertion leading to the soreness of medial pterygoid or because of intra-muscular or supra-muscular injection of contaminated LA solution leading to infection of pterygomandibular space.

3. Transient facial paralysis due to deposition of L.A. solution in body of parotid blocking VII[th] cranial nerve.

4. Prolonged paresthesia along the nerve.

### Infraorbital Nerve Block (Fig. 6)

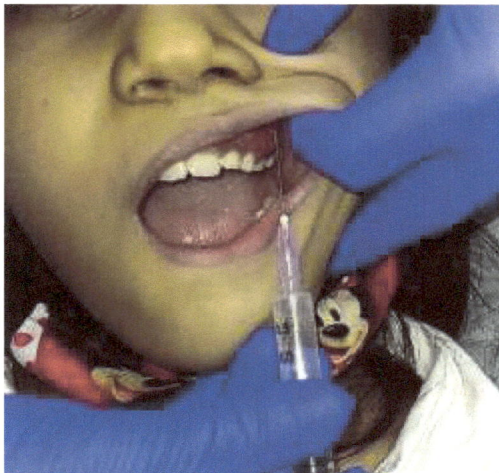

**Fig. (6).** Infraorbital nerve block.

- The infraorbital notch is palpated and the infraorbital foramen is palpated.
- The mucobuccal fold is palpated in the region of the first and second primary molars or premolars and the needle is inserted parallel to the long axis of the teeth to direct the needle towards the infraorbital foramen.
- When the needle hits the bone, it is retracted slightly and aspiration is done
- Slowly inject the solution.

### Greater Palatine Nerve Block (Fig. 7)

The greater palatine or anterior palatine nerve supplies the soft tissue and hard tissue of the palate. It is usually given during raising the palatine mucoperiosteal flaps and extraction of maxillary posterior teeth.

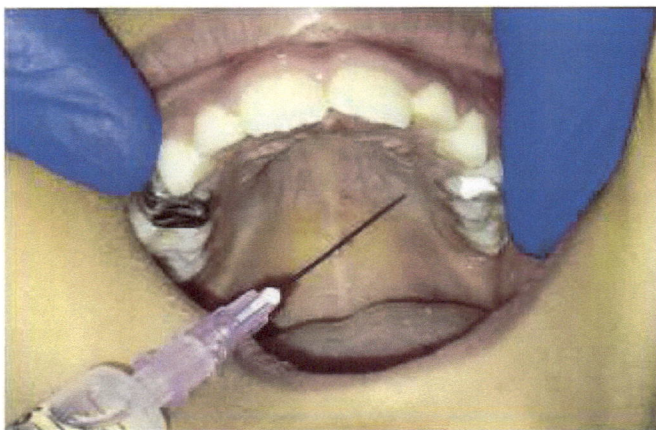

**Fig. (7).** Greater palatine nerve block.

### Alternate Techniques

#### *Intra-ligamentary*

It is a very useful method to limit the extent of anesthesia in children. The LA is directly injected into the periodontal ligament space by placing the needle along the long axis of the root. The insertion point should be in the proximal interdental area on both sides of the root and for each root in the case of multirooted teeth.

#### *Intra Pulpal*

a. A fine needle is introduced in the exposed pulp chamber with the direction of the needle towards the root canal orifice.
b. The child is informed about initial discomfort to avoid sudden movements
c. The needle is penetrated as deep as possible until resistance is felt, and a small amount of solution is deposited under pressure.

d. It is highly effective if performed correctly

e. When the pulpal exposure is too large, the pulp should be bathed with a small amount of LA for a minute before deep insertion of the needle

## *Intraosseous*

This technique may be contraindicated with primary teeth due to the potential for damage to developing permanent teeth. but maybe useful in young permanent teeth

## *Local Anesthesia in Infants*

- Local anesthesia given for complex surgical procedures should be reduced in neonates by around 50% from the equivalent adult dose per kg body weight and should be given slowly in increments [5].
- An infant is at increased risk of amide local anesthetic toxicity. The usual early warning symptoms are not exhibited in the first sign of toxicity may be a Grand-Mal convulsion, apnea, or arrhythmia.
- The risk of convulsion is increased in the presence of hypoxemia, hypothermia, acidosis, and hypercarbia.
- In an acid environment, local anesthetic dissociates from plasma protein increasing the unbound fraction
- Raised cerebral blood flow will increase delivery of LA to the brain
- The blood-brain barrier is not well developed in the neonates
- Decreased plasma protein binding and reduced hepatic clearance result in increased free drug availability

## Complications of LA in Pediatric Dentistry

## *Local Complications*

1. Needle breakage

2. Prolong anesthesia or paresthesia

3. Facial nerve paralysis

4. Trismus

5. Soft tissue injury

6. Hematoma

7. Burning sensation on injection

8. Infection

9. Edema

10. Sloughing of tissues

### Systemic Complications

1. Toxicity

2. Allergy

3. Idiosyncrasy

4. Drug interaction

5. Serum hepatitis

6. Occupational dermatitis

7. Respiratory arrest

8. Cardiac arrest

9. Hyperventilation

### Toxicity (Overdose)

- Absorption, metabolism, and excretion are not fully developed before age 6 [3].
- Children are more likely to experience toxic reactions because of their lower weight.
- The most adverse reaction occurs within the first 5 to 10 minutes.
- There will be high blood levels of anesthetic because of an inadvertent intravascular injection or repeated injection.

### Central Nervous System

LA overdose results in excitation followed by depression.

- The Classic overdose reaction to local anesthetic is generalized tonic and clonic convulsions

### Early Subjective Symptoms

- Dizziness
- Anxiety

- Confusion
- Diplopia
- Tinnitus
- Drowsiness
- Circumoral numbness or tingling

## Objective Signs

- Muscle twitching
- Tremors
- Talkativeness
- Slurred speech
- Shivering
- Seizure
- Unconsciousness
- Respiratory arrest

## Cardiovascular System

Its response to local anesthetic toxicity is also biphasic *i.e.*, stimulation followed by depression.

## Excitation Phase

1. Increase in heart rate and blood pressure

2. Vasodilatation

## Depression Phase

1. Depression of the myocardium with subsequent fall in blood pressure

2. Bradycardia

3. Cardiac arrest

Cardio-depressant effects need a significantly high level of local anesthetics in the blood.

## Management

• When signs and symptoms of toxicity are noted administration of LA should be discontinued.

• Maintain airway, breathing, and circulation

• Administer 100 percent oxygen

• Additional emergency management including activation of emergency medical services is based on the severity of the reaction.

**Prilocaine** is contraindicated in patients with methemoglobinemia, sickle cell anemia or symptoms of hypoxia in patients receiving acetaminophen or phenacetin since both medications elevate methemoglobin levels [4].

## Allergy [9]

• Hypersensitivity reactions are not dose-dependent
• It is an immune system response to a foreign substance

Two types of allergic reactions to a local anesthetic agent may occur

1. Ig E mediated Type 1

2. T-cell mediated type 4

### *Immediate Allergic Reactions (Type 1)*

• They are rare.
• They generally occur within 6 hours (rarely within 6 to 12 hours and no longer than 24 hours) after exposure [6].

### Clinical Manifestations (Type 1)

1. Urticaria

2. Angioedema

3. Bronchospasm

4. Rhinitis

5. Conjunctivitis

6. Gastrointestinal symptoms

7. Anaphylaxis

8. Anaphylactic shock

## Clinical Manifestations (Type 4)

## Eczema

- Eczema occurs within 24 to 72 hours after exposure usually after 6 hours
- Both Type 1 and type 4 allergic reactions are most common with Ester compounds.
- Amides have lower allergic potential and therefore they are preferred in clinical practice

## Dose Calculation

The formula is as follows: - [7]

Maximum allowable dose (mg/kg)x(weight in kg ÷10) x(1 / concentration of LA) = ml lidocaine.

Thus, if maximum dose is 7 mg/kg for LA with epinephrine using 1% lidocaine with epinephrine for a 20kg patient

7 x (20÷10) x (1÷1)

*i.e.*,7 x 6 =14 ml lignocaine.

- The maximum dose of lidocaine without adrenaline is 3 mg/kg
- The maximum dose of lignocaine with adrenaline is 7 mg/kg

## Adrenaline

1. Local anesthetics are vasodilators.

2. Therefore, the addition of vasoconstrictors like adrenaline provides the following advantages: -

  a. Improve anesthetic onset and duration.
  b. Reduces bleeding.
  c. Decreases in systemic absorption rate of local anesthetics.

3. However, adrenaline is unstable and therefore an antioxidant is added to prevent its oxidation.

4. Sodium bisulfite is the preservative most added to local anesthetic.

5. Patients allergic to sulfites will react to LA containing sodium bisulfite [8].

## Dose Calculation of Vasoconstrictors: [10]

• Doses are expressed as a dilution ratio and are not weight dependent.

The most used concentrations of adrenaline are-

1:80000

1:100000

1:200000

The maximum dose of adrenaline in a healthy patient is 0.2 mg for an appointment. However, in medically compromised patients such as those having cardiac risk recommended maximum dosage of adrenaline is 0.04 mg. Hence in cardiac patients, LA without adrenaline should be used.

## ADVANCES IN PAIN CONTROL MEDICAMENTS AND METHODS

### Topical Anesthesia

#### *Lidocaine Patch*

Lidocaine patch is a transoral delivery system of lidocaine *via* a mucoadhesive base attached to the oral mucosa. The anesthetic agent, lidocaine, is absorbed by the mucosa and the reported time to onset of anesthesia is within 2 minutes of application, which may last up to 30 minutes after removal. However, the scientific evidence regarding its minimum effective dose, clinical efficiency, and duration of action are sparse and inconclusive. Lidocaine patches are indicated for superficial mucosal and gingival procedures and topical analgesia before local anesthesia injection. The disadvantages include high cost and poor adhesion to the oral mucosa [11].

#### *EMLA - Cream*

Eutectic mixtures for local anesthesia [EMLA] are the 1:1 mixture of 2.5% prilocaine and 2.5% lidocaine anesthetic agents, aimed for topical anesthesia. These formulations are considered to have lower melting points, which promotes easier absorption in the oral mucosa. Indications for use include the procedures on the oral soft tissues causing minor pain. Following the introduction of EMLA cream, as a topical anesthetic in dermatology, studies have been conducted to evaluate the safety and efficacy of administration to the oral mucosa. The use of EMLA in children has shown satisfactory results. Although some authors have reported no significant difference in efficacy of EMLA and 5% lidocaine. The main concern with the use of EMLA in children is the risk of overdosing and adverse effects [12].

## *Intranasal Spray*

This is a novel technique for achieving local anesthesia of maxillary teeth by infiltration of an anesthetic solution through the nostrils by a metered device. It is hypothesized that the anesthetics spray penetrates the maxillary sinus and anesthetizes anterior superior and middle superior alveolar nerves [innervates maxillary incisor, canine, and premolars. Its composition consists of a mixture of 3% tetracaine hydrochloride and 0.05% oxymetazoline. Besides its anesthetic properties, it also reduces the risk of bleeding due to the shrinkage of regional blood vessels without causing a significant cardiovascular disturbance in healthy patients. Indications for its use are conservative dental manipulations requiring pulpal anesthesia of maxillary frontal teeth, canines, and premolars in adults and children weighing more than 40 kg. The most common side effects include nasal runniness, stuffiness, and stinging. More studies on the effectiveness and safety of the administration of the method for pediatric patients are necessary [13].

## *Cryotherapy*

Ice is believed to help control pain by inducing an anesthetic effect around the treatment area. Investigators have also shown that it reduces edema, nerve conduction velocities, cellular metabolism, and local blood flow. There have been numerous studies in medicine where pre-cooling has been used to relieve pain from a local anesthetic injection and prevent edema. Cooling the injection site before infiltration of local anesthetics for 1 min significantly reduces the pain perceived by pediatric patients. Topical cold application is believed to stimulate myelinated A-fibers, activating inhibitory pain pathways, which in turn raises the pain threshold. It slows the nerve conduction, causing temporary vasoconstriction. Pre-cooling the injection site with ice can be an effective adjunct to topical anesthesia in reducing both subjective and objective pain during local anesthesia administration in children.

**a) *Gebauer's Pain Ease*®** is a topical anesthetic skin refrigerant (vapocoolant) introduced and approved by US Food and Drug administration in the year 2004. It is a proprietary blend of 1,1,1,3,3-pentafluoropropane and 1,1,1,2-tetrafluoro-ethane and is non-flammable. Its onset of action is 4-10 seconds (Fig. **8**).

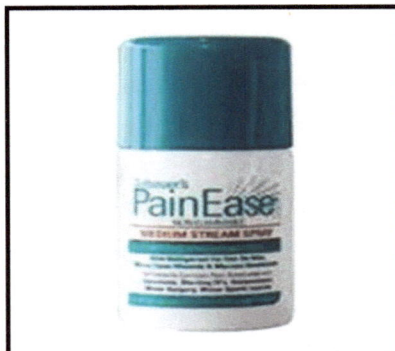

**Fig. (8).** Gebauer's pain ease.

**b)** *__Pharma ethyl__*® (Fig. **9**) introduced by Septodont. It is used in the production of topical cryoanesthesia in the oral cavity and to test pulpal vitality. It is a proprietary blend of 1,1,1,2-tetrafluorethane and dimethyl ether with a natural mint flavor (Fig. **9**).

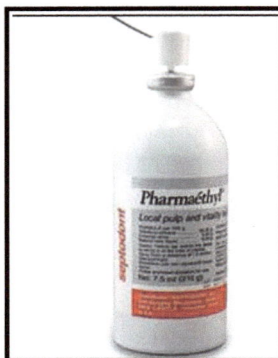

**Fig. (9).** Pharmaethyl.

## Advantages of Precooling

a. It produces immediate anesthesia as it suppresses both pain and pressure
b. It is an easy, reliable, and effective technique.
c. It is comfortable, safe, and physiologically active.
d. Cost-effective.

### Novel Herbal Anesthetic Gels

It is prepared from the roots of Anacyclus pyrethrum DC and fresh flower buds of Spilanthesacmella MURR. A. pyrethrum is a plant that belongs to the Asteraceae family commonly known as Akarkara, in Indian ayurvedic medicine. The cortical portion of the root contains about 5% of the acrid compound called pyrethrin [pellitorine], which is responsible for the various medicinal values of this plant, especially its local anesthetic activity. On chewing the leaves and flowers of this plant, a tingling sensation is experienced followed by numbness of the lips and tongue. The effectiveness of a novel herbal anaesthetic gel used as a topical anaesthetic before an inferior alveolar nerve block in children was found to be effective and safe in reducing the pain from needle insertion [14].

## LA Delivery Systems

### Wand / Compudent System

It is designed to enable the dental practitioner to manipulate the needle placement very accurately and administer the LA with the assistance of a foot-activated pedal. It is designed to be held like a pen, which naturally provides the practitioner with a greater tactile sensation and control compared to the traditional syringe. The delivery of the LA is controlled by a computer resulting in a significantly improved injection experience. Although this device uses standard cartridges, for each patient it requires an additional single-use set consisting of a plastic tube and a needle holder. There is no difference in the pain perception and disruptive behavior in children subjected to computerized or conventional dental local anaesthesia. However, the quality of the available evidence is low.

### Single-Tooth Anaesthesia System [STA]

STA was designed in 2006 by the manufacturers of the Wand. It uses dynamic pressure sensing technology which monitors the exit pressure of the local anesthesia solution in real-time during its administration. It was originally developed to be used in Epidural Regional Anaesthesia; however, it has been adapted for use in dentistry to overcome the issues associated with periodontal ligament [PDL], anterior and middle superior alveolar [AMSA], and palatal anterior superior alveolar [P-ASA] injections. It is also used for traditional intraoral injection techniques. The STA includes a training mode, which verbally explains to the dental practitioner how to use the device properly. The benefits of this system include administration of a greater volume of LA with increased comfort to the patient, as well as less tissue damage, that may otherwise be encountered with the use of traditional syringes or periodontal ligament pressure devices [15].

### Comfort Control Syringe

It is an electronic anesthesia delivery device that administers the solution in two phases. Initially, the anesthetic is injected slowly, and the rate of flow is then increased to a preprogrammed rate chosen by the dentist. The practitioner operates the initiation, termination, aspiration, and flow rate of the injection, using the button on the handpiece.

### Sleeper One

It is designed by Dental HI Tec in Cholet, France. According to the manufacturer, it can be used in regular infiltrative injections as well as intraligamentary, intraseptal, palatal, and nerve block techniques. The device essentially looks like a pen, is gripped like one, has four injection speeds, and the deposition of the anesthetic is controlled by a wireless foot pedal. This ensures higher precision when injecting that of a standard syringe. The sleeper One system mechanism involves Permanent Analysis of Resistance [PAR], which results in constant control and monitoring of tissue resistance. The dose and rate of administration of the anesthetic are controlled in order not to exceed the pain threshold. Regarding intraseptal injection, sleeper One is supplied with a double-beveled needle, which allows easier penetration to the bone. The intercrestal and cancellous bone is thin and sparse in children which enables the needle to be placed into the bone easily and the injection performed with minimal pressure. For this reason, the SleeperOne device is becoming popular in pediatric dentistry. Its use for intraligamentary anesthesia in adults is also indicated, allowing good control of the needle while introducing it into the ligamental space, as well as reducing the number of injections when compared to mechanical intraligamentary syringes (Fig. **10**).

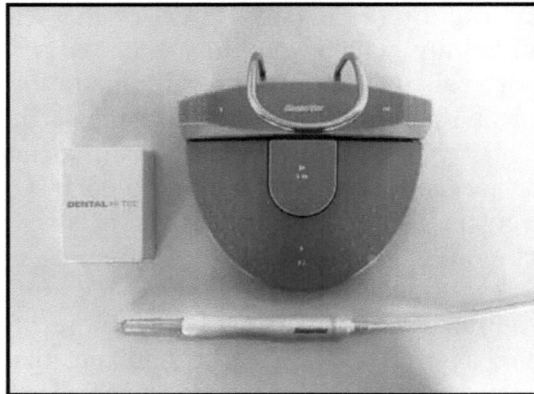

**Fig. (10).** Sleeperone system (Dental HiTec).

### Vibrotactile Devices and the Gate-control Theory

Vibratory stimulation is one of the non-pharmacological techniques used in pain reduction. The brain is only able to perceive one type of sensation from one area at any given time; therefore, when using vibratory stimulation in local anesthesia, that sensation will reach the brain before the pain sensation. Many devices have been developed to take advantage of the 'Gate-control' theory, which suggests that when applying pressure and using vibration; the neural gate can be closed, thereby reducing the perception of itch and pain (Fig. **11**).

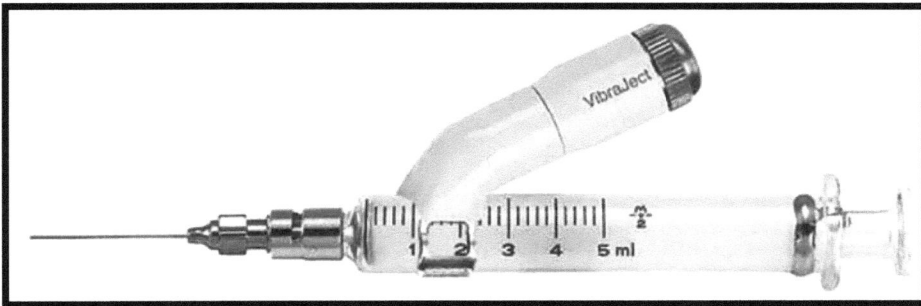

**Fig. (11).** Vibraject system.

i. **Vibraject.** A small, battery-operated device is attached to the standard dental syringe to deliver high-frequency vibrations to the needle.
ii. **DentalVibe.** A cordless hand-held device that works by delivering smooth, pulsating micro-oscillations to the location where the injection is being administered.
iii. **Accupal**. A cordless device that preconditions the oral mucosa by applying pressure and vibrations to the injection site, after which the needle is placed through a hole in the head of the disposable tip attached to the motor.
iv. **Syringe micro-vibrator [SMV].** The SMV motor provides high-frequency vibrations that alleviate pain and its low vibration ensures that the dexterity of the practitioner and accuracy of the injection is not affected. This allows the dentist to perform an accurate pain-free injection. The SMV also reduces the ballooning effect that occurs due to a forceful injection under high pressure, which may lead to swelling or other complications after completing the treatment. The vibrations reduce the size of this balloon effect by enhancing tissue infiltration of the anesthetic solution. Also, the use of SMV eliminates the need and saves the time required for application and onset of topical anesthetics.

## *Buzzy Bee Device*

Buzzy® is an economical versatile, quickly vibrating plastic device designed like a bee, with cooled wings. It is hypothesized to work based on the gate control theory, which proposes that pain is conducted from the peripheral nervous system to the central nervous system *via* modulation through a gating system in the dorsal horn of the spinal cord. The vibration component of this device will excite the A-beta fibers [fast nonnoxious motion nerves], which eventually block the A-delta [afferent pain receptive nerves]. The cold component on the contrary will excite the C fibers; and if applied before the pain stimulus, will block the A-delta pain signal as well. Buzzy® has been shown in some studies to be superior to placebo and vapocoolants and analgesic creams.

**Techniques for Increasing Comfort During Injection of Local Anesthetics**

*Warming the Anesthetic Solution*

Warming the anesthetic solution up to the body temperature [37 °C] before administration of LA is one of the approaches that is recommended for the reduction of pain during LA. However, there is also conflicting evidence. Some research has shown that warming the cartridges to body temperature (37°C) did not significantly reduce the pain associated with intraoral injections. Overheating the local anesthetic may cause discomfort to the patient especially children during deposition of the LA, as well as the destruction of the vasoconstrictor which is heat-labile, thus resulting in the shorter action of the anesthetic. Also, some studies have shown contrary results while comparing warm and room-temperature anesthetics for dental procedures and found no significant differences between the two. More research is required to have conclusive evidence on the benefits of warming anesthetic solutions in dental procedures and their effect on children.

*Buffering of anesthetic solution (Fig. 12)*

LA solutions without vasoconstrictors have a pH of around 6.5. Once a vasoconstrictor, adrenaline, and the antioxidant sodium bisulfite are added, the pH lowers to 2.5 to 3.4. Inside the cartridge of the LA, 2 ionic forms exist: unionized [B] tertiary form and ionized quaternary [BH+] form. The unionized form [B] is more lipid-soluble than the ionized form [BH+]. Therefore, the unionized form [B] of the drug can diffuse across the lipid-rich nerve membrane, where it picks up an H+, and subsequently gets converted to BH+ which enters the sodium channel and blocks the nerve conduction. Recent technical advances have shown that if the pH of the LA solution were to be increased to 7.4 before the injection by alkalization of LA cartridges, both speed of onset and patient's comfort would improve during the injection. Sodium bicarbonate is used as a buffer when administering the LA to alleviate the pain associated with the injection. LAs with a higher pH is more readily accepted by patients. However, there are mixed findings of the efficacy of sodium bicarbonate as a buffer, since there is a big variation in the pH of the sodium bicarbonate solution. Its pH ranges from 7.0–to 8.5. Injections are more comfortable with alkalinized 2% lignocaine when used for the inferior alveolar nerve block; whereas there is no difference in the pain perception between buffered and unbuffered lignocaine [8].

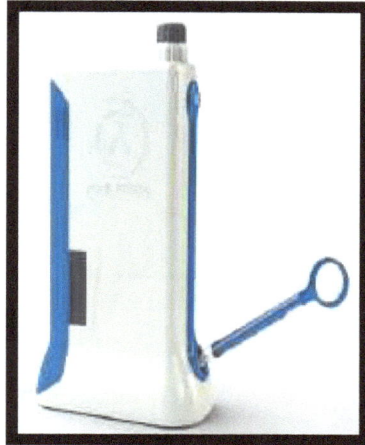

**Fig. (12).** Anutra™ system.

The Anutra™ local anesthetic delivery system. Fig. (**12**) makes buffering simple. By loading an Anutra™ cassette at the beginning of the week clinicians can simply buffer anesthetic for every patient by twisting the knob on the Anutra™ dispenser. Up to 6 milliliters of anesthetic can be drawn in a single syringe. With the Anutra™ the dentist can draw the equivalent of the three traditional 1.8 ml dental cartridges which provides for a more efficient and practical way to administer anesthesia.

## Local Anaesthesia Drugs

### *Articaine*

Articaine is unique among local anesthetics because it is the only local anesthetic that possesses a thiophene group instead of a benzene ring; it is also the only widely used local anesthetic that contains an ester group. These properties account for the better performance of articaine over other local anesthetics. It has been speculated in the scientific literature that the thiophene ring encourages rapid transport across the nerve cell membrane, which may account for the reported faster onset of action and the decreased pain during administration. The clinical effectiveness of articaine as a local anesthetic in pediatric dentistry is better than the gold standard lidocaine.

## *Oraverse (Phentolamine Mesylate Anesthesia Reversal) (Fig. 13)*

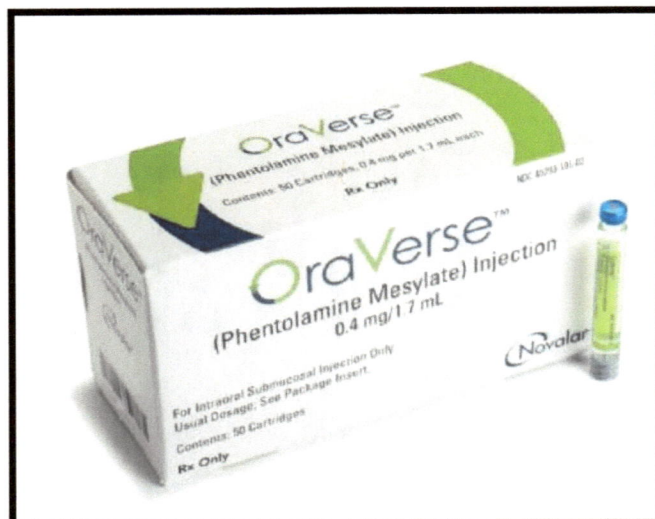

**Fig. (13).** Oraverse.

It is the first and only local dental anesthesia reversal agent in the market proven to accelerate the reversal of anesthetic effect(numbness)after dental procedures [16].

*Action:* Phentolamine is a nonselective α-adrenergic receptor antagonist that competitively inhibits the ability of sympathomimetic amines like norepinephrine and epinephrine to stimulate vascular contraction. The smooth muscles of vascular beds, including those beneath the oral mucosa, contain α -receptors (predominantly α l), and the ultimate effect of the α-receptor blockade is vasodilation.

### *Dosage*

- OraVerse is manufactured in 1.7 mL dental cartridges, each of which contains 0.4mg active drug.
- The dose of oral submucosal injections of phentolamine approved by the FDA is 0.2-0.8 mg.
- It is used in a 1:1 ratio to local anesthetic
- The maximum recommended dose of *OraVerse* is two cartridges in patients aged12 or greater, one cartridge in children aged6-11years and weighing over 66 lbs., and one-half cartridge in children 6-11years and weighing 33-66lbs.

## *Method of Use*

- To administer *OraVerse, the* dentist will inject it into the area of the patient's mouth that has been worked on and is therefore already numb.
- Since the oral injections site will already be numb by the time the *OraVerse* is given, patients will not feel any additional discomfort during this process.
- After *OraVerse* is given, patients can expect their numbness recovery period to be virtually reduced to half the duration of total anesthesia.

## CONCLUSION

Local anesthetics when used carefully with an appropriate technique for the procedure can give multiple benefits in the management of children during dental procedures. The right drug with this correct dosage providing the adequate duration of anesthesia has to be planned and selected in advance. Although many children are apprehensive towards dental treatment due to fear of pain and injection, it is possible to safely administer local anesthesia and improve the patient's co-operative behavior with a truly pain-free experience that allows the child to develop a positive attitude towards future dental visits. The advances in anesthetic drugs and methods of delivery further allow the dental surgeon to tackle pain; the single deterrent that prevents the patients from seeking dental treatment.

## CONSENT FOR PUBLICATION

Not applicable.

## CONFLICT OF INTEREST

The authors declare no conflict of interest, financial or otherwise.

## ACKNOWLEDGEMENTS

Declared none.

## REFERENCES

[1]     Malamed S. Handbook of local anesthesia. 7th ed., Mosby Paperback 2019.

[2]     Herroeder S, Schönherr ME, De Hert SG, Hollmann MW, Warner DS. Magnesium--essentials for anesthesiologists. Anesthesiology 2011; 114(4): 971-93.
        [http://dx.doi.org/10.1097/ALN.0b013e318210483d] [PMID: 21364460]

[3]     Monheim's Local Anesthesia and Pain Control in Dental Practice. Richard Bennett. 7th ed., CBS Publishers 1990.

[4]     Weinberg L, Peake B, Tan C, Nikfarjam M. Pharmacokinetics and pharmacodynamics of lignocaine: A review. World J Anesthesiol 2015; 4(2): 17-29.
        [http://dx.doi.org/10.5313/wja.v4.i2.17]

[5]     Morton NS. Local and regional anaesthesia in infants - Continuing Education in Anaesthesia Critical Care & Pain - Contin Educ. British journal of anesthesia 2004; 4(5): 148-51.
[http://dx.doi.org/10.1093/bjaceaccp/mkh041]

[6]     American Academy of Pediatric Dentistry. Use of local anesthesia for pediatric dental patients The Reference Manual of Pediatric Dentistry. Chicago, Ill.: American Academy of Pediatric Dentistry 2020; pp. 318-23.

[7]     Walsh K, Arya R. A simple formula for quick and accurate calculation of maximum allowable volume of local anaesthetic agents. Br J Dermatol 2015; 172(3): 825-6.
[http://dx.doi.org/10.1111/bjd.13335] [PMID: 25113018]

[8]     Kattan S, Lee SM, Hersh EV, Karabucak B. Do buffered local anesthetics provide more successful anesthesia than nonbuffered solutions in patients with pulpally involved teeth requiring dental therapy? J Am Dent Assoc 2019; 150(3): 165-77.
[http://dx.doi.org/10.1016/j.adaj.2018.11.007] [PMID: 30803488]

[9]     Peroni D, Pasini M, Iurato C, Cappelli S, Giuca G, Giuca MR. Allergic manifestations to local anaesthetic agents for dental anaesthesia in children: a review and proposal of a new algorithm. Eur J Paediatr Dent 2019; 20(1): 48-52.
[http://dx.doi.org/10.23804/ejpd.2019.20.01.10] [PMID: 30919645]

[10]    Moodley Desigar. Local anaesthetics in dentistry - Part 3: Vasoconstrictors in local anaesthetics. SADJ: journal of the South African Dental Association 2017; 72: 176-8.

[11]    Bai Y, Miller T, Tan M, Law LS-C, Gan TJ. Lidocaine patch for acute pain management: a meta-analysis of prospective controlled trials. Curr Med Res Opin 2015; 31(3): 575-81.
[http://dx.doi.org/10.1185/03007995.2014.973484]

[12]    Milani AS, Zand V, Abdollahi AA, Froughreyhani M, Zakeri-Milani P, Jafarabadi MA. Effect of Topical Anesthesia with Lidocaine-prilocaine (EMLA) Cream and Local Pressure on Pain during Infiltration Injection for Maxillary Canines: A Randomized Double-blind Clinical Trial. J Contemp Dent Pract 2016; 17(7): 592-6.
[http://dx.doi.org/10.5005/jp-journals-10024-1895] [PMID: 27595728]

[13]    Capetillo J, Drum M, Reader A, Fowler S, Nusstein J, Beck M. Anesthetic Efficacy of Intranasal 3% Tetracaine plus 0.05% Oxymetazoline (Kovanaze) in Maxillary Teeth. J Endod 2019; 45(3): 257-62.
[http://dx.doi.org/10.1016/j.joen.2018.12.003] [PMID: 30803532]

[14]    Mohite V, Baliga S, Thosar N, Rathi N, Khobragade P, Srivastava R. Comparative evaluation of a novel herbal anesthetic gel and 2% lignocaine gel as an intraoral topical anesthetic agent in children: Bilateral split-mouth, single-blind, crossover *in vivo* study. J Indian Soc Pedod Prev Dent 2020; 38(2): 177-83.
[http://dx.doi.org/10.4103/JISPPD.JISPPD_226_20] [PMID: 32611865]

[15]    Baghlaf K, Elashiry E, Alamoudi N. Computerized intraligamental anesthesia in children: A review of clinical considerations. J Dent Anesth Pain Med 2018; 18(4): 197-204.
[http://dx.doi.org/10.17245/jdapm.2018.18.4.197] [PMID: 30186967]

[16]    Hanadi A, Majid A, Hamdi A. The Unaddressed local anesthesia reversal Action of Phentolamine Mesylate after Plain Mepivacaine. Eurasian Journal of Biosciences 2021; 14: 3883-8.

# CHAPTER 2

# Extraction, Minor Oral Surgeries, and Implants in Children

**Deepashri Meshram**[1,*], **Abdulkadeer M. Jetpurwala**[2] and **Amit Jain**[3]

[1] *Department of Oral and Maxillofacial Surgery, Nair Hospital Dental College, Mumbai, India*

[2] *Department of Pediatric Dentistry, Nair Hospital Dental College, Mumbai, India*

[3] *Consultant Implantologist, Mumbai, India*

**Abstract:** Surgical procedures in children are often required for alleviation of pain, or removal of pathologic or aberrant entities from the oral cavity. The general principles for surgical management are relevant in children as well. Due to behavioural and cooperation problems in children the minor surgical procedures should be planned well, taking into consideration all aspects. Extraction of primary teeth must be commonly done due to extensive dental caries. Minor surgeries like cyst enucleations, frenctomies, mucoceles *etc.* require proper planning and execution for successful results.

The advent of dental implants has opened new vistas in rehabilitation of adult patients. However, the use of implants in pediatric dentistry has not been extensively used due to the growth and developmental changes in chidren. There is a limited scope for implants in dentistry hence it has been covered. If used judiciously implants can be an important addition to the field of work of pediatric dentists.

**Keywords:** Dental implants, Extraction of Primary teeth, Minor surgeries.

## INTRODUCTION

Dental extractions are often required in children due to extensive caries, traumatic injuries or for guidance of eruption of the permanent teeth. The children and parents get equally anxious when face with the need for extractions or any surgical procedures in their children. Minor oral surgical procedures are the procedures of small duration and can be done under local anesthesia or in combination with LA and sedation or inhalational anesthesia. These procedures will always remain a challenge especially in pediatric patients due to the young age and lack of cooperation.

---

[*] **Corresponding author Deepashri Meshram:** Department of Oral and Maxillofacial Surgery, Nair Hospital Dental College, Mumbai, India; E-mail: 24deemes@gmail.com

In pediatric dentistry minor procedures that can be carried out under local anesthesia are shown in Fig. (**1**):

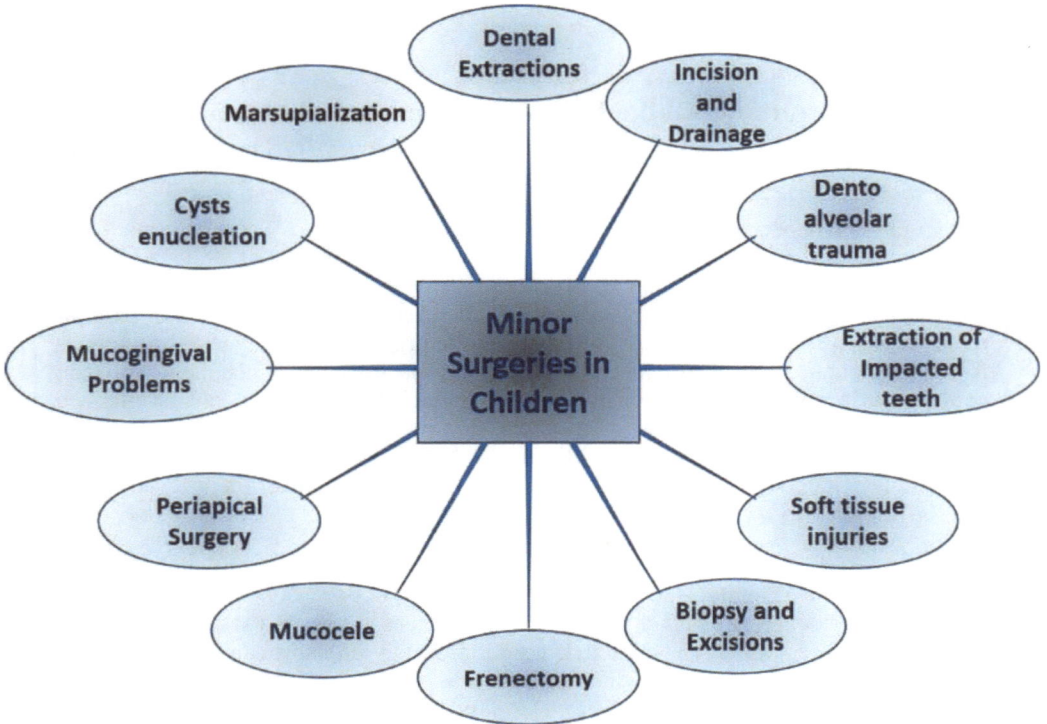

**Fig. (1).**  Minor surgeries in children.

## Preoperative Consideration

1. Informed consent

2. Medical evaluation

3. Dental evaluation

4. Growth and development

5. Behavioral evaluation

## Peri and Postoperative Considerations

1. Pain and infection control

2. Metabolic management of children following surgery

3. Calorie intake

4. Fluid and electrolyte management

5. Blood replacement in case of blood loss.

**Extraction of Erupted Teeth**

*Indications*

Dental extractions are indicated in following:

1. Caries – extensive decay of the crown or root rendering the tooth non restorable

2. Periapical abscess

3. Failed pulpotomy or pulpectomy

4. Orthodontic correction

5. Over-retained teeth

6. Acute trauma

7. Root resorption

8. Serial extraction

9. Teeth associated with cyst and tumors of the jaw

Dental caries remains the most common reason for dental extraction and the first primary molars and maxillary central incisors are the most frequently extracted teeth.

*Contraindications*

Dental extraction has relative contraindications in following conditions and should be done carefully: -

1. Acute dental infection

2. Cyanotic congenital cardiac disorders

3. Blood dyscrasia

4. Bleeding and clotting disorders

5. Juvenile diabetes mellitus

6. Recently irradiated bone

7. Cancer chemotherapy

## Armamentarium Used for Extraction of Teeth

The instruments used for extraction of primary teeth are as follows

1. Moon's Probe
2. Elevators
   3. Straight elevator
   Angle apexo elevators – pair
3. Forceps
   a. Maxillary (Fig. **2**)
   b. Anterior
   c. Posterior
   d. Root
   e. Mandibular (Fig. **3**)
   f. Anterior
   g. Posterior
   h. Root

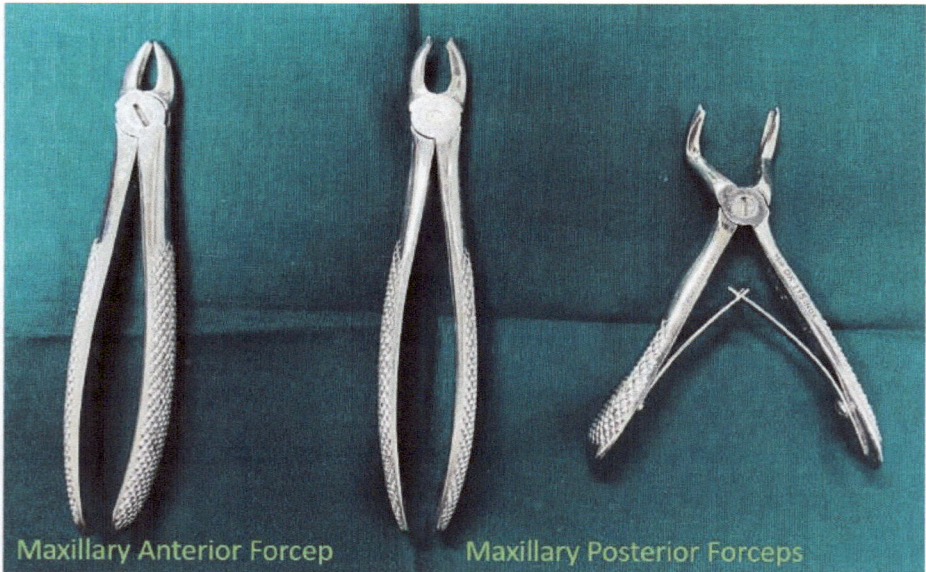

**Fig. (2).** Pediatric maxillary forceps.

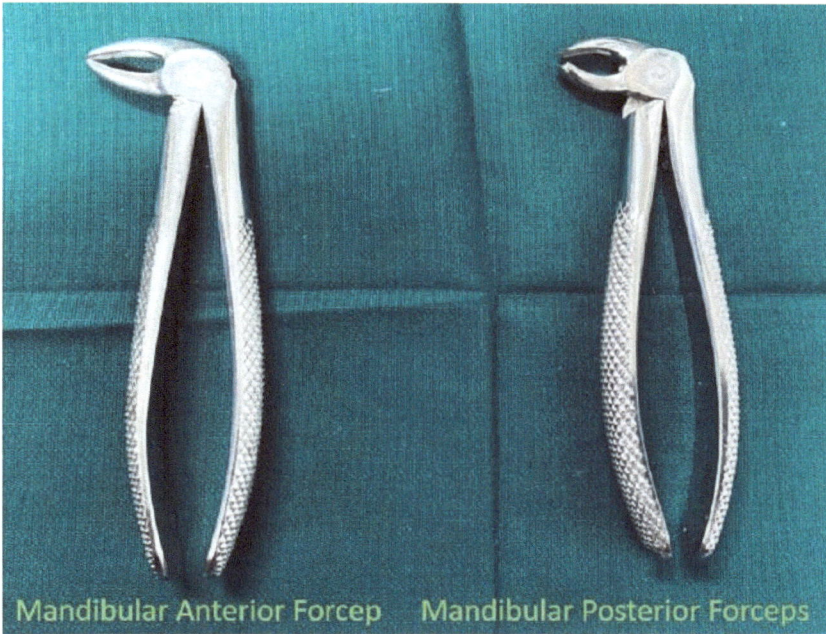

**Fig. (3).** Pediatric mandibular forceps.

Instruments used for extraction of permanent teeth are:

1. Moon's probe (Fig. **4**)

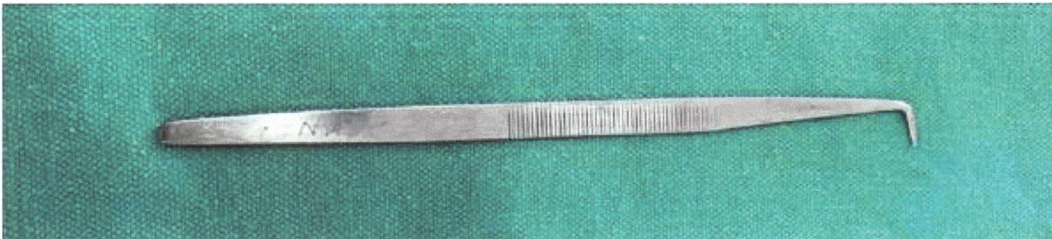

**Fig. (4).** Moon's probe.

2. Forceps
    a. Maxillary (Fig. **5**)
        i. Anterior
        ii. Premolar
        iii. Molar – pair
        iv. Cow horn – pair
        v. Root

    b. Mandibular (Fig. **6**)
      i. Anterior
     ii. Premolar
    iii. Molar
    iv. Cow horn
     v. Root

3. Elevators
   Straight elevator (Fig. **7**)
   Angle apexo elevators – pair (Fig. **7**)
   Winter-Cryer elevators – pair (Fig. **8**)

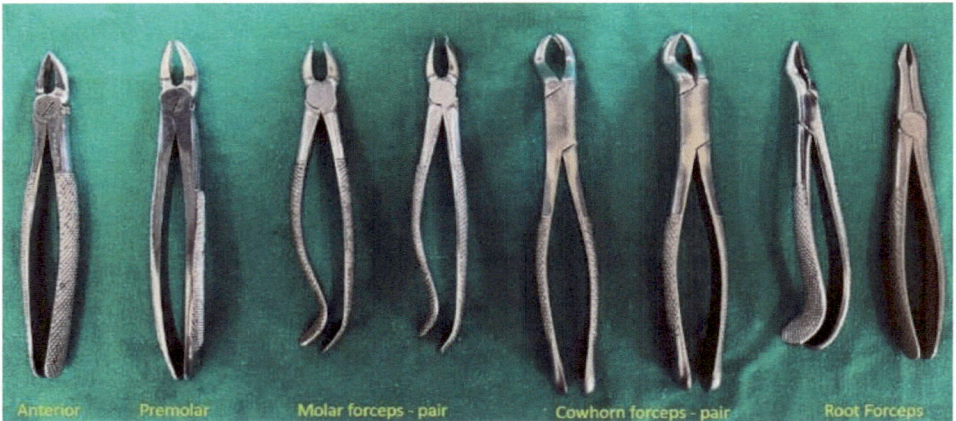

**Fig. (5).** Permanent maxillary forceps.

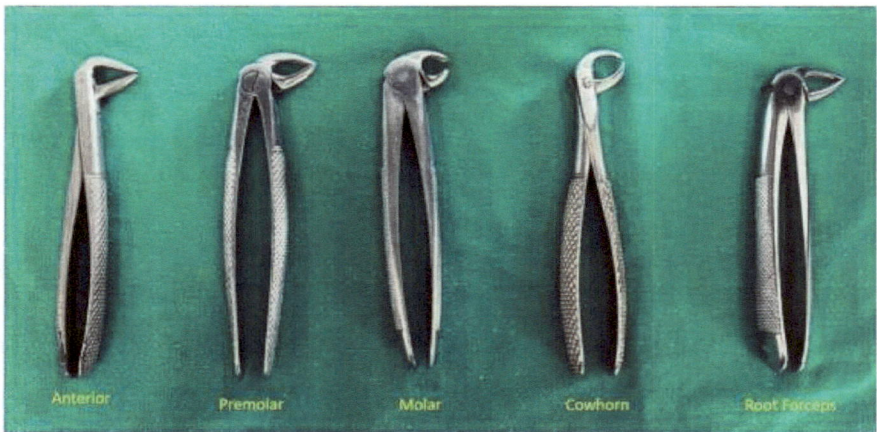

**Fig. (6).** Permanent mandibular forceps.

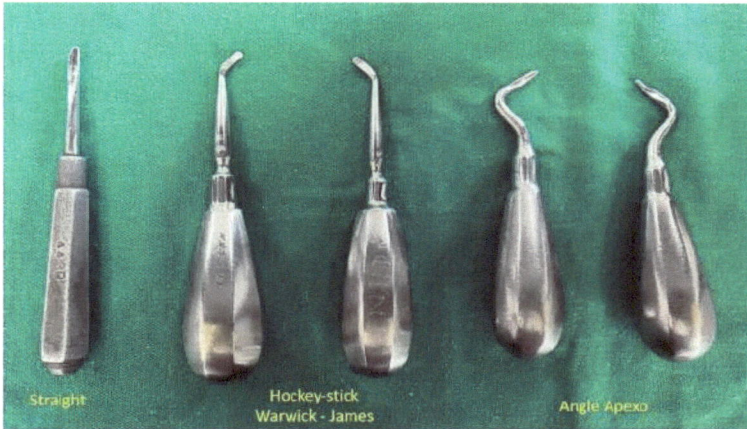

**Fig. (7).** Elevators.

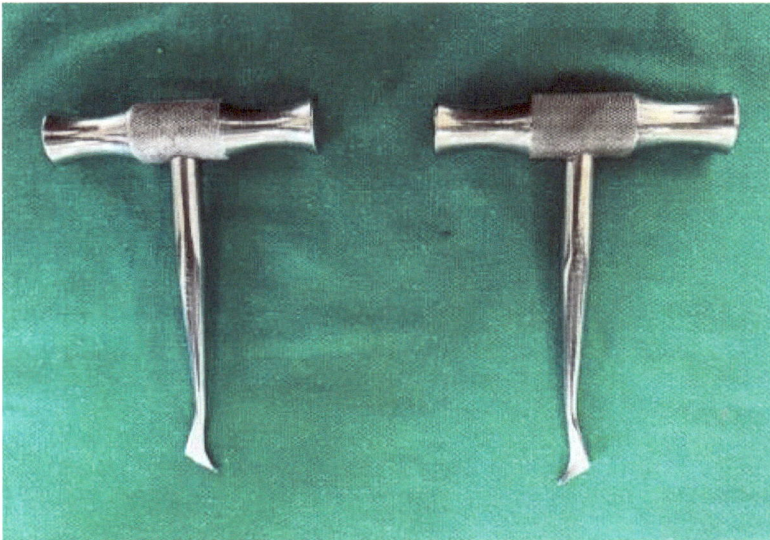

**Fig. (8).** Winter cryer elevators.

## Forceps

Parts of a forceps:

1. Handle
2. Hinge (joint)
3. Beaks.

The hinge (joint) will act as a fulcrum. To exert more force during extraction procedure the grip should be taken as far as possible from the fulcrum or hinge.

Inadvertent forces during extraction will lead to fracture of tooth, alveolar bone or maxilla or mandibular bone.

## Elevators

Elevators are designed to impart forces at the fulcrum (between bone and root) to sever the periodontal ligament and luxate the tooth.

### Parts of elevator:

1. Handle

2. Shank

3. Blade

### Elevation of a Tooth

Elevation of a tooth is indicated for the luxation of a firm permanent tooth. It is rarely indicated for extraction of primary teeth due to presence of permanent tooth bud below. Instruments like a straight elevator (universal elevator) or winter's elevator are used to elevate a tooth by breaking periodontal ligament and expanding the bony socket. Certain conditions need to be followed while elevation of a tooth: -

1. While elevation anterior adjacent tooth should preferably be present and the interdental bone on the mesial side is used as a fulcrum.

2. The instrument should be guarded by finger to prevent any soft tissue injury due to slippage.

3. The flat surface or the concave surface of the elevator should be facing towards the tooth to be elevated.

The elevators work on following principles:

1. Lever principle – It has three basic components that is effort, resistance, and fulcrum. The effort arm is longer while the resistance arm is shorter, and the fulcrum is placed between two (Class I lever).

2. Wedge principle – the force is used apically at the junction of interdental bone and root of the tooth with the help of elevators at $45^0$ angulations thus tearing off the periodontal membrane and luxating the tooth.

3. Wheel and axle- The force is applied to the circumference of the wheel which turns the axle to raise the weight or the tooth.

4. Combination of these principles.

## Preparing the Tooth for Extraction

- The tooth indicated for extraction should be re-examined and confirmed, all available investigations like IOPA, OPG should be rechecked.
- Re-evaluate the medical history including history of previous extractions and allergies.
- The patient's general condition should be evaluated
- Enquire whether the child has had a meal
- Ascertain whether any premedication prescribed has been taken by the patient
- Seat the child in a comfortable position according to the tooth that needs to be extracted
- Thoroughly clean the extra oral and intra oral soft tissues with betadine
- Administer adequate local anesthesia and check subjective and objective signs
- Reflect the gingival from the cervical region of the tooth with a Moon's probe

### *Maxillary and Mandibular Anterior Teeth Extraction*

- Most primary and permanent maxillary with mandibular central incisor, lateral incisors and canines have conical single root.
- In most cases extraction of anterior teeth is accomplished with the rotational movement due to their single root anatomy.
- The beaks of the forceps should be paced as deep as possible to grip the tooth
- Care should be taken to avoid placing any force on adjacent teeth that could become luxated or dislodged easily due to their root anatomy.

## Maxillary and Mandibular Molars Extraction (Fig. 9)

- Primary molar roots are smaller in size and more divergent than permanent molars.
- Root fracture in primary molars is common due to their characteristics flared appearance as well as the potential weakening of the roots caused by the eruption of their permanent successors
- While extraction of primary molars pressure should be avoided in the furcation area to protect the developing permanent tooth.
- Apply a gentle bucco palatal/lingual movement to mobilize the tooth
- Take a firm grip and maintain pressure throughout the extraction

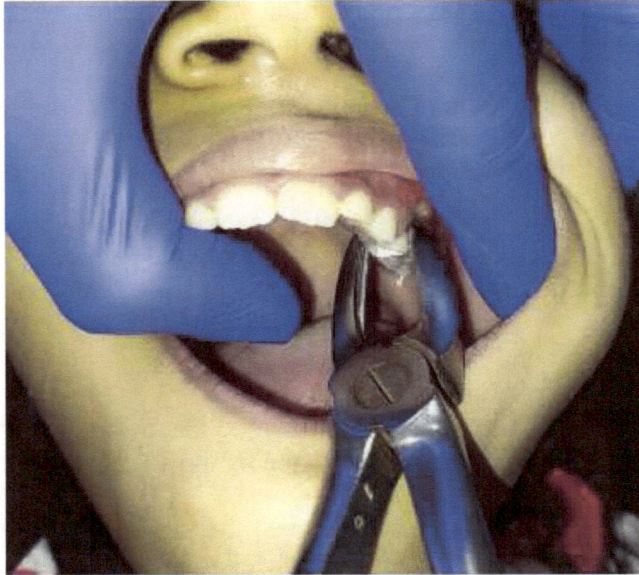

**Fig. (9).** Extraction of primary maxillary molar.

## *Fractured Primary Tooth Roots Extraction*

The general opinion suggests that if the fractured root tip can be removed easily, it should be removed. If the root tip is small, located deep in the socket, situated near permanent successor or unable to be retrieved after several attempts, it its best left to be resorbed. The parents must be informed, and documentation should be done. The patient should be kept under observation at appropriate intervals. The root segment may spontaneously erupt closer to the eruption of the permanent tooth, or it may get resorbed.

## *Unerrupted and Impacted Teeth*

**Impaction**: - It is a condition in which a tooth fails to erupt completely usually because of crowding or lack of space in bone. It may also be associated with certain disorders.

## *Eruption Disorders*

1. Syndromic

2. Non-syndromic

3. Ankylosis

4. Tooth impaction or primary eruption failure

## Impacted Canines

1. Permanent maxillary canine teeth are second to third molars in frequency of impaction.

2. Extraction of primary canine is the treatment of choice to correct palatally displaced permanent canines or to prevent resorption of teeth.

3. If no improvement in permanent canine position occurs in a year, surgical or orthodontic treatment is advised.

## Impacted Premolars

1. Premolars may occasionally get impacted due to space loss in the mixed dentition.

2. Early loss of deciduous molars causes space loss and mesial drifting of distally located tooth.

3. Arch size tooth length discrepancies may also cause premolar impaction.

### Supernumerary Teeth

1. They are thought to be related to disturbances in the initiation and proliferation stages of dental development.

2. Although some supernumerary teeth maybe syndrome associated (*e.g.*, cleidocranial dysplasia) or a familial inheritance pattern.

3. Supernumerary teeth can occur in either the primary or permanent dentition.

4. The maxillary anterior midline is the most common site for supernumerary tooth known as mesiodens.

5. The second most common site is maxillary molar area, the para molars.

### Management

Surgical treatment should be planned by establishing the diagnosis of impacted or supernumerary tooth with

1. Radiographs.

2. Taking two periapical radiographs using either two projections taken at right angles to one another or the tube shift technique (buccal object rule or Clark's rule).

3. Three dimensional investigations.

4. Core beam computed tomography (CBCT) (Fig. **10**).

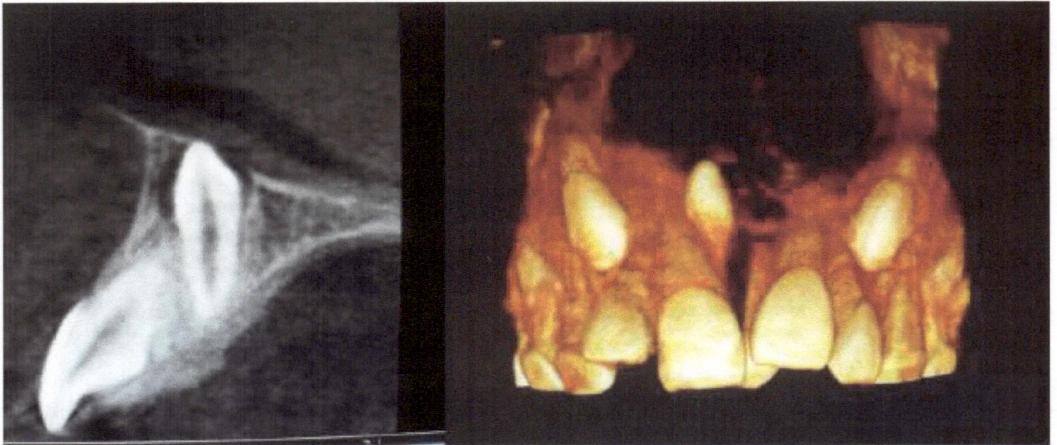

**Fig. (10).**  CBCT and 3-D imaging of inverted and impacted supernumerary tooth.

Imaging techniques like 3D imaging ang CBCT provide an accurate spatial representation and can help to identify intricate details of the position of the impacted tooth in relation to other teeth and important anatomical structures. Fig. **(10)** shows an inverted impacted supernumerary tooth with the crown in close relation with the nasal floor. Such teeth require planning and need to be approached with proper understanding of the orientation of the tooth and its proximity to important anatomical structures.

### *Treatment Objective*

1. The objective for removal of a non-erupting permanent mesiodens is to minimize eruption problems for the permanent incisors.

2. The treatment objective for a non-erupting mesiodens in the primary dentition differs in that the removal of these teeth usually is not recommended as the surgical intervention may disrupt or damage the underlying developing permanent teeth.

3. Erupted mesiodens in the primary dentition may be easily extracted.

4. Prevent potential formation of cyst and tumors of odontogenic origin due to the impacted teeth.

## Odontogenic Infection

A child presenting with facial swelling or fascial cellulitis secondary to an odontogenic infection should receive prompt dental attention or surgical intervention. Odontogenic infection arises mainly by the direct entry of bacteria into the pulpal tissue through carries, exposed pulp for dentinal tubules, crack into the dentin and defective restorations or periodontal infections. The upper face infection (orbits, paranasal sinuses, maxillary teeth, and cheeks) affects mostly the younger children group. While lower face infections (Mandibular teeth, submental, sublingual, and submandibular structure) occur more frequently in older children [1]. The infection tends to spread through areas of least resistance beyond the alveolar bone involving facial spaces around the face and oral cavity. In maxilla the alveolar bone is weakest at buccal side while in mandible the buccal bone is weakest in anterior region and lingual bone is weakest in molar region.

### Classification of Facial Spaces

1. Canine space

2. Buccal space

3. Temporal space

4. Infratemporal space

5. Submental space

6. Submandibular space

7. Sublingual space

8. Masseteric space

9. Pterygomandibular space

10. Para – pharyngeal (lateral) space

### Signs and Symptoms of Odontogenic Infection

1. Fever

2. Malaise

3. Facial swelling

4. Lymphadenopathy

5. Trismus

6. Tachycardia

7. Dysphagia

8. Respiratory distress

## *Investigation*

1. Complete blood examination

2. C-reactive protein

3. Blood cultures

4. Bacterial culture and sensitivity

## Cellulitis

Cellulitis of odontogenic origin is an acute, deep, and diffuse inflammation of the subcutaneous tissue that spread through the spaces between tissue cells to several anatomic regions, tissue spaces and throughout the aponeurotic plane because of the infection of one or several teeth or due to dental or supportive tissue associated pathologies. In the inflammatory process, the condition may be complicated depending on the relevance of the microbial aggression and the body's defense ability. This may cause a systemic inflammatory response which sometimes leads to septic shock, multiple organ failure and finally death. Oral infections may be bacterial, fungal, or viral. Odontogenic infections tend to be mixed (aerobic and anaerobic) and bacterial growth and dissemination are observed to be faster in systemically compromised patients.

## *Clinical Features of Cellulitis Include*

1. Swelling

2. Pain

3. Redness of skin

4. Raised local temperature

5. Fever

6. Dysphagia

7. Dyspnea

8. Skin dimpling

## Treatment of Odontogenic Infection and Cellulitis

The pressure of tooth germs, the large amount of cancellous bone with wider medullary spaces and the presence of bone growth centers make infection spread more rapidly in children than in adults. The treatment of such infection is based on two essential principles that is elimination of the underlying cause and local draining or debridement together with the use of oral or parenteral antibiotics [2].

### Mild Odontogenic Infections

Oral Amoxicillin + Clavulanic acid

### Cellulitis

Oral Amoxicillin + Clavulanic acid / Clindamycin (If infection progress rapidly)

### Severe Facial Cellulitis

IV Amoxicillin + Clavulanic acid at 100 mg/kg/day

### Complications of Odontogenic Infections

1. Ludwig's angina

2. Cavernous sinus thrombosis

### Frenectomy

It is the complete removal of the frenulum including its attachment to the underlying bone under local anesthesia (Fig. **11**).

### Diagnosis is Based on

1. Tension test: - While applying pressure over frenum, the interdental papilla shifts when the frenum extended.

2. Blanch test: - When the lip is pulled outward blanching occurs between two Central incisors.

3. Limited mobility of tongue due to thick and tight lingual frenum attachment from bottom of body of tongue to the mandibular bone. In children or adults also evaluate the possibility of the tongue to touch with its tip the retro mesial papilla in palate (Ankyloglossia / tongue tie).

## Techniques for Frenectomy

- Conventional technique - involves excision of the frenum by using a scalpel.
- Electrocautery.
- Lasers.

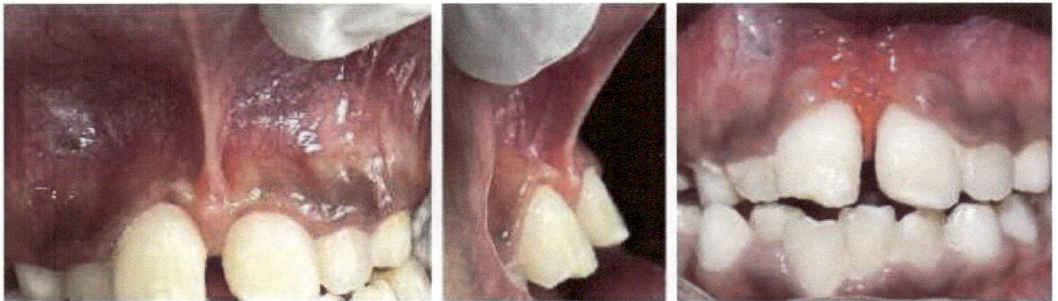

**Fig. (11).** Frenectomy.

## Mucocele

It is the most common lesion of the accessory (minor) salivary glands affecting all genders in all age groups with peak incidence between 10-29years.It is a benign lesion characterized by an extravasation or retention of mucus in sub-mucosal tissue from minor salivary glands. Mucoceles are known to occur most commonly on lower lip followed by floor of the mouth and buccal mucosa. Trauma and lip biting are main cause for these types of lesions. It is rarely observed in infants. These lesions are short lived and burst spontaneously (Fig. **12**).

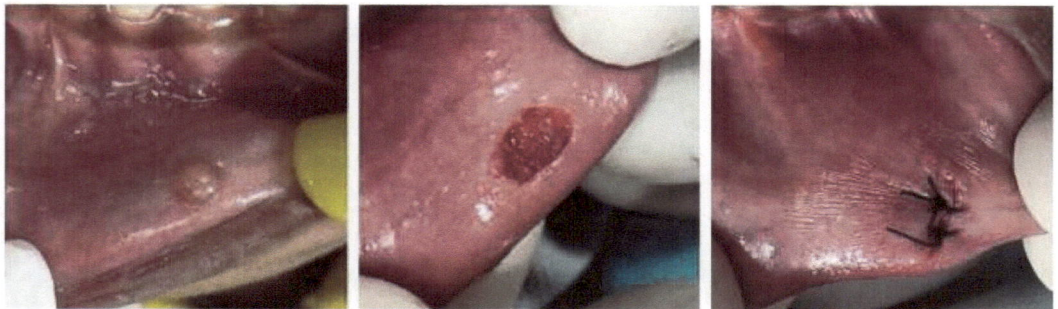

**Fig. (12).** Excision of mucocele.

## Management

1. Excision by electro surgery / scalpel.

2. Vaporization by ($CO_2$) laser.

3. Cryosurgery.

4. Sclerotherapy.

5. Micro marsupialization.

6. Intralesional injection of sclerosing agents or corticosteroid [3].

## Clinical Features

1. They present as a soft painless swelling ranging from deep blue to normal pink colour.

2. The variation in colour depends on the size of the lesion, its proximity to the surface and the elasticity of the overlying tissue.

## Diagnostic Tools

1. Ultrasonography

2. Computed tomography(CT)

3. Magnetic resonance imaging (MRI)

## Surgical Management

- An elliptical incision is placed around the lesion followed by surgical excision of respective minor salivary gland.
- Micro marsupialization- It is draining the accumulated saliva and creating a new epithelialized tract along the path of sutures.

## Eruption Cyst (Eruption Hematoma)

It is an unusual lesion occurring within mucosa over teeth that are about to erupt. It appears as a dome shaped lesion of the alveolar ridge having a pale or bluish translucent soft consistency.

According to WHO classification of epithelial cysts of jaws, eruption cyst is a separate entity [4]. It may be associated with natal or neonatal teeth. Its occurrence on alveolar ridge may be due be due to secondary trauma leading to hematoma or accumulation of blood within the lesion resulting its blue, black, or brown color of the lesion.

### Treatment

- Basically, the tooth erupts through the lesion and no treatment is required.
- If the lesion does not rupture spontaneously or becomes infected, then and micro marsupialization may be planned.

### Soft Tissue Lesions

1. Irritation fibroma

2. Verruca vulgaris

3. Squamous papilloma

4. Localized juvenile spongiotic gingival hyperplasia

5. Pyogenic granuloma

### Fibroma [5]

It is a benign neoplasm of fibrous connections tissue in response to local irritation or trauma (irregular restoration margin, cheek bite, deep bite). It may have sessile or pedunculated base with soft consistency and normal colored mucosa (hyperplasia). Systemic diseases - considered with multiple small fibromas are Cowden syndrome or fibromatosis.

### Recurrence of the Fibroma is Attributed to Two Possible Reasons

1. Non removal of the irritant

2. Incomplete surgical excision of the lesions

### Treatment

1. Excision biopsy

2. Removal of irritant

### Differential Diagnosis

1. Neurofibroma - tongue, buccal mucosa, and another site as well.

2. Neurilemmoma - tongue with associated pain.

3. Lipoma – has yellow hue due to lipid content

4. Peripheral ossifying fibroma- occurs on gingiva and is hard in consistency due to calcific nature of lesion

5. Fibrosarcoma – rare, but all soft tissue tumors must be ruled out.

## *Verruca Vulgaris*

It is an uncommon lesion caused by HPV (human papilloma virus). They are commonly seen on skin and occasionally appear in oral cavity and associated with HPV 6 and 11. These are the benign painless lesions and treated by surgical excision.

## *Squamous Papilloma*

They present as an exophytic mass (papillary lesion) of benign origin found on tongue, soft palate, uvula, and vermilion border of lip. Surgical excision is the treatment of choice long with other treatment modalities like laser surgery, electrocauterization and cryosurgery.

## *Gingival Hyperplasia*

The child may present with gingival hyperplasia associated with eruption gingivitis, poor oral hygiene, and acute myeloid leukemia. The gingival hyperplasia may be hereditary, syndromic, or non-syndromic, drug induced and idiopathic. Before institution of any kind of treatment a proper history related to family, underlying medical condition and drugs should be noted.

## *Treatment Modalities*

1. Improve oral hygiene

2. Gingivectomy through surgical incision, lasers, or cryosurgery

3. In drug induced or syndromic gingival hyperplasia the medical personnel should be consulted before implementation of treatment plan.

## *Pyogenic Granuloma*

It is a commonly found benign tumor like growth of the oral cavity present in aggressive or non-aggressive form. It is also called as hematogenous granuloma and granuloma telangiectatic. It is found to be a red colored, localized (exophytic growth), ulcerative and vascular lesion.

## Treatment

During treatment planning age consideration of child is necessary due to tendency of the lesion to bleed. Indicated treatment is the excision of the growth. Small size lesions in pediatric patients can be managed with local anesthesia but large size lesions will need general anesthesia.

### Dentoalveolar Trauma

1. Soft tissue injury

2. Hard tissue injury

Dental trauma in children is most associated with falls and sports.

### Soft Tissue Injury Types

1. Abrasion

2. Contusion

3. Laceration

4. Avulsion

5. Hematoma

In soft tissue injuries consideration should be given to the child's age and development. Lips should be examined for possible embedded tooth fragments. Immediate treatment is given by controlling pain with a pain killer, ice application at the injured area and suturing of open wounds. A tetanus booster may be required if environmental contamination of the wound has occurred. Antibiotics should be given in cases of infection.

### Hard Tissue Injury

Simple mandibular fracture or dentoalveolar fractures can be reduced, stabilized, and immobilized under local anesthesia. Majorly displaced fractures need to be treated under General anesthesia.

### Periapical Lesions (Fig. 13)

It is an inflammatory lesion present at the apical end of a tooth caused by deep dental caries, tooth trauma, abrasion or erosion of tooth, and periodontal infection leading to pulp necrosis and infection. Osmotic fluid formed by microorganisms gets accumulated in the periapical area of a tooth giving rise to periapical lesion. On radiograph they present as loss of laminadura in periradicular region or a well-defined radiolucency around the root.

They are classified as -

1. Periapical granuloma

2. Periapical cyst (radicular cyst)

Periapical granulomas are usually composed of solid soft tissue whereas cysts are semisolid tissue surrounded by an epithelium.

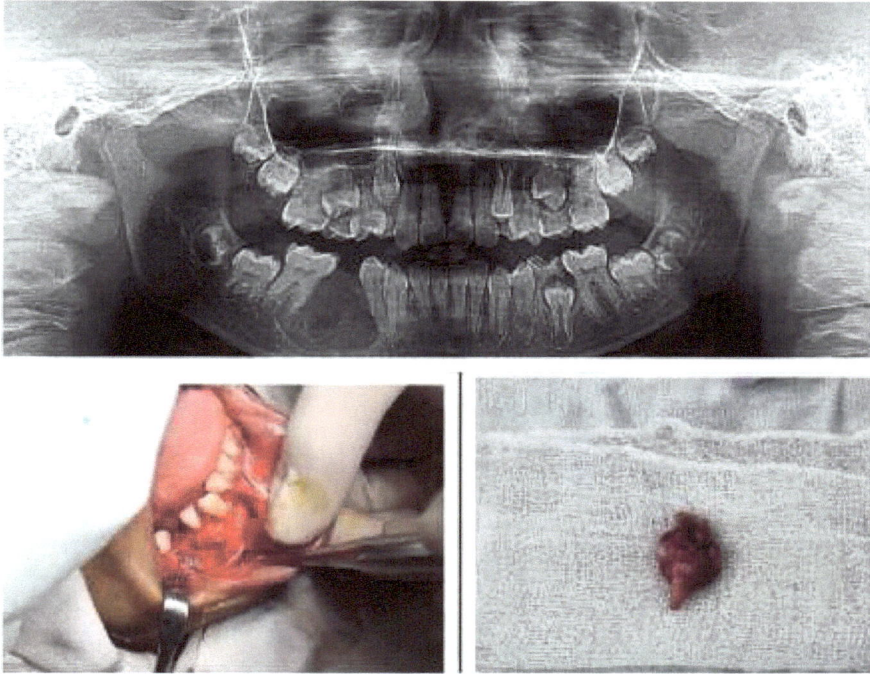

Fig. (13). **a** – OPG of cystic lesion; **b** – Enucleation of cyst; **c** - Cyst lining removed.

## *Treatment*

Majority of small periapical lesions heal subsequently following endodontic treatment. Some lesions may need enucleation and curettage along with endodontic treatment. Large lesions like radicular cyst need surgical intervention (enucleation or marsupialization) under General anesthesia along with either extraction or endodontic treatment of the offending tooth. Release of osmotic fluid pressure helps in the healing of the lesion.

## *Armamentarium for Minor Surgery (Fig. 14)*

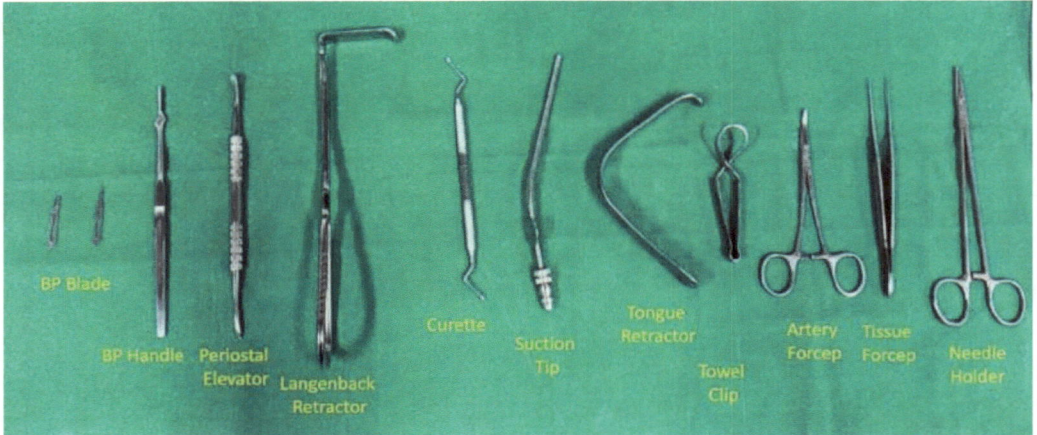

**Fig. (14).** Set of surgical instruments.

## A. Scalpel and Blade

Parts-

1. **Blade**: available as different shapes and sized (#11, #12, #15).

2. **Handle:** also called as BP handle (Bard Parker). Available in different sizes (#3, #4, #7) and may be disposable or sterilizable.

Uses - Surgical incision & Dissection

## B. Periosteal Elevator

It is a double ended instrument having a sharp edge on one side and a flat blade on the other side. It is used to raise a mucoperiosteal flap after incision.

## C. Lagenback Retractor

They are available in varying length

Use:

It is used to separate the edges of the surgical incision to access area or tissue under the incision.

## D. Curette

It is a straight instrument and like small scoop, hook, or gauge at its tip.

Use:

It is a surgical instrument designed for debridement or curettage of biological tissue.

## E. Suction Tip:

It is used for suctioning the secretion or irrigation solutions present at the surgical site. Thus, provide a clear field for surgery.

## F. Tongue Depressor

It is used to retract tongue away from the surgical site.

## G. Towel Clip

Use:

Used to hold sterile drapes in place as close to the incision as possible.

And to fix suction tubes, diathermy wires to sterile drapes.

## H. Artery Forceps

It belongs to a group of surgical instruments called hemostats.

They are held in place by their locking mechanism.

They are of two types: -

A. Mosquito artery forceps – These have a short, slender, and curved tip.

B. Straight artery forceps

Use:

It is used for grasping and compressing an artery to control bleeding

## I. Tissue Forceps

They are of two types

1. Toothed

2. Plain

Use:

They are used for grasping tissue and objects.

## J. Needle Holder (Fig. 15)

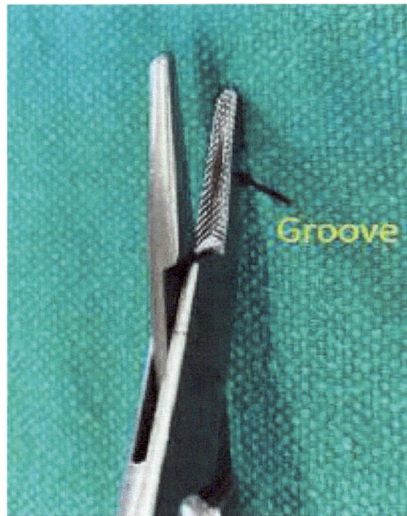

**Fig. (15).** Needle holder.

Parts

1. Jaws - It has groove for firm grip of needle

2. Joint

3. Handle

4. It has a clamp that locks the needle in place.

Use:

It is used to hold suture needle while suturing.

## Rongeur

The instrument looks like a plier having a handle and beaks (Fig. **16**). It is used to trim sharp bony margins or spicules.

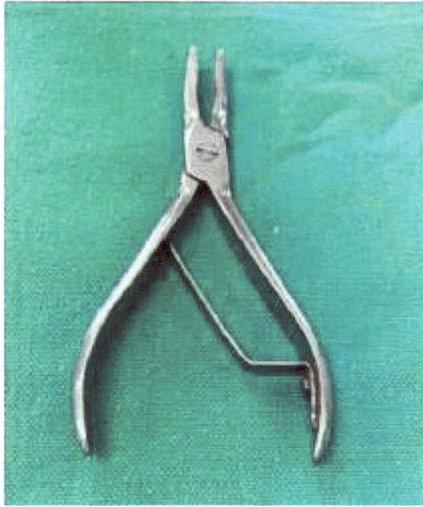

**Fig. (16).** Rongeur forceps.

## Bone File

It is a double ended instrument with serrations on a flat blade like blunt surface. The serrations are used to scrape over sharp bony spicules to smoothen them. They are moved using a pull stroke over the bone (Fig. **17**).

## Surgical Needle:

It has three parts

1. The point- the point penetrates the tissue

2. Body

3. Swage (eye) - the swage holds the suture material

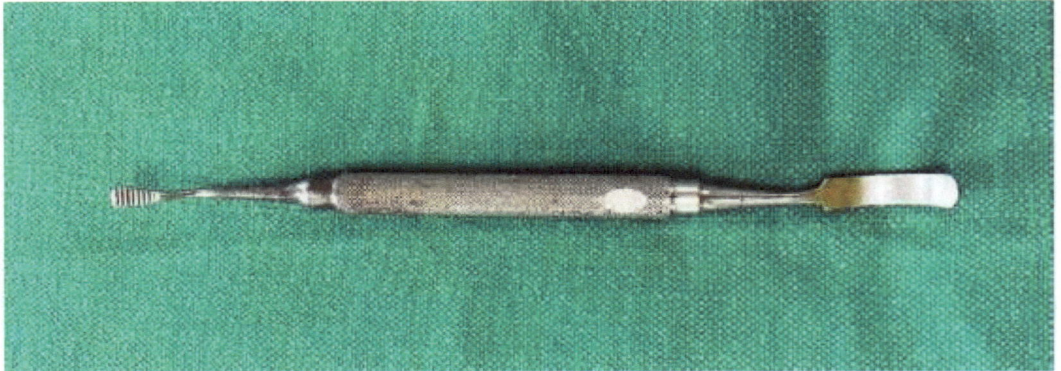

**Fig. (17).**  Bone file.

## Types of Surgical Needles

1. Straight

2. One fourth circle

3. 3/8 circle

4. 1/2 circle

5. 5/8 circle

6. Compound curve

7. Half curve

8. Half curve at both ends of straight surface

### *Needles May Also be Classified by their Point Geometry*

1. Taper

2. Cutting

3. Reverse cutting

4. Round body

Permanently swaged needles are traumatic.

## *Sutures*

## *Types*

a. Absorbable *e.g.*, vicryl
b. Non absorbable *e.g.*, silk
c. Synthetic / natural silk
d. Monofilament - nylon, PDS or Proline
e. Multifilament - braided silk or vicryl

The diameter of suture material will affect its handling properties and tensile strength.

The larger the size ascribed to the sutures, the smaller the diameter is *i.e.*, *e.g.*, 5-0 suture is smaller than 1-0 suture.

## *Syringe*

It is a kind of small pump used to administer injection. It has measuring markings in milliliters (ml).

## *Parts of Syringe*

1. Barrel

2. Plunger

3. Needle adapter

4. Luer lock- locking, slipping

## *Types of Syringes*

1. Disposable syringe - It is made up of plastic and has a rubber seal at one end. It is disposed of after one use thus reducing the risk of spreading blood - borne diseases like HIV and Hepatitis B.

2. Non- disposable syringe- It is made up of glass and can be reused and sterilized in an autoclave.

3. Cartridge- It consists of a metal syringe and a glass carpule containing anesthetic solution and the carpule can be refilled.

## Arch Bar and Wires (Fig. 18)

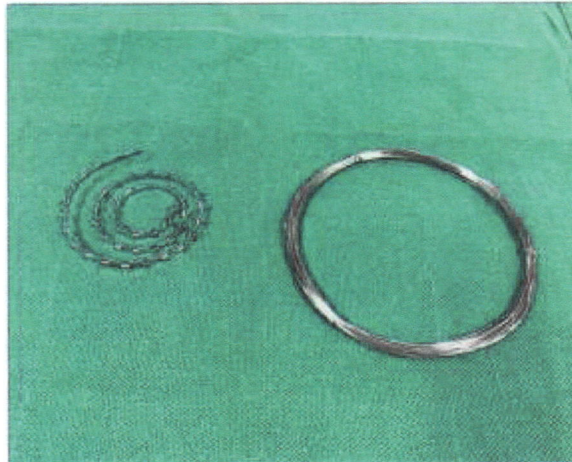

**Fig. (18).** Arch bar and wires.

They are made up of stainless steel and are semirigid.

Use:

They are used for the stabilization of maxillofacial fractures.

### Dental Implants in Pediatric Dentistry

*Introduction*

**Dental implants:** They are the surgical load bearing component, or an artificial root used to replace the missing tooth or teeth and provide strength and stability to the artificial dentition while chewing food and support facial structures also prevent bone loss and maintain strength of the jaw.

*Osseointegration*

It is a process by which an implant anchors to the bone. Osseointegration was discovered in 1962 by Per-Ingvar Branemark of Sweden. It is regarded as a foreign body reaction with bone formed to shield off the foreign material from the tissue [6].

The success of dental implant depends upon various factors:

1. Quality and quantity of bone

2. Oral hygiene

3. Underlying medical issues

4. Treatment planning

5. Patient's compliance

In pediatric patients the dental implant outcome is less predictable due to their ongoing dental and skeletal growth. Children need special consideration given long term morbidity concerns, requirement of growth, manual dexterity, and coping skills [7].

### Growth and Development in Children

Skeletal growth in children follows a general pattern except in syndromic patients. Before planning a dental implant in a pediatric patient, it is imperative to study and understand the growth and development pattern of the face.

Human face grows in four distinct planes [8]: -

1. Mid sagittal plane (MSP): - the midline of face divides bilaterally into left and right sides.

2. Midfacial plane (MFP): - it divides the face into superior and inferior (or lower and upper) halves.

3. Transverse nasal plane (TNP): - it is the horizontal plane parallel to MFP.

4. Trans Glabellar plane (TGP): - it is parallel to TNP and MFP passing through glabella.

### Growth of Maxilla

- Maxilla grows in downward and forward projection with steady /passive growth until age 5 years (85%).
- The maxilla then increases its growth pace until age 11 years and coincides with tooth eruption pattern.
- Also, there is a rapid maxillary expansion up to the age of 10 years.
- Growth of maxillary tuberosity in a posterior direction result in the whole maxilla being carried anteriorly.
- The growth of the cranium base leads to vertical maxilla by displacing the naso-maxillary complex downward and forward.
- The transverse growth of maxilla is facilitated by growth at the median sutures. This leads to forward and downward relocation of the maxilla.

- Sagittal growth occurs by surface remodeling of the anterior surface of maxilla, bringing maxilla even more downward and forward.
- Vertical growth occurs by bone deposition on the palatal side and bone resorption on the lateral wall of the nose and floor of nasal cavity.
- Deepening of the palate occurs around the eruption of the second molar.
- There will be an increase in alveolar bone height with eruption of teeth.

## *Growth of Mandible*

- Ramal lengthening occurs due to bone resorption on anterior part of ramus and bone deposition on posterior part of ramus along with flaring of angle of mandible.
- Lingual tuberosity also moves posteriorly.
- Resorption in the lingual tuberosity forms lingual fossa.
- The alveolar height increases with eruption of mandibular teeth.
- There is bone deposition at the condylar region which reaches its peak between 12-14 years.
- The coronoid process grows following 'V' principle.
- Transverse bone growth ceases before eruption of permanent canine.

The overall skeletal growth ceases around 15 years in females and 17 years in males. Every child's face grows at a different pace and velocity as compared to children of the same age. For evaluation of growth chronological height and age are not appropriate determinants. Skeletal age has relatively a better relationship with the growth of jaws [9].

## *Dento-alveolar Ankylosis*

Periodontal membrane acts as a physiologic barrier and protects the root from potential bone – in growth and subsequent root resorption. When the periodontal ligament is severely injured following dental trauma (avulsion or infusion of tooth) the protective mechanism will no longer function and the bone – in growth to the dental tissue (ankylosis) may occur. This condition is called as dentoalveolar ankylosis. Considering placement of implant early diagnosis of ankylosis is necessary for treatment planning and timing.

## *Classification of Implants*

1. Depending on placement with the tissues
    i. Epiosteal implants
    ii. Transosteal implants
    iii. Endosteal implants
2. Depending on material used

1. Metallic implant (titanium, titanium alloy, cobalt chromium, molybdenum alloy)
2. Nonmetallic implants (ceramic, carbon)
3. Depending on their reaction to bone
   i. Bio- active (hydroxyapatite)
   ii. Bio inert implant
4. Depending upon treatment options

According to Misch (1988), the first three are fixed prosthesis (partial or complete) which may be cemented or screw- retained. The remaining two are removable prosthesis based on support derived.

## *Indications of Dental Implants*

1. Anodontia: - it is a complete absence of teeth

2. Hypodontia: - missing teeth less than six.

3. Oligodontia: - missing six or more teeth

4. Trauma: - avulsion

5. Dental caries (extraction)

6. Ectodermal dysplasia

## *Bone Assessment will be done with*

1. Radiographs (OPG)

2. Cephalometric analysis (in children)

3. CBCT

## *Steps in Placing an Implant (Fig. 19)*

1. Extraction of decayed tooth

2. Alveolar bone preparation (bone augmentation may be needed)

3. Placement of implant surgically

4. Osseointegration around implant

5. Placement of an abutment (a connection between an implant and artificial tooth)

6. Cementation of an artificial tooth over the abutment.

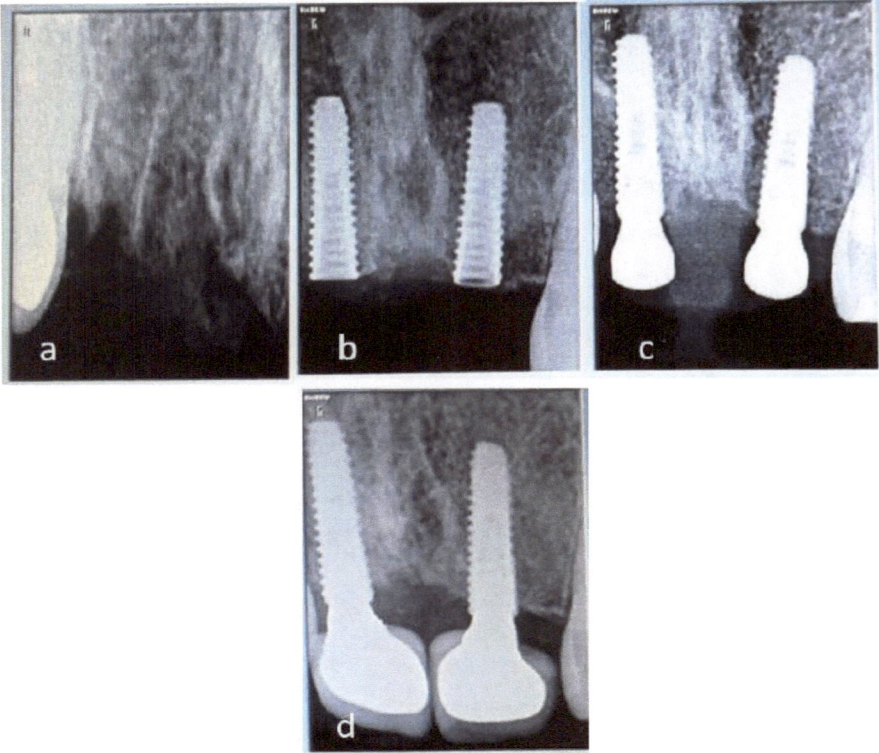

**Fig. (19).**  Steps in implant placement – **a:** Extraction of decayed teeth; **b:** Placement of implants; **c:** Gingival attachments; **d:** Prosthetic rehabilitation.

## *In Pediatric Patient, Placement of Implant Needs*

- A multidisciplinary approach, involving a prosthodontist, orthodontist, periodontist, and a maxillofacial surgeon.
- Pre assessment of skeletal growth, anatomy of adjacent structures (maxillary sinus, nerves etc.), gingival condition and underlying medical conditions.
- Once the treatment plan is decided, the surgical procedure is preceded with anesthesia followed by an incision over gingiva of alveolar ridge to expose underlying bone (crestal/ paracrestal incision).
- The size of the implant is decided according to the mesiodistal and buccolingual size of the ridge and proximity to the vital structures.
- Physiodispenser is a machine with high torque at varying rpm having an attachment for handpiece and irrigation is used during implant placement.
- As far as possible an implant should be placed as close as the natural position of a tooth.

- For maxillary central incisors implants should be placed slightly distal to the center of the final mesiodistal length of crown and slightly palatally due to resorption pattern of maxilla.
- While in mandible the implants should be placed slightly buccally due to resorption pattern of mandible.
- In case of a sharp alveolar ridge, sharpness should be reduced before osteotomy.
- Implants should never be placed in bony suture areas as it may cause expansion of sutures.
- If the implant is placed below the alveolar crest it may lead to peri – implantitis.
- In pediatric patients the bone is very soft therefore the under preparation of the implant site is helpful to achieve stability.
- The initial osteotomy cut is given with the help of a small round bur or spiral drill followed by a 1.5mm diameter drill at 2500 rpm.
- Then guiding pins or paralleling pins of same diameter are placed to assess the direction of axis.
- A larger diameter drill with less rpm (500-600) is then used to increase the depth and width of the site.
- After final drilling, 1.5 – 2mm of bone should be present around an implant.
- In case of multiple implants adjacent implants should be placed 3-4mm away from each other to accommodate crowns over it.
- An implant is placed in the prepared surgical site with the help of a handpiece with speed as low as 25 rpm or by hand with a wrench.
- A cover screw is placed over the implant and the wound is sutured.
- Time required by bone to heal is 5-6 months in maxilla and around 3-4 months in mandible.
- Healing period may extend if the quality of bone is poor.
- Once the healing (hard tissue) is achieved the implant is exposed surgically and the cover screw is replaced by the gingival former (Fig. **19c**) that helps in contouring gingiva around the implant.
- Later the gingival former is replaced by an abutment and a crown is cemented over it (Fig. **19D, 20 a,b,c,d**).
  - During masticatory function, occlusal force distribution over an implant depends upon the position of the implant. Therefore, implants with deviation more than $25^0$ leads to failure.

In children because of less bone height, width and the softness of bone smaller implants will be used. In special cases of tooth agenesis like Ectodermal Dysplasias implants should be planned once the skeletal growth is completed. Implants placed in cases where the skeletal growth is still ongoing will cause discrepancy in occlusal plane as the teeth eruption process is responsible for alveolar bone growth and an implant will remain inside as an ankylosed root. Also implant failure will be more in children due to softness of bone and skeletal growth.

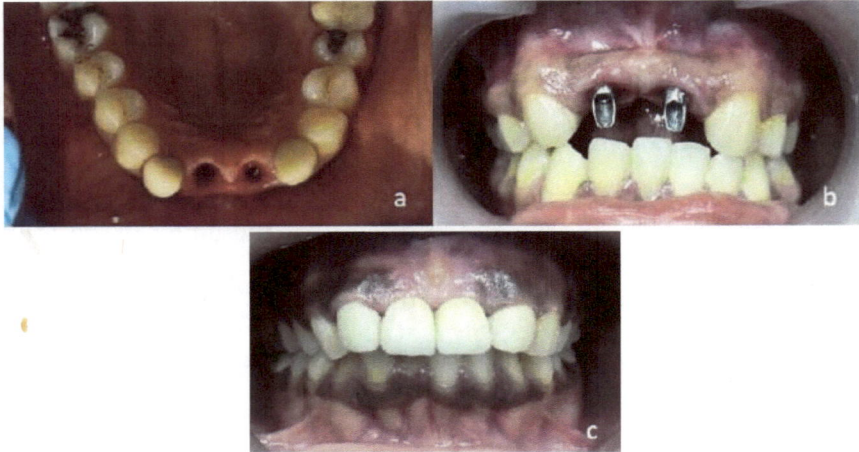

**Fig. (20). a** – Implants placed *in situ*; **b** – Abutment fixed over implants; **c** – Implant with prosthesis.

## *Mini Implants*

Implant dentistry has significantly changed over a period and there is an introduction of mini-implants an alternative to traditional dental implants. These implants are either self-driving or self-tapping small size implants suitable for pediatric patients. They consisted of a one-piece screw that is less than 3 mm in diameter and a ball at top protruding in the oral cavity or supragingivally. Their length is decided according to the bone height and surrounding vital structures. They are placed over the alveolar ridge under local anesthesia and a flapless surgery. No sutures are needed. The mini-implants have a diameter ranging from 1.8mm - 3mm and the pilot hole for the mini-implants is made with 1.2mm pilot drill (approximately half of the size of the diameter of mini-implant) using sterile surgical technique. Osseointegration period required for mini-implants are shorter than conventional implants. It is a minimally invasive procedure and success rate of these implants is more in mandible as compared to maxilla [10,11].

## CONCLUSION

Extraction of teeth when required should be done keeping in mind the age of the child followed by appropriate care for space maintenance. Delay in extraction of decayed teeth can often lead to serious spread of infection in the Oro-facial region.

Minor oral surgical procedures when planned for various conditions decrease the morbidity during adolescence and adulthood. Children are usually very apprehensive about dental treatment and parent too may show anxiety when faced with a situation requiring surgical intervention of their children. Hence a dental surgeon should follow an empathetic approach towards children and their parents who require minor surgical intervention.

Teeth lost due to dental caries, trauma or other reasons can be replaced using dental implants if the parents are explained about the interim nature of the procedure and a thorough understanding of the growth and development of the jaws. They can give acceptable esthetic a functional rehabilitation of children during their formative years.

## CONSENT FOR PUBLICATION

Not applicable.

## CONFLICT OF INTEREST

The authors declare no conflict of interest, financial or otherwise.

## ACKNOWLEDGEMENT

Declared none.

## REFERENCES

[1]     Dodson TB, Perrott DH, Kaban LB. Pediatric maxillofacial infections: A retrospective study of 113 patients. J Oral Maxillofac Surg 1989; 47(4): 327-30.
        [http://dx.doi.org/10.1016/0278-2391(89)90331-5] [PMID: 2926541]

[2]     GiuntaCrescente C. Medical-dental considerations in the care of children with facial cellulitis of odontogenic origin. A disease of interest for pediatricians and pediatric dentists Arch Argent Pediatr 2018; 116(4): e548-53.
        [http://dx.doi.org/10.5546/aap.2018.eng.e548]

[3]     Chalathadka M, Ranganathan A, Pb R, Abraham A, Gera M, Unakalkar S. Management of Mucocele. RE:view 2019; 227-34.

[4]     Navas A. Ramón & Mendoza, María & Leonardo, Mário & Silva, Raquel & Herrera, Henry & Herrera, Helen. 2010.

[5]     Kajal A, Tandon S, Rai TS, Mathur R, Kajal A. Recurrent Irritation Fibroma—"What Lies Beneath": A Multidisciplinary Treatment Approach. Int J Clin Pediatr Dent 2020; 13(3): 306-9.
        [http://dx.doi.org/10.5005/jp-journals-10005-1769] [PMID: 32904090]

[6]     Albrektsson T, Chrcanovic B, Jacobsson M, Wennerberg A. Osseointegration of Implants – A Biological and Clinical Overview. JSM Dent Surg 2017; 2(3): 1022.

[7]     Brahim Jaime S. Dental Implants in Children. Oral and Maxillofacial Surgery Clinics 17(4): 375-81.
        [http://dx.doi.org/10.1016/j.coms.2005.06.003]

[8]     A Midori Albert, Amanda L Brady s. Craniofacial changes in children - birth to late adolescence. ARC Journal of Forensic Science 2019; 4(1): 1-19.

[9]     Das S. Dental Implants in Pediatric Dentistry: A Review Article. Indian Journal of Forensic Medicine

& Toxicology 2020; 14(4): 9183-6.
[http://dx.doi.org/10.37506/ijfmt.v14i4.13181]

[10]   Arun T. PonnuduraiArangannal, Jeevarathan J, AmudhaS, AarthiJ, Vijayakumar M. Dental implants in pediatric dentistry: A Review. Eur J Mol Clin Med 2020; 7(2): 6497-501.

[11]   Shatkin, Todd &Petrotto, Christopher.. Mini dental implants: a retrospective analysis of 5640 implants placed over a 12-year period. Compendium of continuing education in dentistry 2012; 2-9.

# CHAPTER 3

# Sedation & General Anaesthesia in Pediatric Dentistry

**Alka Halbe**[1,*] and **Falguni Shah**[2]

[1] *Breach Candy Hospital Trust, Mumbai, India*

[2] *Lilavati Hospital and Research Centre, Mumbai, India*

**Abstract:** Managing a child for dental treatment is one of the most challenging tasks for both anaesthesiologists & pediatric dentists alike. The goal is to provide safe, painless, anxiety-free, prompt & appropriate treatment in the minimum number of sessions. To achieve this, children need to be given Monitored Anaesthesia Care (MAC), Sedation, Anxiolysis or sometimes complete general anaesthesia (GA) by appropriately trained specialists in day-care & ambulatory services settings with better advances in anaesthesia, dentistry, pharmacology, monitoring devices, better understanding of paediatric airway anatomy & physiology, paediatric dental anaesthesia has become safe over the last few years. This chapter overviews the various aspects of Pediatric dental anaesthesia & sedation and highlights the significance of specialised infrastructure, personnel, & protocols.

**Keywords:** General Anaesthesia, Nitrous Oxide, Pediatric Dental Anaesthesia, Sedation.

## INTRODUCTION

Managing children for various dental procedures in free-standing ambulatory clinics or hospitals. Careful & sensitive planning of the system & anaesthesia, if necessary, is vital to develop a positive attitude towards dental treatment [1]. Depending on the child's emotional maturity, physical, psychological & mental ability & skills, the usual behavioural control techniques may or may not offer adequate efficacy & safety for dental treatment [2].

There are various reasons for stress, fear & anxiety in children, exposure to strange environments, noises of mechanical dental instruments, injections pain, parents' visible stress, and parental separation [3]. In these situations, alter-

---

\* **Corresponding author Alka Halbe:** Breach Candy Hospital Trust, Mumbai, India; E-mail: arhalbe@breachcandyhospital.org

nate & more invasive methods like sedation or GA (general anaesthesia) may be necessary for optimum treatment.

## Objectives of Sedation & Anaesthesia

1. Patient Safety- **"primum non Nocera** *"* ("first, do no harm")

2. Control of anxiety, fear, and psychological trauma

3. Pain control and amnesia of the event

4. Movement restrains

5. Minimise oral secretions

6. Patient and operator comfort so that procedure is completed successfully & in a minimum number of sessions.

## Different Methods of Sedation and Anaesthesia for Paediatric Dental Treatment

Behaviour management can be pharmacological or non-pharmacological in paediatric dental patients [1]. However, some children may need sedation or GA during dental treatment due to their inherent anxiety, fear, nature & length of treatment, various congenital or acquired medical conditions *etc.* Noticeably young children perceive any kind of stimulus as pain and keeping them quiet in a dental chair to complete the procedure safely & adequately becomes difficult. Thus, the anaesthesia requirement in pediatric dental patients may vary from monitored anaesthesia care (MAC) to sedation to general anaesthesia (GA) [4].

Challenges for anaesthesia care providers in dental practice is regarding sharing the airway with the pediatric dentist. The patient's ability to control the airway may be impaired due to pharmacological override of normal protective airway reflexes like swallowing& coughing. This increases the chances of blood, water, saliva, and dental debris aspiration. The level of analgesia and sedation needs to be controlled carefully as inadequate sedation will increase secretions, may cause masseter spasms or clenching and more primitive reflexes like laryngospasm can be activated [1]. Untreated or prolonged laryngospasms can result in hypoxia &long-term brain damage or even death in rare cases. Deeper levels of sedation may precipitate respiratory depression, airway obstruction, if it goes unnoticed, may culminate into hypoxia and hypercarbia, leading to long term morbidity and rarely even mortality.

Stimulating the trigeminal nerve during the dental procedure under lighter planes of sedation or anaesthesia may be implicated in the increased incidence of ventricular arrhythmias. This incidence may be exacerbated by accompanying hypoxia, hypercarbia, and the presence of inhalational anaesthetic agents like halothane. Local infiltration can significantly reduce this incidence [5].

## Non-Pharmacological Methods of Behavior Management

Nonpharmacologic methods include behavioural and cognitive approaches like a distraction, desensitisation, relaxation, reinforcing and strengthening positive behaviour. These procedures complement pharmacologic interventions; however, sedation or GA may not be needed in some mature children if these methods are adequate.

Parental presence in the treatment room helps ease anxiety and improve cooperation. Besides baby, when allowed to remain in the arms of the mother, venepuncture or mask acceptance becomes more manageable. However, anxious parents can transfer their anxiety to the child, and parents can be a hindrance [6]. For older children playing music through headphones, video games, video, or virtual reality goggles works well as a distraction technique. Subsequent visits also become more accessible, and the sedation requirement goes down. It is worth a try [7 - 9].

## Pharmacological Methods

Procedural sedation has become the standard of care for managing pain and anxiety in children in the dental chair and for short diagnostic and therapeutic procedures in children outside the operation theatre. The increasing grades of sedation ultimately lead to GA like state. The American Academy of Pediatrics (AAP), the American Society of Anaesthesiologists (ASA), the American Academy of pediatric dentistry, and the Joint Commission use the following definitions to describe the depth of sedation [7, 8].

1. Analgesia- Pain relief with or without altered mental status due to the drug's effect.

2. Minimal Sedation is a state of depression of the central nervous system in which cognitive function and coordination may be impaired. It enables treatment to be carried out without losing verbal contact with the patient. Patients retain their protective airway reflexes and cardiovascular functions. It's a state of 'Anxiolysis'.

3. Moderate Sedation or Analgesia is a controlled, pharmacologically induced, minimally depressed level of consciousness that retains the patient's ability to maintain a patent airway independently and continuously and respond appropriately to physical and verbal command. Cardiovascular and respiratory functions are supported and do not require any intervention.

4. Deep Sedation- It is a steady, pharmacologically induced state of depressed level of consciousness from which the patient is not easily aroused and may be accompanied by a partial loss of protective reflexes, including the ability to maintain a patent airway independently and respond purposefully to physical stimulation or verbal commands. May require assistance to maintain an airway and adequate ventilation. Cardiovascular function is usually held.

5. General Anaesthesia (GA) – A reversible state in which the patient cannot be aroused often requires assistance to maintain airway and ventilation. Cardiovascular function may be impaired. It is accompanied by reflex suppression and muscle relaxation.

Personnel administering either sedation or General anaesthesia to children for their dental treatment should be trained adequately to manage laryngospasm, airway obstruction & apnoea.

"Conscious sedation" is a term that is sometimes used to refer to minimal or moderate sedation. Because effective sedation usually impairs consciousness, this term has been abandoned when referring to sedation states [8].

## *Monitored Anaesthesia Care (MAC)*

Monitored anaesthesia care (MAC) is a type of anaesthesia service in which an anaesthesia clinician performs the peri-procedural assessment and understands the patient's coexisting medical conditions, continuously monitors, supports the patient's vital functions, diagnoses and treats clinical problems that occur, administers sedative, anxiolytic, or analgesic medications as needed; and converts sedation process to general anaesthesia if required.

## *Sedation Techniques*

The various sedation techniques described can be titratable & non-titratable (Table 1). However, during routine clinical practice, both methods are usually used.

**Table 1. Sedation techniques.**

| Non-Titratable | Titratable | Combinational |
|---|---|---|
| Oral | Inhalational | Most followed |
| Subcutaneous | Intravenous | |
| Intramuscular | - | |
| Intranasal | - | |
| Submucous | - | |

## *Commonly Used Drugs for Sedation*

Following are the routinely used drugs in clinical practice (Table **2**).

**Table 2. Commonly Used Drugs for Sedation.**

| Hypnotics | Chloral Hydrate |
|---|---|
| Benzodiazepines | Diazepam (oral), Midazolam |
| Phencyclidine | Ketamine |
| IV Anaesthetics | Methohexitone, Propofol, Etomidate |
| $\alpha_2$ Agonist | Dexmedetomidine, Clonidine (oral) |
| Opioids | Fentanyl, Remifentanil, Morphine, Pentazocine |
| Antihistamines | Hydroxyzine, Promethazine |
| Inhalational Agents | $N_2O$, Sevoflurane, Desflurane |
| Antisialogouges | Glycopyrrolate, Atropine |

The various routes of administration for these medications can be oral, nasal, intramuscular, inhalational, intravenous, *etc.*

## *Oral Route*

Advantages of this route are ease of administration, cost-effectiveness, no need for special skills or equipment & parental participation. In younger children, acceptance rate is high. However, absorption of the medication from the stomach can be erratic & hence onset and duration of action may not be predictable. The exact route cannot extend the period of activity. It must be complemented by other ways like intravenous (IV) or inhalational. The oral approach works well in younger children and allows easy parental separation, IV access, and mask acceptance if planned inhalational sedation.

**Oral Chloral Hydrate** was routinely used in the past. But it has a bitter taste; it gives gastric irritation and, at times, excessive sedation. With the availability of better options, this drug is rarely used nowadays.

**Triclofosis**: specially used for inducing sleep in dental and other OPD procedures in children. It is the monophosphate sodium salt of trichloro ethanol (the pharmacologically active metabolite of chloral hydrate). It is available as 50mg/ml soln. The dose is 75 mg/kg of body weight. This dose induces sleep within 10 min, and sleep lasts over 1 hr in nonpainful conditions. It has good quality palatability and more minor gastric irritation than Chloral Hydrate. Respiratory depression is not known when used in the dosages mentioned above. As the half-life of this drug is long, the child may remain drowsy but arousable for long& hence instructions for post-procedure care need to be given accordingly to a responsible adult at the time of discharge. Triclofos is cost-effective and does not have other systemic side effects [10].

**Midazolam** is a short-acting benzodiazepine with a wide toxic/therapeutic ratio and safety margin [11]. It does not produce prolonged sedation associated with other drugs mentioned earlier. When taken orally, midazolam is rapidly absorbed from the gastrointestinal tract. It has its peak effects in a relatively shorter time of about 30 minutes, with a half-life of about 1.75 hours [11]. When administered in doses between 0.5 to 0.75 mg/kg of body weight, oral midazolam has also produced sedation, anxiolysis, and excellent anterograde amnesia. It is a valuable sedative agent for pediatric dental patients. Midazolam is a short-acting agent; its action lasts for a short duration, requiring intra venous or inhalational supplementation of sedation. Midazolam has anticonvulsant properties too. It is beneficial to terminate and prevent seizures in the dental chair (Fig. **1**).

**Ketamine** is a Phencyclidine derivative. It is a dissociative anaesthetic and analgesic used as a sedative, palliative, and analgesic drug. It maintains the muscle tone, and the respiratory system's protective reflexes and circulation are also supported. However, ketamine is known to cause hallucinations and nightmares during the recovery period in older children and adults, especially after prolonged administration and excessive dosage. Still, these side effects are rarely seen in younger children [12]. Excessive oral secretions may become troublesome, requiring anti sialagogue medications (*e.g.*, atropine, glycopyrrolate [13].

No oral formulations of ketamine hydrochloride are available. Intravenous preparations are used orally. However, the Intravenous preparation has a bitter and astringent taste. To make it palatable by the oral route, it is often mixed with cola, honey, apple juice, yoghurt, paracetamol syrup, sugar cubes to suck, *etc.* of course, the bioavailability of such preparation is not studied [14]. The oral dose is 3 to 6 mg/kg of body wt. It induces sleep within 5 to 10 min.

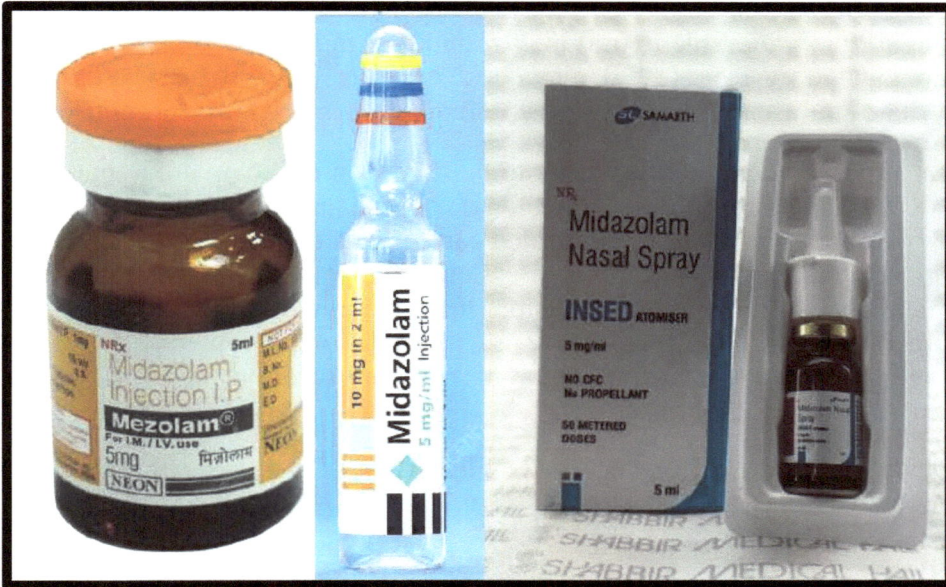

**Fig. (1).**  Midazolam im/iv, vial-1mg/ml; ampoule-5mg/ml, nasal spray 0.5mg/puff.

Hydroxyzine is an antihistaminic agent with sedative and anxiolytic properties and a bronchodilator. It is used as a premedication before surgery. The syrup is palatable and available in good flavour. The onset of action is almost 30 min. Earlier it was used with Chloral Hydrate. It is used with Midazolam syrup in doses of 1 to 2 mg/kg. This combination works within 10 minutes, but action lasts for about 30 – 40 minutes. More prolonged procedures require supplementation. Respiratory depression to be watched out for [15].

## *Intranasal Route*

The intranasal route is predictable specific and gives faster action with sedatives. Nasal mucosa being vascular, the area being wider, absorption of the drug is more instantaneous, reducing the time of medication delivery. It bypasses the stomach & there is direct transmucosal absorption. Hence drug requirement is less. Concentrated solutions are required as there is a restriction on the total volume of drugs that can be instilled. No pain due to injection is an added advantage. Intranasal drug administration thus is an effective method for delivering analgesia [16].

Intranasal Dexmedetomidine has been used as an alternative to usual oral sedatives like midazolam. It is a good anxiolytic in the dose 1µgm /kg. Adequate sedation for IV cannulation is achieved in about 25min and last up to 80 to 100min in 62% of children [17, 18]. Intranasal Dexmedetomidine in the dose of 0.5–1 µg/ kg is preferable to oral midazolam (0.5 mg/ kg) in producing a state of sedation, and drowsiness [19]. Up to a dose of 2.0 µg/ kg may be used intranasally safely. The atomiser administration is preferable to drop by drop administration.

Midazolam is a versatile drug that can be used as a sedative and hypnotic along with Ketamine, Propofol and Fentanyl or Inhalational sedation. Intranasal Midazolam sedation needs to be titrated carefully as there can be a sudden loss of control of the airway, respiratory depression, cardiovascular depression & delayed recovery. The child may feel exhausted, tired, or weak for 1 or 2 days afterwards on rare occasions. Small kids may not be able to hold themselves or walk. Midazolam Sprays are available for nasal administration. One puff from the container is 0.5mg of Midazolam.

Although it appears easy and simple to administer, parents and children prefer the oral route to the nasal. Dose used is 0.2 - 0.3 mg/kg intranasally [20].

Ketamine has been used intranasally to induce analgesia and sleep for procedural sedation in children and anaesthesia in higher doses. The recommended range of Dose – is 0.5mg to 10 mg/kg of body weight. There is no special nasal preparation of ketamine for clinical use. Hence intravenous medication is routinely used nasally. It is known to produce cardiac stimulation vomiting. Sedation quality is inferior to that of Dexmedetomidine or Midazolam. However, ketamine can come in handy during emergencies [21, 22]

Ketamine and Dexmedetomidine, along with or without Midazolam, have been used for paediatric procedural sedation by nebulisation. The drugs are diluted in 0.9% N Saline to 30ml. Nebulised using $O_2$ at six lit/min, either with a mouthpiece or Face Masks. Both the drugs have good bioavailability by this route. The large droplets get deposited in the oropharynx, Nares, and Nasopharynx depending on the droplet size. Most of the drug thus deposited, little of the medication is carried to lungs. Dexmedetomidine produced good sedation, allowing easy parental separation, IV cannulation, mask acceptance, immobility, and minimal side effects post-procedure. The known side effects of Dexmedetomidine, *i.e.*, Bradycardia and hypotension are rarely seen with intranasal administration [19, 23, 24] (Fig. **2**).

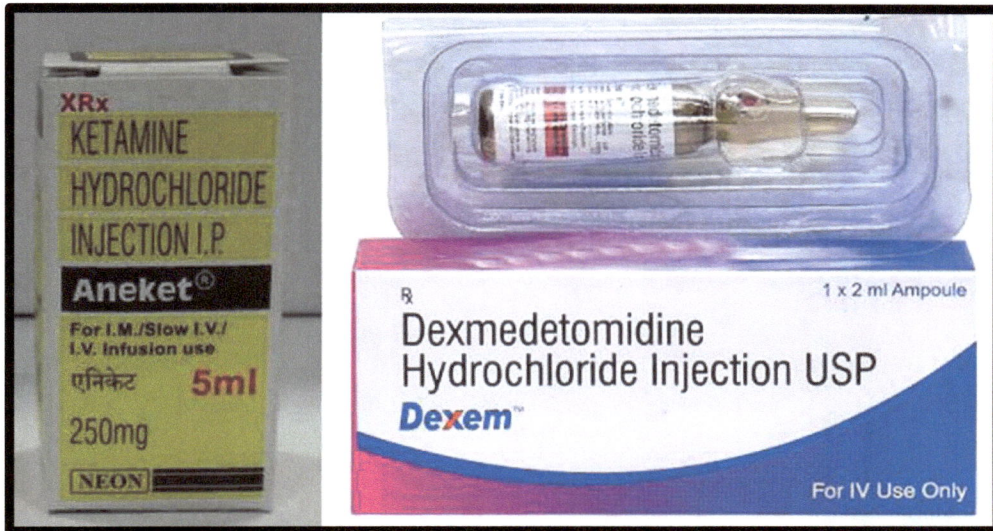

Fig. (2). Ketamine 50 mg/ml, im/iv; Dexmedetomidine 100 µgm/ml iv.

Intranasal Sufentanil has an onset of action in about 5-10 min with a maximum sedative and analgesic effect at about 20-25 min. Doses: 0.7-1 µg/kg. There is an increased incidence of respiratory depression, breath-holding, *etc*. Also, a higher incidence of vomiting during immediate and 1st postoperative day [12] is commonly not preferred in day-care settings.

## *Intramuscular Route*

IM route requires a trained person to administer the drug. Acceptance by children is extremely poor. But the action is faster, and effects are generally predictable. The intragluteal injection is usually preferred to intra deltoid injections.

Ketamine is frequently used in dental sedation procedures by this route. Besides sedation, it offers good analgesia as well. There is a need to combine it with anti-sialagogue like glycopyrrolate as it causes an excessive increase in oral secretions. Tachycardia, cardiac arrhythmias, and increased blood pressure are some of the other side effects. High doses over an extended period can precipitate the emergence of delirium and irrational behaviour. These side effects can effectively be curtailed by supplementing with Midazolam and Propofol.

Doses of ketamine- Intramuscular – 5.0 – 10.0 mg/kg, Intravenous- 0.25 – 0.5 mg/kg (Sedation)1.0-2.0 mg/kg (Induction of Anesthesia [25] Midazolam- IM and IV- 0.03 to 0.05mg/kg.

## *Intravenous Administration*

Propofol is a short-acting hypnotic agent with fast onset. Pain on injection is known as a significant side effect. It is due to a preparation containing long-chain triglycerides as a vehicle. To reduce the pain, pre-treatment with Lignocaine is recommended by manufacturers. Recently, Propofol-LCTA new formulation of propofol (a mixture of long-chain and medium-chain triglycerides in the carrier emulsion; Propofol-MCT/LCT) reduces the incidence of pain on bolus injection (Fig. **3**).

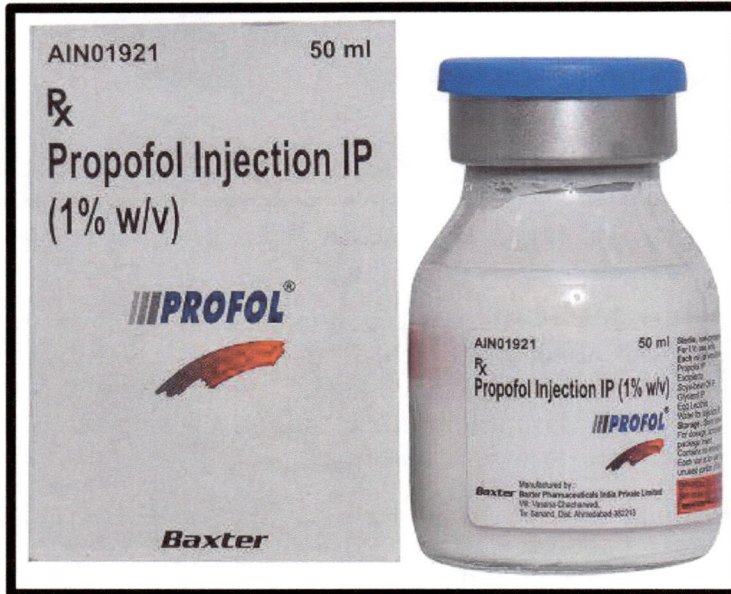

**Fig. (3).** Propofol- 1%w/v 10mg/ml, 2% w/v 20mg/ml,mct/lct.

Other side effects are apnea/ breath-holding, bradycardia, hypotension, muscular movements, rarely delayed effects like skin rashes & allergy. Prolonged& repeated boluses can lead to delayed recovery from the sedation.

Recommended dose is: 2.0 – 2.5 mg/kg (Induction); 0.5 – 1.5 mg/kg sedation (Sub anesthetic dose), Infusion- 4 to 6 mg /kg /hr. The infusion is the preferred method rather than giving intermittent boluses. Infusion should be given through syringe pumps or infusion pumps for the proper administration of correct dosage to get desired effects Combination with Ketamine – 1:1 in the same syringe or sequence to reduce possible side effects &to give better analgesia. One mg Propofol to one mg ketamine in the same syringe (Fig. **4**). This combination takes both drugs' side effects, maintaining cardiovascular and respiratory status. It is sometimes labelled as Ketofol [25]. Qualified, trained Anesthesiologists should always use propofol.

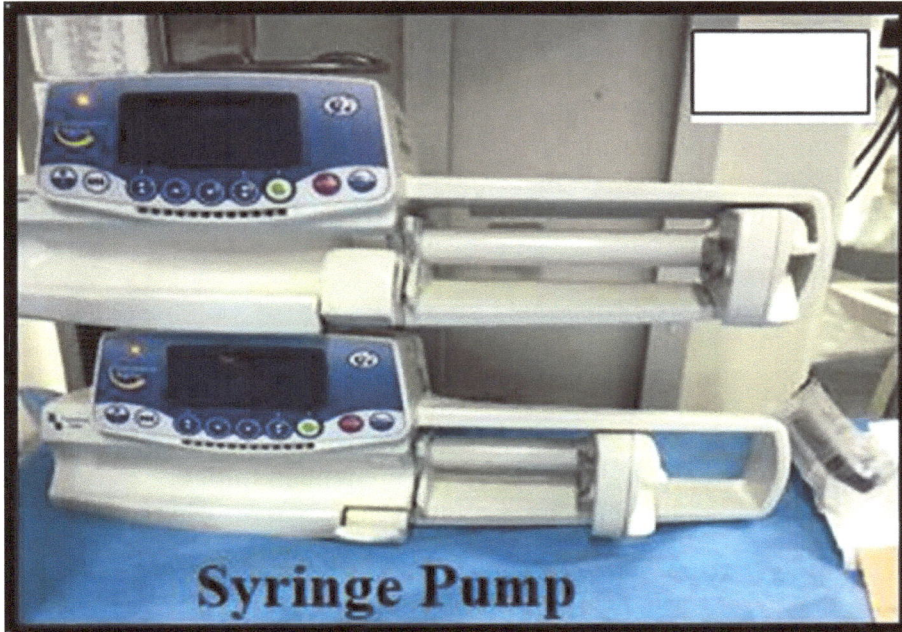

**Fig. (4).** Syringe pump.

Midazolam is often used in combination with other Ketamine, or $N_2O$ inhalations is rarely used as a sole agent. With higher doses, the incidence of breath-holding leading to desaturation is known. Similarly, loss of airway due to muscle relaxation hypotension is also known. Combining with Ketamine takes care of the side effects of both drugs. Recommended dose: Midazolam: 0.05- 0.1mg/kg; Ketamine:0.5mg-1.0mg/kg.

Fentanyl is an opioid analgesic agent. It is used in combination with the above drugs. Respiratory depression is common to all opioids with bradycardia, itching, nausea & vomiting, drowsiness & fatigue. Rarely, it is known to cause spasms of chest wall muscles leading to difficulty in breathing and ventilation. It is a narcotic agent. The regulations for narcotic drugs use must be followed strictly while using fentanyl. Dose: 1 to 2 µgm/kg [12].

Intravenous Methohexital is a short-acting and effective sedative that was immensely popular in the past for dental procedures in adults and children.

Methohexital has lost its place since drugs with better pharmacokinetics and pharmacodynamics are available.

## *Reversal Agents*

Naloxone hydrochloride is an opioid antagonist & should be available if fentanyl is used. It reverses the respiratory depression consequence of Fyl and neutralises the analgesic effects. In larger doses, it can cause respiratory depression. Quantity: 0.1 mg in children. The result is seen within a few minutes. Half dose can be divided and given slowly if there is no effect. Naloxone can be injected intravenously, intramuscularly, subcutaneously, and even intranasally in babies [24].

Flumazenil is a Benzodiazepine antagonist. It reverses benzodiazepine induced CNS depression. Flumazenil produces a rapid and dependable reversal of unconsciousness, respiratory depression, sedation, amnesia, and psychomotor dysfunction. It also reverses the anticonvulsant effects of Benzodiazepines, due to which the child may suddenly start convulsions. It should be introduced intravenously at incremental doses. The recommended initial dose is 0.01 mg/kg (up to 0.2 mg) in children, administered intravenously over 15 seconds.

Suppose the desired level of consciousness is not obtained after waiting for a minute. In that case, further injections of 0.01 mg/kg (up to 0.2 mg) can be given at 60-seconds intervals to a maximum total dose of 0.05 mg/kg or 1 mg, whichever is lower. Resedation with respiratory depression occurs especially with longer-acting benzodiazepines [24] (Fig. **5**).

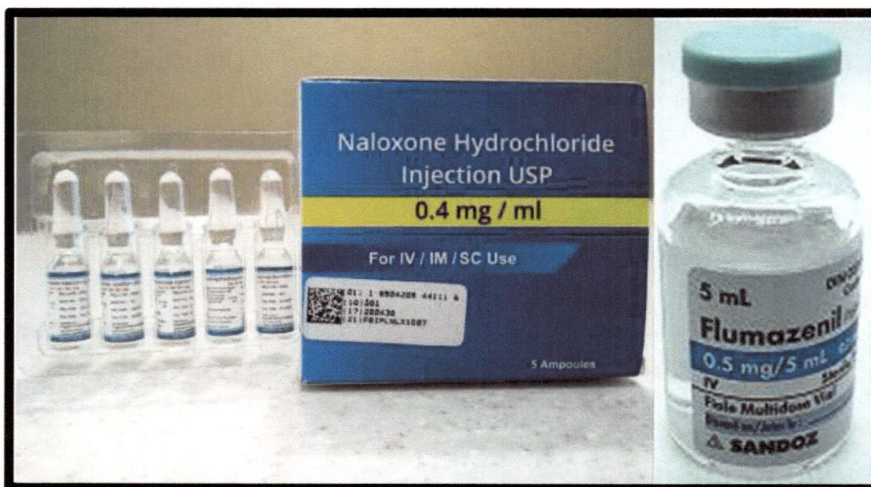

**Fig. (5).** Reversal agents- Naloxone 0.4mg/ml, Flumazenil 0.1mg/ml.

## Newer Drugs for Sedation

Remimizolam besylate (CNS 7056) is a benzodiazepine introduced in Japan in January 2020 as a drug for procedural sedation. It has several advantages over current IV sedatives like midazolam, propofol, *etc.* Its metabolism is organ independent—no pain on injection, no respiratory depression or loss of airway, no nausea vomiting. Rare side effects of Remimizolam are like that of midazolam, *e.g.*, headache, drowsiness, changes in heart rate, blood pressure, *etc.*, but these are reversed by flumazenil. However, its use in children is still under study [27] (Fig. **6**).

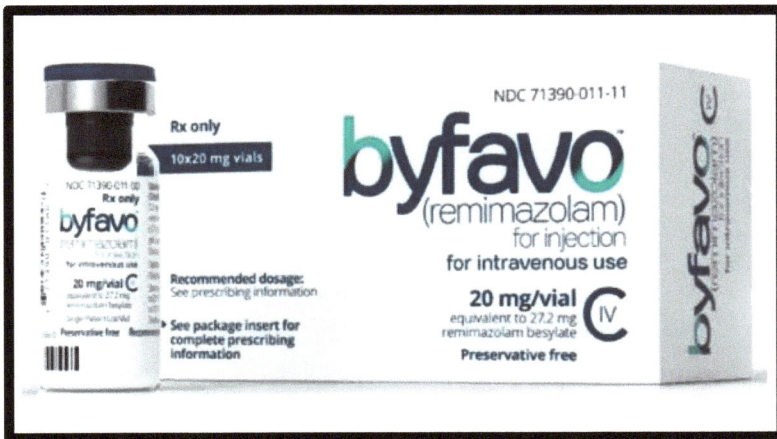

**Fig. (6).**  Remimizolam Besilate (cns 7056), 2mg/ml.

ADV6209 **(**gamma-cyclodextrin-Midazolam): is 2mg/ml solution of Midazolam with cyclodextrin. It was introduced in September 2018. It is palatable provides good sedation, anxiolysis, and amnesia. A dose of 0.3mg/kg gives moderate sedation for pediatric procedural sedation [27].

## Inhalational Sedation

$N_2O$ is a top-rated sedative inhalational agent in dental anaesthesia. The hallmark of $N_2O$ is quick induction and fast emergence. It is the oldest drug still used in anaesthesia & is safe for daycare use. $N_2O$ offers excellent analgesia and good amnesia too. There are no significant side effects. $N_2O$ may be used from 30% to 70% in oxygen either alone or with Propofol, ketamine, midazolam *etc.* $N_2O$ has low potency, MAC (Minimum Alveolar Concentration) =104. In sub-MAC doses, it gives excellent anxiolysis and analgesia. It is known to give rise to postoperative nausea and vomiting. The point to be kept in mind is since it is 30 times more soluble than nitrogen, it diffuses inside the cavity faster than nitrogen can diffuse out. Hence air-filled cavities can expand, *e.g.*, pneumothorax, gas-filled abscess cavities, *etc* [28].

$N_2O$ in Oxygen is used in varying concentrations up to 70% $N_2O$. As $N_2O$ concentration increases, analgesia and amnesia increase. However, there is also an increase in uncoordinated movements, clenching of the jaw, loss of verbal contact with the patient and increased risk of nausea and vomiting in the chair. Hence it is prudent to stay around 45 to 50% $N_2O$ in $O_2$.

$N_2O$ is administered from 50:50 $O_2$: $N_2O$ premixed cylinder called Entonox or is given with a particular dental machine which delivers only 50% $N_2O$ as maximum concentration. Additional inhalational agents like Sevoflurane or Desflurane may be used along this delivery system. Matrix MDM is a pneumatically operated $N_2O$ sedation machine (Fig. **7**). It is small and compact. It works with the non-rebreathing circuit. It has built-in pressure and flow compensation. The minimum concentration of $O_2$ given is 30%. There is an $O_2$ fail-safe system, *i.e.*, if $O_2$ flow falls, $N_2O$ will fall in the same proportion or will not be delivered. In that case, the automatic Air Inlet Valve opens, and room air is sucked in so that patient gets some $O_2$ from the perspective. The machine has an $O_2$ flush, which delivers 20 lit of $O_2$/ min when activated. The device is mounted on a 5-legged stainless-steel stand, making it steady, stable, and portable [29, 30].

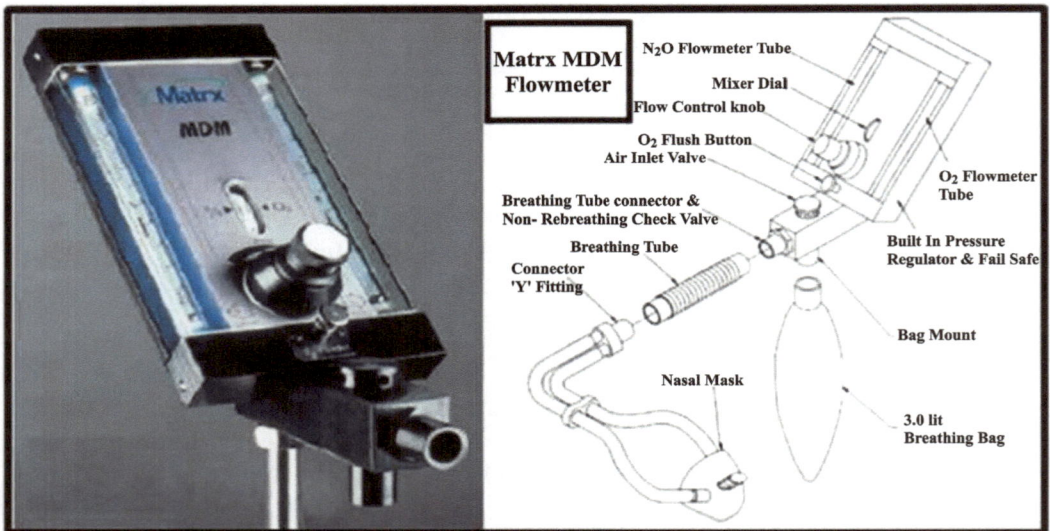

**Fig. (7).** Matrix MDM Flowmeter.

Matrix digital MDM machines require an electric current to work. The front panel has an on/ off button; gas flow indicators, % of $O_2$ and Flow are indicated, which can be adjusted by up and down keys. $O_2$ flush delivering 20 lit/min is also present. The air inlet valve is also provided to enter the room air in case of gas failure. Room air will have 21% $O_2$. The gas supply comes from the back of the unit. This machine also works with a non-rebreathing circuit, as seen in Fig. (**8**).

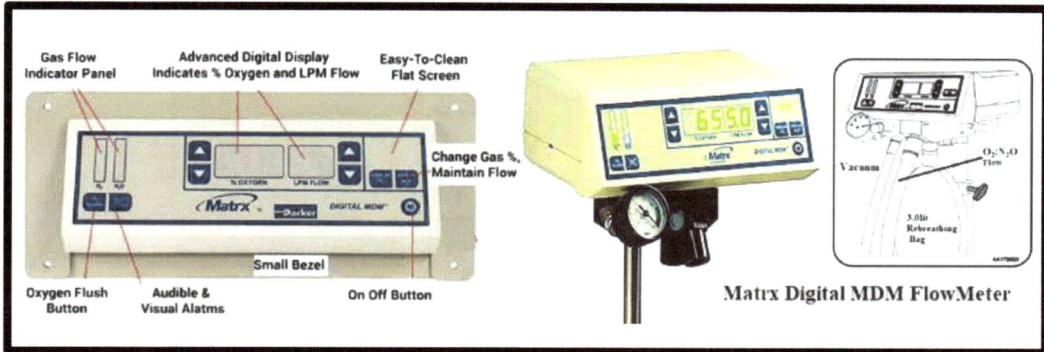

**Fig. (8).**  Matrix Digital MDM Flow Meter.

$N_2O$ is administered through the nasal mask so that mouth remains open and accessible for dental treatment. The Nasal Masks used for Dental Analgesia are usually double masks. The Outer one is called Nasal Hood and are triangular; inner cover, called liners, are softly pliable, creating a comfortable and tight seal around the nose. The masks are made of soft silicon rubber, durable and latex-free. Both the nasal hood and liners, after use, are to be washed with soap and water and then autoclaved.

The breathing system has two coaxial tubings. One carries Fresh gases from the machine to the inner mask, and $2^{nd}$ tubing carries exhaled gases to the vacuum and scavenging system (Fig. **9**). The patient inhales gases from the inner cover through the nose during inspiration. When the child exhales, expired gases through the Flapper valve on the inner surface or liner are collected in the outer hood along with some fresh gases. The expired gases are now taken to vacuum or Scavenging system away from the patient through the second coaxial tube. In addition, due to the gap between the inner liner and outer hood, any pollution caused by mouth breathing or speaking can be lessened, as some of the waste gases are 'sucked' back into the hood and exhausted *via* the vacuum hose (Fig. **10**) [29 - 31].

In a single mask system, the expired gases are vented to the atmosphere to flap the valve causing aerosol generation and theatre pollution. So, the Single nasal mask is no longer popular or used (Fig. **11**).

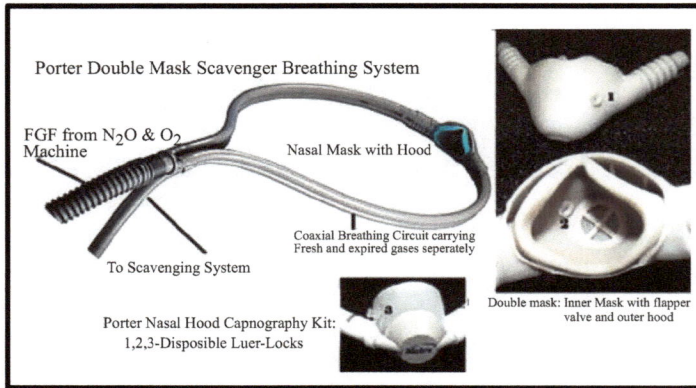

**Fig. (9).** Porter double mask scavenger breathing systems.

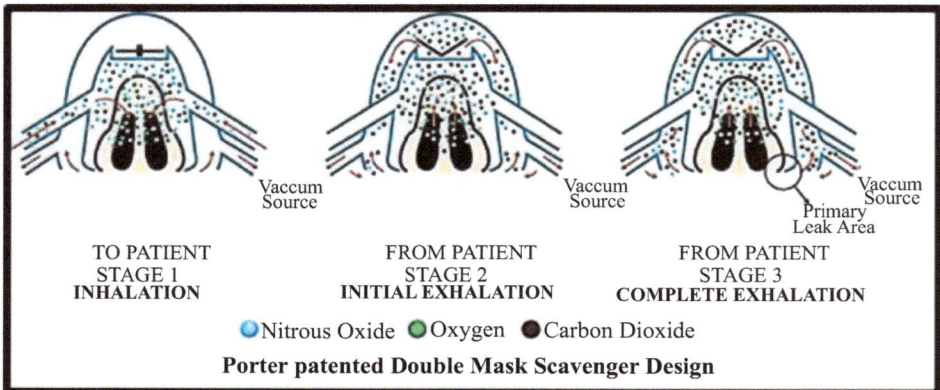

**Fig. (10).** Porter Patented double mask scavenger design.

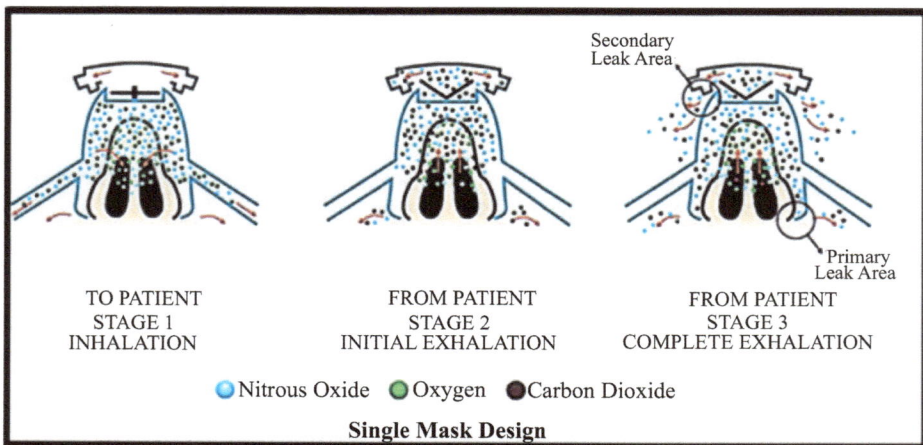

**Fig. (11).** Single mask design.

For small children, unique scented masks with cartoons figures are also available so that the acceptance of masks is better (Fig. **12**). They are single-use systems, so they do not require cleaning or Autoclaving. A breathing system available with a mask can be retrofitted to any $N_2O$ sedation machine. Children are pleased to carry home the sticker on the mask [29 - 31].

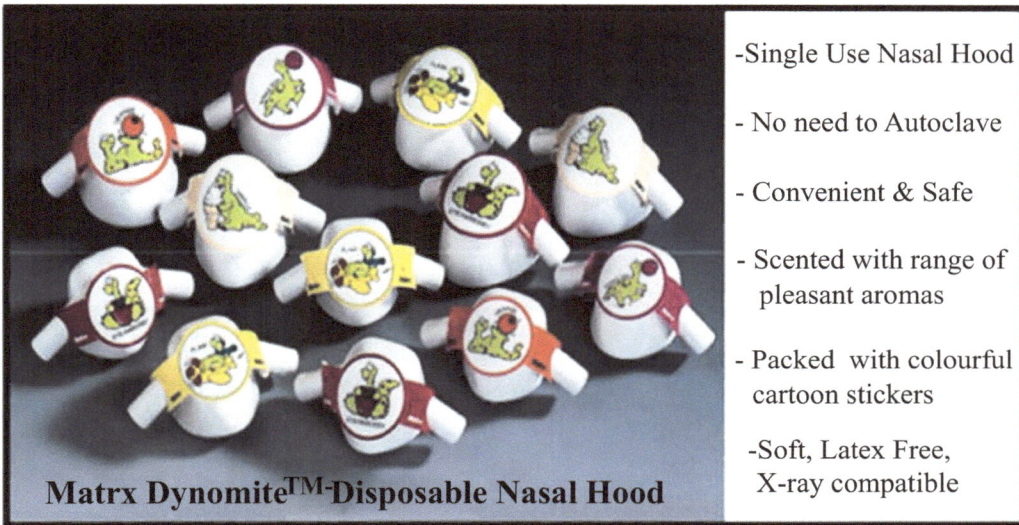

-Single Use Nasal Hood

- No need to Autoclave

- Convenient & Safe

- Scented with range of pleasant aromas

- Packed with colourful cartoon stickers

-Soft, Latex Free, X-ray compatible

**Matrx Dynomite™-Disposable Nasal Hood**

**Fig. (12).** Matrxdynomite™disposable nasal hood.

Some newer masks have been introduced in recent years, out of which Silhouette Masks (Fig. **13A**) have become popular. Masks and circuits are for single-use hence disposable. No sterilisation is required. It has an adhesive strip at the edge, and it snuggly fits around the nose hence there is no leak around the nasal mask. So, reasonable, predictable $N_2O$ sedation is obtained, and $N_2O$ pollution is minimised. It is lightweight and smaller in size, providing better access to the oral cavity. A specially designed nasal cannula is placed at the angle inside so that gases are effectively introduced inside the nostril (Fig. **13B**) [27]. The cannula has fenestrations on the upper surface (of tubing, from where the exhaled gases are sucked by Vacuum to scavenger system. The Enhanced scavenging system reduces $N_2O$ exposure of operator and theatre personnel.

The tubings are connected to fresh Gas and vacuum tubes. Adult, as well as paediatric sizes, are available along with sizers to determine proper fitting mask (Fig. **14**). It is possible to monitor End-tidal $CO_2$ (capnography). According to the recent monitoring guideline of ASA- American Society of Anaesthesiologists, it is now mandatory to monitor $EtCO_2$ during MAC, Analgesia and Anaesthesia procedure.

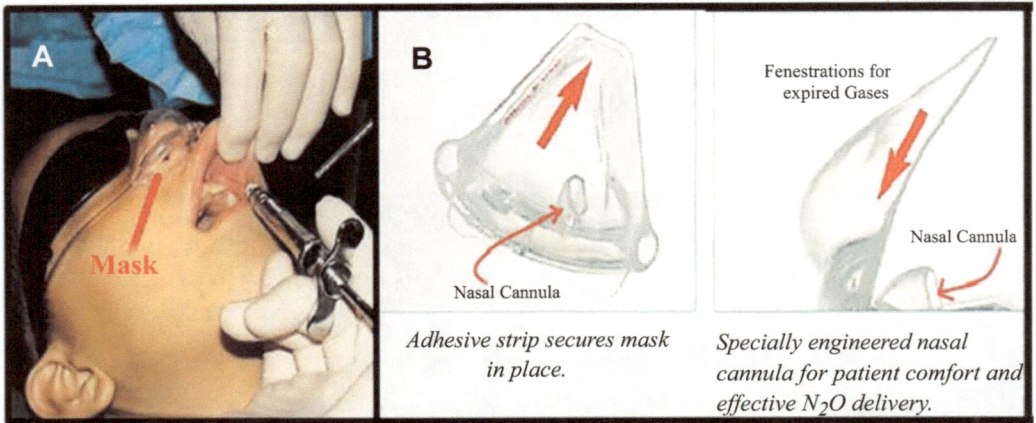

**Fig. (13).** A- easy access with silhouette mask, B- details of silhouette mask.

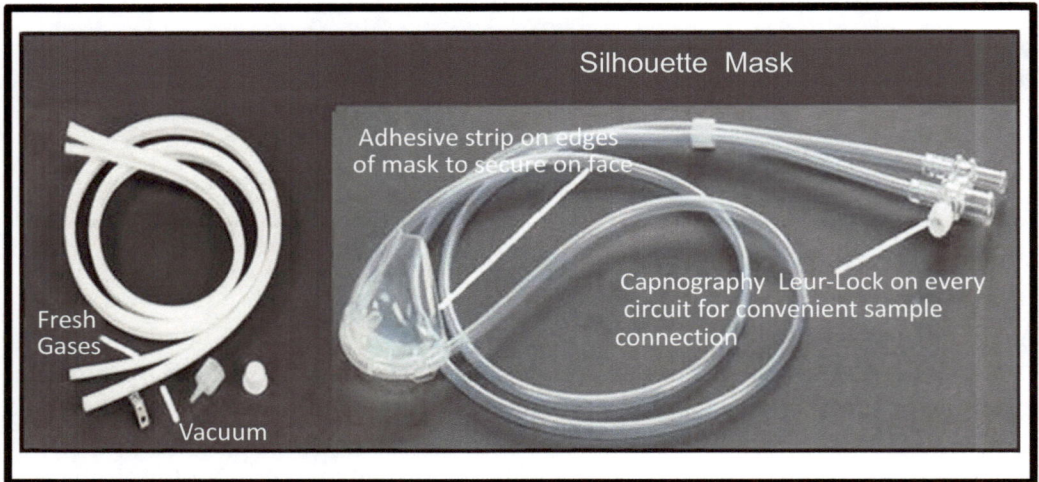

**Fig. (14).** Silhouette mask.

To isolate the oral cavity to minimise aspiration, various objects are used- throat pack, Rubber Dam assembly, *etc* (Fig. **15**). Besides separation of oral cavity and oropharynx, Rubber dam *etc*, prevents mouth breathing and dilution of gases given nasally. To maintain patent airways, nasopharyngeal airway or nasal trumpet may be used. The area is actively sucked, and minimum use of Air – Saline is undertaken.

If airway obstruction or respiratory depression and apnoea or laryngospasm occur, prompt detection & management is mandatory [Flowchart 1]. Such flow charts prove extremely useful and should be placed on the dental clinic or treatment room wall for easy reference.

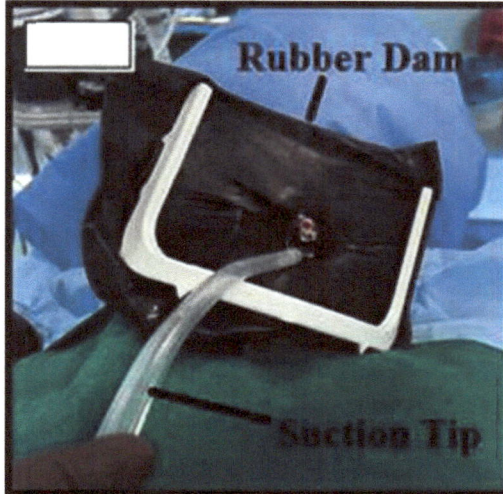

**Fig. (15).** Separation device 'rubber dam'.

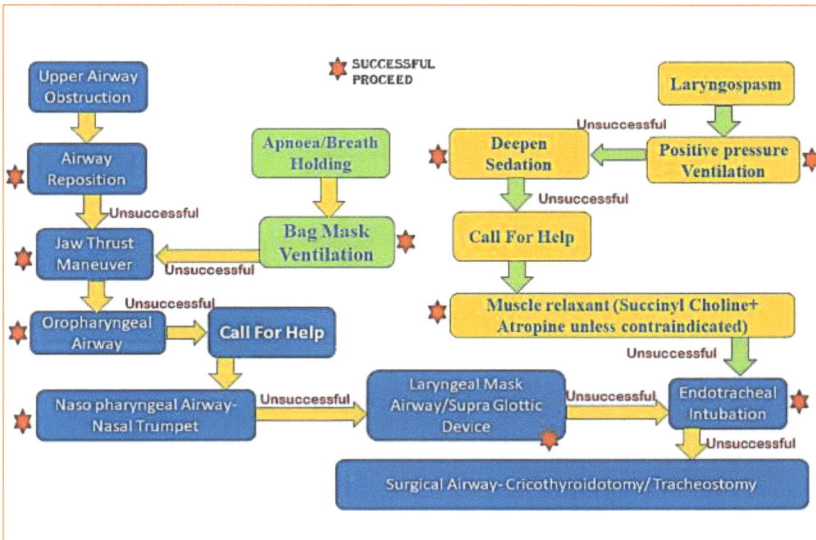

**Flow chart 1:.** Suggested treatment for upper airway obstruction, breath-holding/ apnea, laryngospasm.

***Diffusion Hypoxia***: At the end of the procedure, $N_2O$ administration is discontinued. The partial pressure of $N_2O$ is high in the blood. $N_2O$ diffuses rapidly from blood to alveoli, thus decreasing the $O_2$ concentration in alveoli. In minutes hypoxia may develop. It is called diffusion hypoxia. It is rarely seen with

$N_2O$ through the nasal mask but may be seen at the end of GA. To prevent this, it is safer to give 100% $O_2$ for at least 5 minutes or more under mask after discontinuing $N_2O$.

***Sedation Protocol:*** Under sedation, every child undergoing the dental procedure should undergo a thorough preoperative assessment (steps discussed further in the chapter). According to the child's weight and selected route of administration, sedation should be administered to the child. Children, along with the parents, should wait in the holding area and be left undisturbed. $SpO_2$ to be monitored throughout and watched for signs of sedation.

Following are the signs of the onset of sedation.

- Glazed look or vacant look
- Delayed eye movement, inability to focus the gaze
- Lack of muscle coordination
- Slurred speech
- Sleep after 30 minutes of drug administration, level sedation should be assessed according to the Ramsay Scale of Sedation [32] (Table **3**).

**Table 3. Ramsay sedation scale.**

| 1 | Patient is anxious and agitated or restless, or both |
|---|---|
| 2 | Patient is co-operative, oriented, and tranquil |
| 3 | Patient responds to commands only |
| 4 | Patient exhibits brisk response to light glabellar tap or loud auditory stimulus |
| 5 | Patient exhibits a sluggish response to light glabellar tap or loud auditory stimulus |
| 6 | Patient exhibits no response |

## *Signs of adequate $N_2O$ Sedation*

- Light-headedness and a lightness of body as if floating or flying in space.
- Tingling in hands, feet and around the mouth and tongue. At this stage, the child may open the mouth and try to roll the tongue.
- May breathe hold if breathing was too fast to start with. However, regular breathing starts once adequate depth achieved
- Eyes come in the centre, and pupils may slightly dilate. The gaze is steady.
- Sense of wellbeing prevails.

## *Signs of Deep Sedation*

- Inability to follow instructions
- Eyes close, swallowing will stop.
- Body becomes relaxed
- Breathing can get obstructed.
- Reducing $N_2O$ concentration lighter levels can be achieved easily.

## *Monitoring during the procedure*

Clinically watching colour- Nails, conjunctiva and tongue, Respiration rate and breathing, pulse rate. Eye movements, lacrimation, salivation will tell the level of analgesia, adequacy of oxygenation and ventilation [33, 34].

*Monitoring:* of ECG, $SpO_2$, $EtCO_2$, Non-invasive Blood pressure measurements. Monitoring the level of analgesia can be done with Bispectral Index (BIS). Multipara monitors with all mentioned parameters along with a vigilant anaesthesiologist will help to achieve patient safety during the procedure.

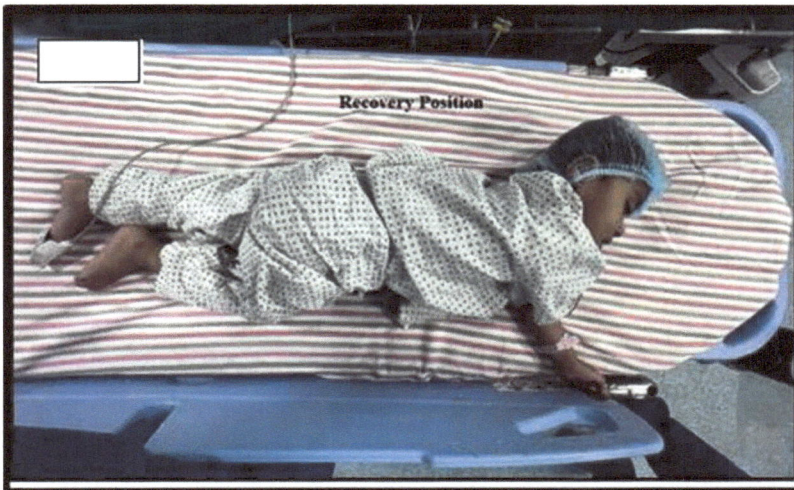

**Fig. (16).**  Recovery position.

Recovery: Inclined dental chair or bed or couch to keep the patient post-procedure till the child recovers well. Child to be placed in the recovery position. (Fig. **16**) Turned on one side, the lower hand is outstretched to stabilise the body and prevent rollover. Lower leg to be placed stretched straight. The upper leg is flexed at 90 degrees, and the body is rolled over on the side of the outstretched hand till the flexed knee touches the bed or couch. The head is extended slightly upwards so that the upper airway remains unobstructed. The upper hand has to be placed under the chin to maintain the lead in this position. In this position, blood saliva drains out of the oral cavity from the dependent angle of the mouth. Breathing remains unobstructed. In this recovery, position abdomen remains free. $O_2$ may be supplemented, and $SpO_2$ monitoring to be continued

### ***Pre-requisites for Sedation / General Anaesthesia: [2]***

1. Well-equipped set up.

2. Qualified personnel for anaesthesia – trained in BLS - Basic Life Support and PALS- Paediatric Advanced Life Support [7].

3. Peri-operative monitoring based on ASA (American Society of anaesthesiologist) & ISA (Indian society of anaesthesiologist) guidelines &its documentation.

4. Careful selection of patient.

5. Thorough preoperative assessment & planning.

6. Adequately trained support staff.

7. Emergency drugs, crash cart including defibrillator & protocols (Figs. **17,18**).

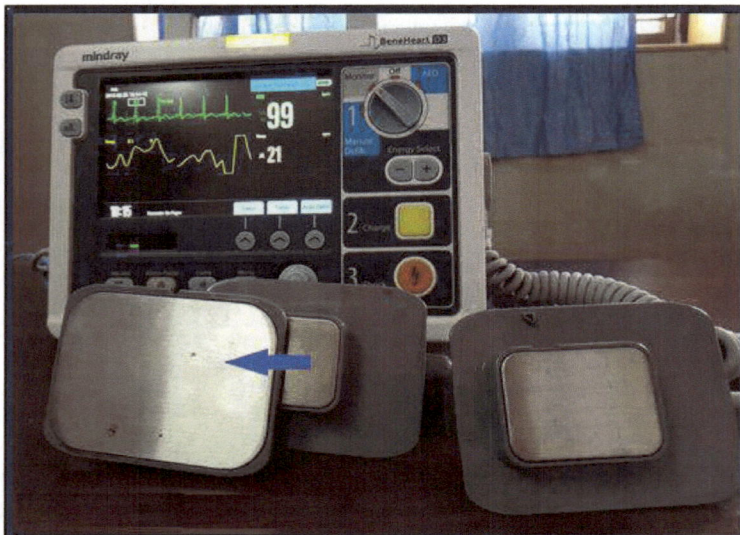

**Fig. (17).** Defibrillator with pediatric paddles.

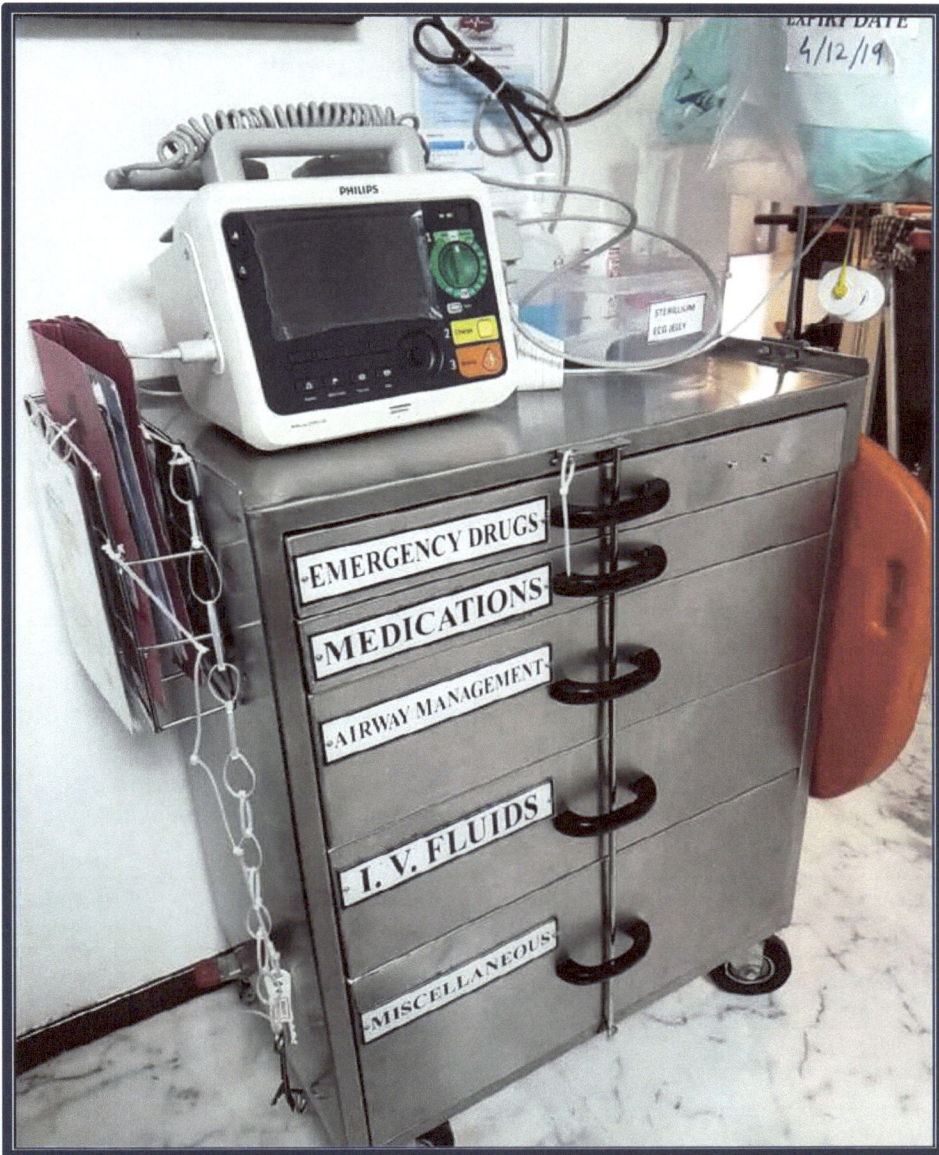

**Fig. (18).** Emergency crash cart with a defibrillator.

8. Recovery & discharge criteria protocols.

9. Provision for peri-operative instructions to patients / legal representatives.

## *Fasting Guidelines*

Fasting guidelines need to be strictly adhered to while treating these children either on OPD or Indoor basis (Table **4**).

**Table 4. Fasting guidelines.**

| Ingested Material | Minimum Fasting Period |
|---|---|
| Clear Liquids* | 2hrs |
| Breast Milk | 4hrs |
| Infant Formula | 4hrs |
| Nonhuman Milk** | 6hrs |
| Light Meal *** | 6hrs |
| Fried, fatty food, Meat | More than 8 hrs |

The fasting period applies to all age groups. *Clear Liquids- Water, Fruit Juice without pulp, Clear Tea & Coffee without Milk. ** Nonhuman milk is equivalent to solids. So, the amount consumed should be noted. The higher the quantity longer is the starvation time. *** Light meal typically includes Toast and clear fluid.

## *Local Anaesthesia with or without Monitored Anaesthesia Care (MAC):* Local

Anaesthetics (LA) are widely used for Dental Procedures in children with or without sedation. Commonly LA is used as nerve blocks and local infiltrations. A variety of Amide and ester groups of drugs are available. For Dose and volume of LA referred to Table (**5**).

**Table 5. Commonly used local anaesthetic agents for nerve blocks or infiltration: doses, duration, & calculations.**

| Local Anaesthetic | Maximum Dose With Epinephrine* (mg/kg) | | Maximum Dose Without Epinephrine (mg/kg) | | Duration of Action** (min) |
|---|---|---|---|---|---|
| - | Medical | Dental | Medical | Dental | - |
| *Esters* | | | | | |
| Procaine | 10.0 | 6.0 | 7.0 | 6.0 | 60-90 |
| Chloroprocaine | 20.0 | 12.0 | 15.0 | 12.0 | 30-60 |
| Tetracaine | 1.5 | 1.0 | 1.0 | 1.0 | 180-600 |
| *Amides* | | | | | |
| Lidocaine | 7.0 | 4.4 | 4.0 | 4.4 | 90-200 |
| Mepivacaine | 7.0 | 4.4 | 5.0 | 4.4 | 120-240 |
| Bupivacaine | 3.0 | 1.3 | 2.5 | 1.3 | 180-600 |
| Levobupivacaine | 3.0 | 2.0 | 2.0 | 2.0 | 180-600 |
| Ropivacaine | 3.0 | 2.0 | 2.0 | 2.0 | 180-600 |

*(Table 5) cont.....*

| Local Anaesthetic | Maximum Dose With Epinephrine* (mg/kg) | | Maximum Dose Without Epinephrine (mg/kg) | | Duration of Action** (min) |
|---|---|---|---|---|---|
| Articaine *** | ---- | 7.0 | ---- | 7.0 | 60-230 |

*These are maximum doses of LA combined with epinephrine; lower doses are recommended when used without epinephrine. Doses of amides should be decreased by 30% in infants younger than six months. When lidocaine is administered IV (*e.g.*, intravenous regional anaesthesia- IVRA), the dose should be decreased to 3-5 mg/kg; long-acting LA agents should not be used for IVRA**Duration of action is dependent on concentration, total dose, site of administration, use of epinephrine & patient's age***use in paediatric patients under four years of age is not recommended.

Local anaesthesia (LA) is a temporary loss of sensation, including pain in the part of the body produced by a topically applied or injected agent without the depressing level of consciousness [5]. All the professionals involved in paediatric dentistry should be aware of the proper dosage of various local anaesthetics to minimise the risk of toxicity & prolonged duration of effects which can result in the self-inflicted tongue or soft tissue injury [27].

**Table 6. Treatment of LA toxicity.**

## Treatment of LA toxicity:

1. **Call for help.**
2. **Ventilate with 100% $O_2$. Alert facility with Cardio-Pulmonary Bypass facility.**
3. **Resuscitation- Chest Compressions, Airway/ Ventilation**
4. **Avoid drugs- More LA, β blockers, Ca channel blockers, Vasopressin**
5. **Reduce doses of Epinephrine if possible. Prolonged resuscitation may be necessary.**
6. **Benzodiazepines for seizure management- IV Midazolam 0.1 to 0.2mg/kg. Propofol (1 to 2.0 mg/kg) to be avoided in case of hemodynamic instability.**
7. **Administer 20% Lipid Infusion at 1.5ml/kg over one minute to trap unbound Amide Local Anaesthetics. Repeat the bolus once or twice if cardiovascular collapse continues**
8. **Start Lipid infusion (20%) @ 0.25ml/kg /min, double if cardiovascular collapse continues**
9. **Continue infusion at least 10 min after circulation restores, dose of lipid**

The only absolute contraindication for LA use is documented allergy to LA in the past. True allergy to an amide LA is extremely rare. Allergy to one amide does not rule out the use of another amide, but allergy to one ester LA rules out the use of another ester. Usually, the patient is allergic to preservatives & stabilisers.

*LA Toxicity:* Local Anaesthetic Systemic toxicity LAST is a life-threatening situation. The presently reported incidence is 0.03% or 0.27 episodes /1000 nerve blocks. Tingling & numbness initially around lips, slowly spreading over the rest of the body, bitter taste in mouth, lightheadedness, ringing in ears/blurring of vision, and muscular twitching are some of the prodromal symptoms and signs, which can lead to convulsions, respiratory arrest, and cardiovascular collapse [26].

Each dental set-up should be geared to detect & treat Local Anaesthetic toxicity. The management guidelines for LA toxicity (LAST) are as mentioned in Table. (**6**).

### General Anaesthesia (GA)

Dental treatment under GA may be provided in the dental clinic on the dental chair (Chair-side) or in the hospital operating room (OR) [1]. The dental clinic should be well equipped in terms of both workforce & devices, for all monitoring and resuscitative needs.

### Indications for GA [1, 2]

**1.** Noticeably young Children who cannot cooperate (usually < 4 years) [2].

**2.** Extremely fearful & anxious children.

**3.** Children with complex medical/physical/mental conditions (ASA 3 or 4).

**4.** Need for extensive/lengthy surgical treatment.

**5.** Allergy to local anaesthetics [5].

**6.** Language barrier preventing communication.

**7.** Have to travel long distances to receive speciality dental care.

### Advantages of Chair-side GA [1]

1. Cost-effective.

2. Decongestion of busy hospital beds & ORs.

3. Less risk of nosocomial infection.

4. Semi-supine position prevents pooled saliva & blood from trickling in the hypopharynx [5].

5. Early recovery in a home environment with family.

6. Better acceptance by children & parents due to less disruption to the daily routine.

7. Familiar environment for the dentists in dental clinics.

However, appropriate equipment for sedation, GA, monitoring, resuscitation, qualified anaesthesiologist & trained support staff is a must for treating these small patients for their dental needs (Fig. **19**). The Professional providing dental treatment should be PALS (Paediatric Advanced Life Support) certified. As, in case of emergency, skilled help can be rendered without wasting valuable time [35].

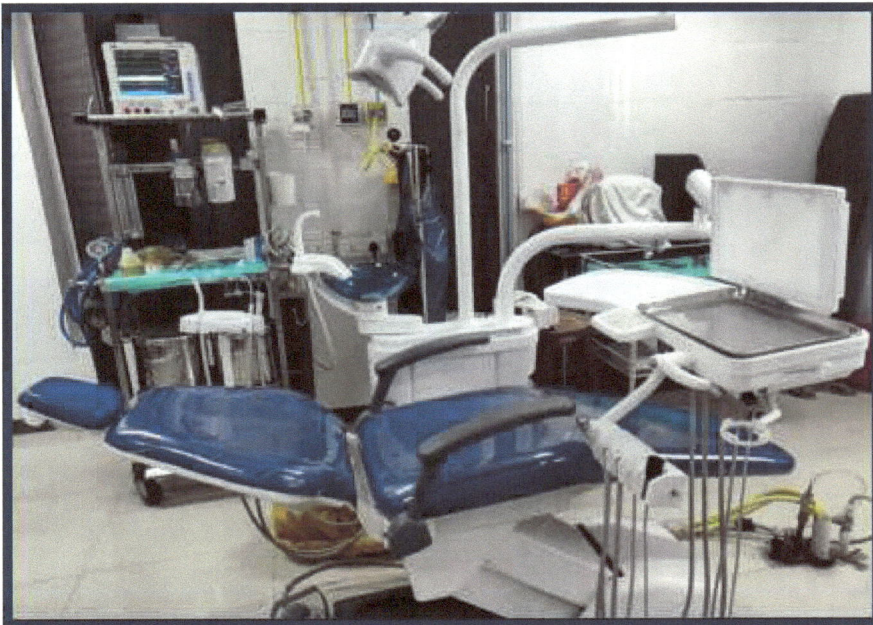

**Fig. (19).** Anaesthesia set up for chair-side general anaesthesia & sedation.

## *Disadvantages of Chair-side GA [1, 5]*

1. Upright position predisposes to postural hypotension.

2. Greater risk of hypoxia to the brain if unrecognised fainting.

3. Chances of aspiration are higher with debris, the blood passing over the posterior tongue into the oropharynx and down.

4. Provision for head-down tilt in the dental chair in case of power failure is mandatory.

5. May need wooden board or arrangement to modify chair to an OT table for safe GA (Fig. **20A & B**).

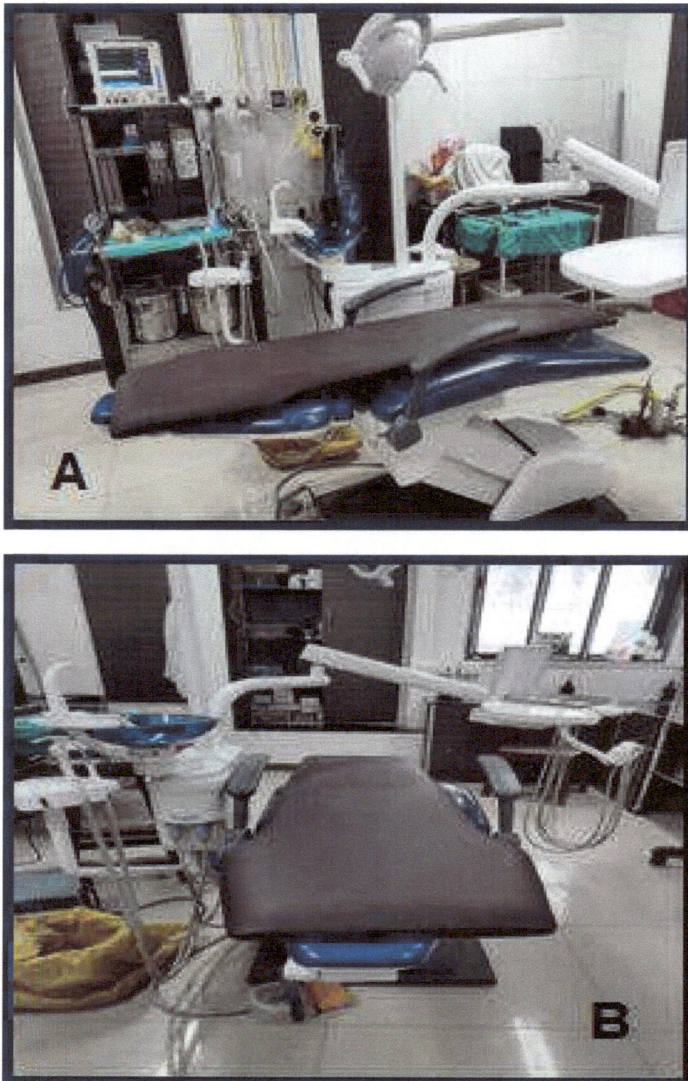

**Fig. (20). A & B** Converting dental chair into OT table with specialised board.

## Preoperative Assessment

GA should be planned for carefully selected children. Children need complete preoperative assessment just like any other surgery under GA.

A child's birth history, developmental milestones, previous illnesses, previous surgeries & anaesthesia details, emotional & psychological status& routine physical examination should be performed [5]. Food & drug allergies & any adverse drug reactions are to be noted in detail. Special considerations to be given to patency of external nares (use of a nasal mask or nasal intubation for sedation / GA), deviated nasal septum, repeated sinusitis, presence of upper or lower respiratory infection, adenoid hypertrophy, enlarged tonsils, Mallampatti grading *etc.* as a part of airway assessment. A history of snoring, sleep-disordered breathing, or obstructive sleep apnoea is noted [4]. Children with severe OSA who have experienced desaturations during sleep may have altered mu receptors resulting in excessive sensitivity to opioids & other sedative agents [36]. Lower& titrated doses of these medications need to be used in such children. Details of pre-existing medical conditions & drug therapy should be obtained if the child is on anti-convulsant, therapeutic levels to be assessed & treatment to be continued till the day of the procedure.

Children who are ASA Gr 3 or 4 have congenital syndromes, congenital heart defects, coagulation defects should be treated in hospital settings only [4, 37].

Blood & biochemical investigations are required for any other surgery under GA. The aim is to optimise the child medically if indicated & counsel the child & the parents for the procedures ahead.

Detailed discussion & communication with the dental surgeon about the procedure helps to plan anaesthesia.

## Preoperative Instructions to Parents

1. Child should wear loose, comfortable & front open clothing [4].

2. Child should be accompanied by a responsible adult, preferably two if one will drive the child home.

3. Fasting guidelines, as mentioned earlier, to be followed strictly.

4. If a child develops respiratory tract infection, be informed & treated immediately.

5. If a child is on anti-seizures medication, to be continued on the day of the procedure.

6. Children with congenital heart diseases to be given Infective endocarditis prophylaxis as per cardiology advice as dental treatment & nasal intubation can cause transient bacteraemia.

### *Premedication*

Premedication children before GA aims at alleviating anxiety, causing amnesia, easing parental separation, decreasing the pain of venepuncture, reducing secretions, decreasing oedema post-procedure, avoiding nausea & vomiting& analgesia postoperatively. The various agents used are Midazolam (oral, nasal or IV), Fentanyl (IV or transmucosal lollipops) or Remifentanil, EMLA (eutectic mixture of local anaesthetics) cream for local application before venepuncture, ketamine (IV, IM, Oral), Glycopyrrolate, Atropine, Dexamethasone, Ondansetron, NSAID (oral, IV, suppository), *etc.*

### *Monitoring*

All standard monitors are attached once a child is taken to the procedure room. ISA (Indian society of anaesthesiologist) & ASA (American Society of anaesthesiologist) recommends the use of pulse oximeter, blood pressure, ECG & capnography (end-tidal $CO_2$) as minimum mandatory monitoring during all cases undergoing general anaesthesia (Fig. **21**). Temperature monitoring should be done, especially in children as they are more prone to hypothermia during general anaesthesia. Warming measures like convective warmer blankets, warming mattresses, fluid warmers should be available in ORs for children. Bispectral index monitoring (BIS), an EEG-based analysis of a patient's depth of sedation & anaesthesia, can be done whenever feasible & indicated (Fig. **22**). BIS helps titrate drugs to achieve adequate depth of sedation and anaesthesia and ensures faster recovery.

### *Induction & Maintenance [4]*

Induction of anaesthesia should be preferably done on the parent's lap whenever feasible. If needed, various distraction techniques should be used until IV cannulation is secured or inhalational anaesthesia is instituted [38 - 40]. Regardless of the induction method, IV access should be considered in all cases and obtained at the earliest opportunity. In cases where securing an intravenous route before inhalational induction is necessary, EMLA (lidocaine .5% and prilocaine 2.5%) application on the skin 60 min prior is applicable. The duration of action is 1-2 hr. after the cream is removed. Its adverse reactions include erythema, itching, rash and rarely methemoglobinemia.

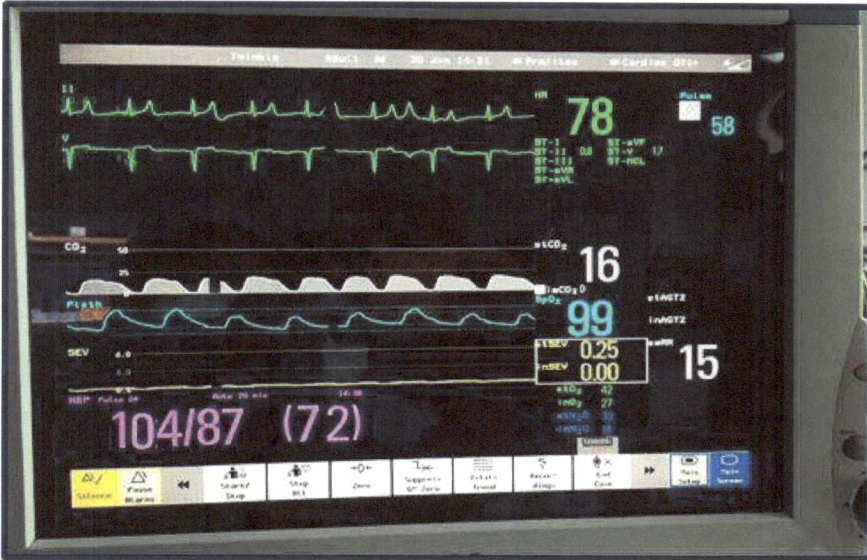

**Fig. (21).** Multiparameter monitor with ECG, Pulse oximeter, Blood pressure & Capnograph (ETCO$_2$).

For induction of anaesthesia, short-acting fast emergence agents, *e.g.*, Propofol, Sevoflurane, Atracurium, are used unless contraindicated.

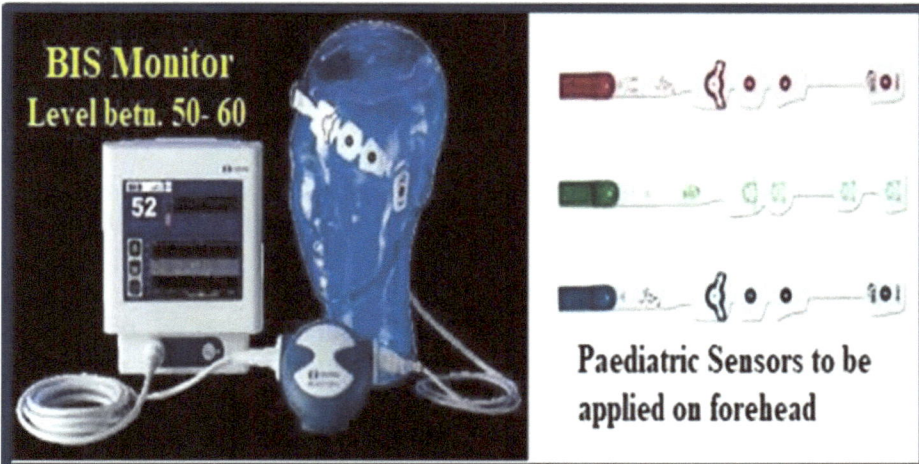

**Fig. (22).** Bispectral index monitor & sensors (bis value of 40- 60 is required for adequate depth of General anaesthesia).

## *Airway*

Securing and maintaining the airway throughout the procedure is of prime concern for these children as dental surgeons and anaesthesiologists share the airway. The airway is connected either with an oral or nasal endotracheal tube or flexo metallic Laryngeal mask airway (LMA). A child with a recognised syndrome associated with a difficult airway should be best managed in an operation room where fibreoptic bronchoscopes or video laryngoscopes are readily available. It may be wise also to ensure the availability of an ENT surgeon competent to perform an emergency tracheostomy (Surgical Airways) in extreme difficult airways.

Nasal intubation is preferred as it provides stability and unobstructed access (Figs. **23** & **24**) to all four quadrants of the mouth, allowing the evaluation of tooth alignment and occlusion. Epistaxis during nasal intubation is the most common complication with an incidence of 80%, and adequate nasal preparation is necessary to prevent bleeding. Several methods have been described to reduce the incidence of traumatic nasal intubation, including selecting the more patent nostril, using lubricating gel, progressive dilatation with nasopharyngeal airways, and thermosetting of the tube, telescoping the tracheal tube into catheters, *etc.* Manually assisted ventilation after applying lidocaine jelly and Xylometazoline drops ensure adequate nasal spread. Lidocaine gel decreases systemic absorption of vasoconstrictor and reduces post-operative nasal pain. North pole RAE tube (Fig. **20**) is preferred. A conventional endotracheal tube with Magill's connector and catheter mount connected to the pediatric circuit may be used if not available. There should be no pressure around external nares while fixing the tube. Eye pads to be used to prevent injuries. One needs to be vigilant as this arrangement's chances of disconnection are high. Silicone-based tubes may be superior to PVC tubes in the prevention of epistaxis. A correct size uncuffed tube starts to leak at a positive airway pressure of 20cm $H_2O$. Usually, an endotracheal tube 0.5-1mm less than that used for oral intubation is recommended for smooth and atraumatic passage of the nasal tube. This could result in an inadequate airway seal. The formation of air bubbles in the oropharynx during the use of the irrigation drill may be disturbing to the pediatric dentist. This can be overcome by using a larger endotracheal tube, repacking the pharynx, or using a micro cuffed tube. Whenever a throat pack is inserted, there should be visual and documented evidence of its presence & its removal on completion of the procedure.

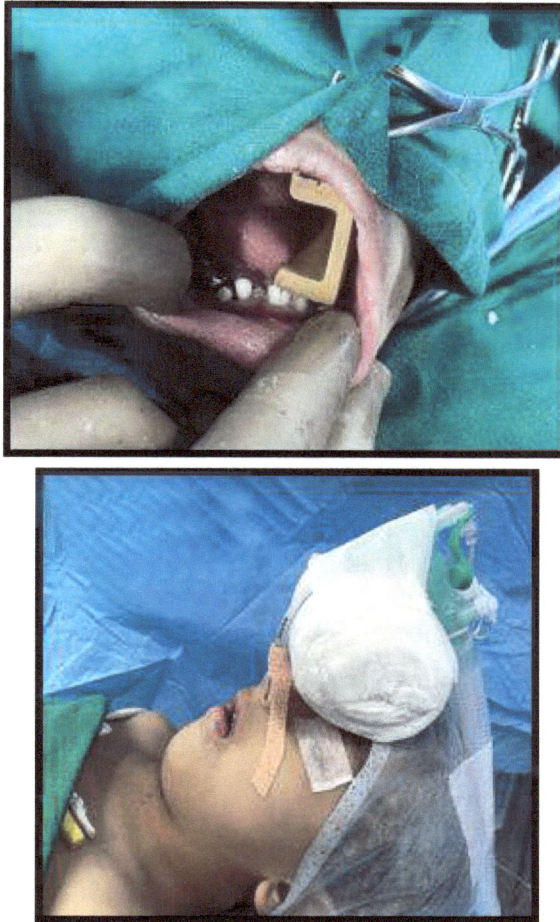

**Fig. (23 & 24).** Nasal intubation allowing unobstructed access.

The oral route may be used when nasal intubation is contraindicated or to avoid trauma to adenoid tissue in younger children. Performed oral south pole RAE tube (Fig. **25**) provides access to either side of the mouth. The preformed orotracheal RAE's tube is designed to be a midline tube; moving it to either side of the mouth may cause an eccentric position within the trachea. Reinforced tube resists kinking but is expensive. A conventional endotracheal tube may prevent endobronchial intubation as the tube is moved from one angle to the other during dental procedures in various mouth quadrants.

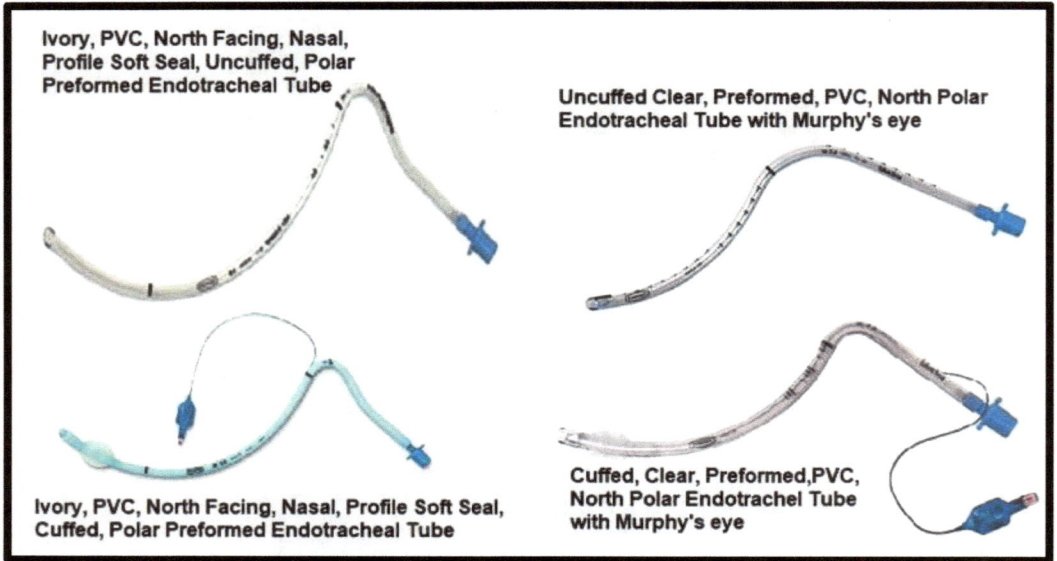

**Fig. (25).** North pole performed nasal endotracheal tube.

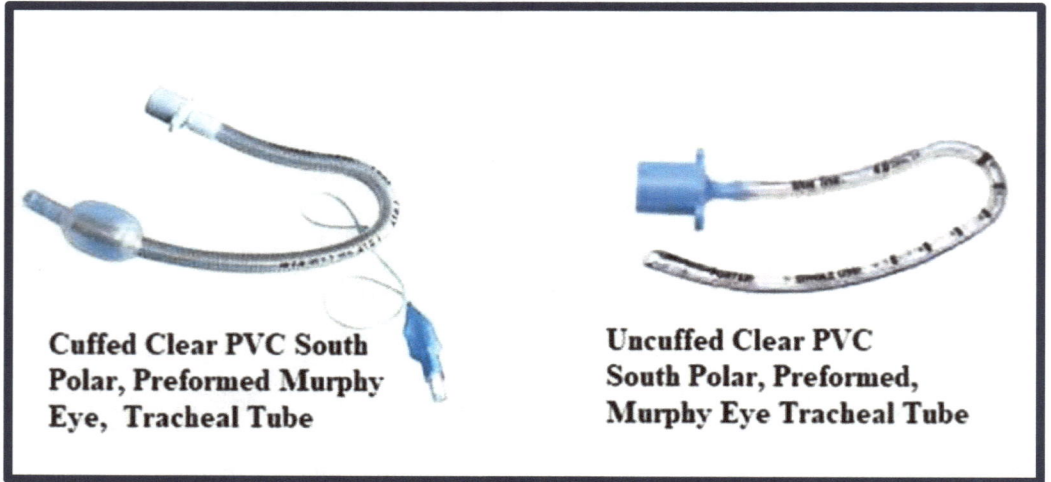

**Fig. (26).** South pole performed oral endotracheal tube.

Increased risk of laryngeal oedema risk of laryngospasm & coughing due to endotracheal tubes (ETT) makes LMA a helpful alternative in many cases [3].

However, ETT prevents aspiration of saliva, mucus, gastric contents into the lower respiratory tract (Fig. **26**).

## Supraglottic Airway Device / Laryngeal Mask Airway (LMA)

LMA makes the surgery difficult because it leaves little space for the dental drill and suction. Although it protects the larynx from the contents of the oropharynx to some extent, a throat pack is still required to absorb any blood and particulate matter. Displacement of the LMA may occur after insertion of the throat pack or positioning of the mouth prop. The flexible LMA is sometimes more difficult to insert in children; however, this device allows more versatility and better access to teeth (Fig. **27**). For short procedures and in cases where airway problems are anticipated, this anaesthesia technique allows maintenance of spontaneous ventilation. Oxygen with nitrous oxide and sevoflurane usually suffices. Incremental doses/continuous/target-controlled propofol infusions can be used to maintain anaesthesia. It is better to use muscle relaxants and control ventilation for extensive and complicated restorations.

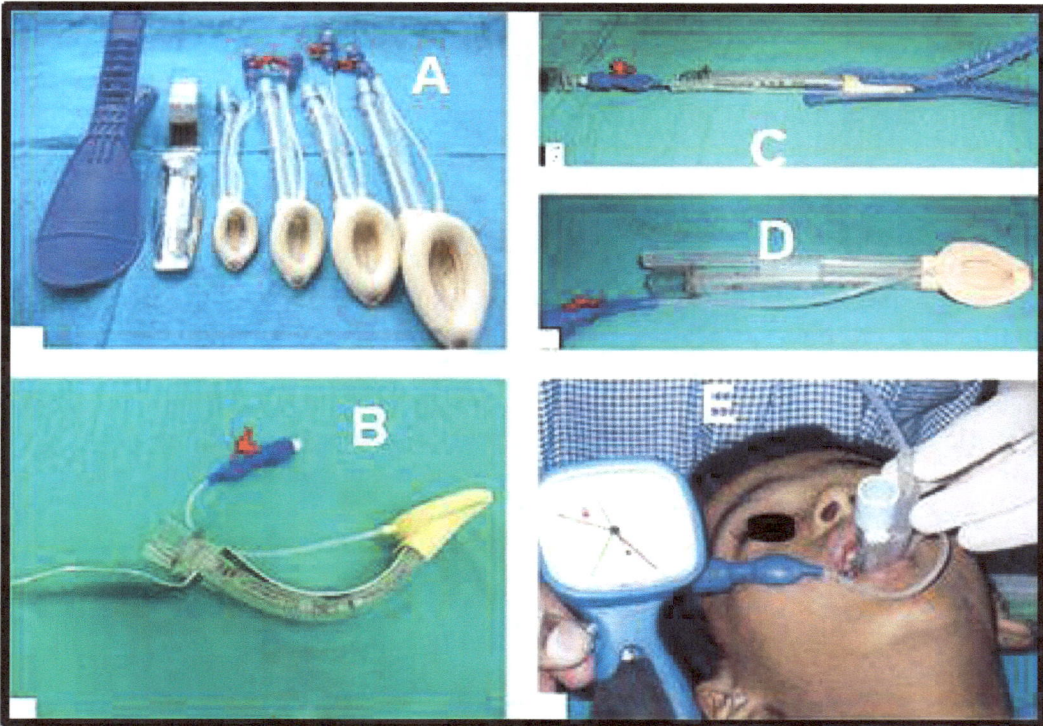

**Fig. (27).** Supraglottic laryngeal mask airway.

## Estuation

It is preferable to extubate the child (after administering reversal agents like neostigmine as needed) completely awake & in the lateral position after the cough reflex has returned. Intravenous dexamethasone (0.4 mg/kg) and Inhaled epinephrine may be used to reduce airway oedema if suspected following extubation. Removal of the LMA, while the child is still deeply anaesthetised, has been associated with lower oxygen saturation in dental patients. Classic recovery position without a pillow is ideal for keeping the airway open and preventing aspiration of blood and debris. Gauze, which is left inside the dental cavities for haemostasis, should be taped to the cheeks following extubation.

## Post-operative Analgesia

Painful procedures like extraction of permanent teeth where a gingival flap and bone drilling are needed can be given opioids intraoperatively, and paracetamol with NSAIDS continued orally in the post-operative period. Acetaminophen suppository (30-40 mg/kg) given shortly before the end of the procedure confers analgesia with minimal side effects. The nonsteroidal anti-inflammatory agent ketorolac (0.5-1.0 mg/kg) given IV as a single dose may be helpful. Once a child is on orals, oral NSAID syrups should suffice. Regional blocks performed intra-operatively will alleviate immediate postoperative pain. A long-acting local anaesthetic, *e.g.*, bupivacaine is not recommended for the child or the physically or mentally disabled patient since the prolonged numbness may increase the risk of tongue &soft tissue biting & injury.

## Recovery & Discharge

The child should be carefully monitored during the recovery phase after general anaesthesia. Recovery position (Fig. **11**) with oxygen supplementation as described earlier is recommended. A study of morbidity & deaths related to dental anaesthesia found that more than half of complications occurred in recovery [4]. Significant desaturation is common after briefing dental anaesthesia, and the principal cause is airway obstruction. Oxygen supplementation lessens the severity of desaturation but does not prevent it. No oral fluids are given for 2-3hr to avoid vomiting and aspiration. Ondansetron 100-150 mcg/kg effectively lessens the severity of PONV.

## Recommended Discharge Criteria after Sedation/ GA are [5]

1. Cardiovascular function & airway patency is satisfactory & stable.

2. Child should be easily arousable & protective airway reflexes are intact.

3. Child can sit unaided, walk, talk, *etc.*, if age-appropriate.

4. Adequate hydration & ability to pass urine confirmed

5. For a young child or infant & for a child with a disability who is incapable of the usual expected response for that age, the pre- sedation /pre-GA level of responsiveness or a level as close as possible to the average level for that child should be achieved.

Several recoveries & discharge scales & tools are available [5]. A simple evaluation tool may be the ability of the infant or the child to remain awake for at least 20 min in a quiet environment.

## Children with Special Needs

Paediatric dental clinics often receive patients with various disabilities or children with special needs like cerebral palsy, Down's syndrome, people with epilepsy, cardiac disorders, *etc.* When needed, these children are safer to be treated in a hospital setting in operating rooms with indoor admissions. Children with Treacher Collins syndrome, Pierre's robin syndrome, facial trauma, temporomandibular ankylosis, obstructive sleep apnoea (OSA) *etc.*, pose a difficult airway management challenge (Fig. **28A & B**). Securing airway with ETT in these babies need advanced skills and equipment like video laryngoscopes (Fig. **29**), fibreoptic bronchoscope, *etc.*. In extreme cases, front of neck access like cricothyrotomy or tracheostomy may be warranted.

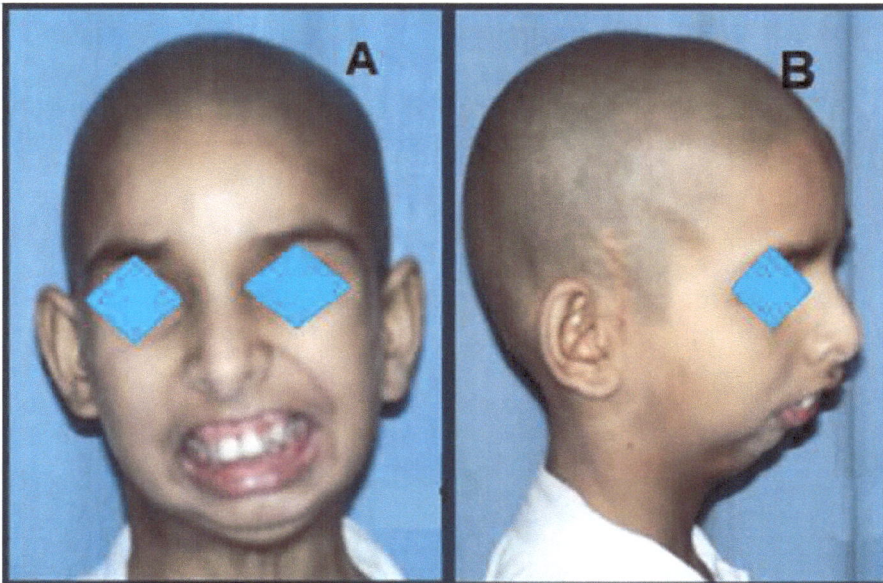

**Fig. (28A &B).** Child with severe mandibular deformity, TMJ ankylosis & restricted mouth opening.

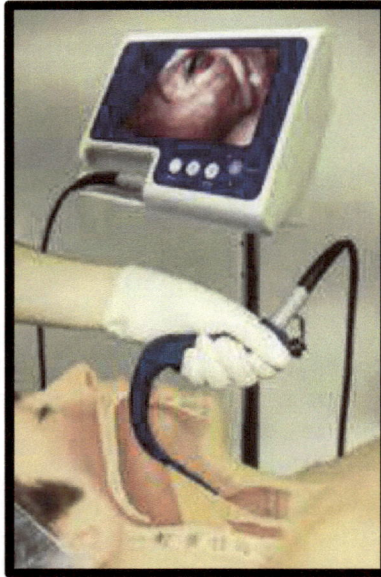

**Fig. (29).** Video laryngoscope.

Cerebral palsy children may pose anaesthesia challenges due to intravenous access, dehydration, spasticity, difficult dental chair or table positioning, altered gastric emptying, multiple medications, convulsions, *etc* [4].

Down's syndrome children may have macroglossia, altered gastric emptying, inability to communicate adequately, difficulty mask ventilation & intubation, *etc.*

Children with Congenital cardiac disorders will need preoperative cardiac workup. Risks & benefits of the procedure & anaesthesia are to be discussed with parents and, if necessary paediatric cardiologist [4]. Infectious endocarditis prophylaxis should be given before procedures with bacteraemia risk in doses appropriate for the child's weight.

Approximately 30% of these children coming for dental work under GA have coexisting epilepsy. Anti-convulsant should be continued till the day of the procedure. Certain inhaled volatile anaesthetics (Sevoflurane), local anaesthetics (Lidocaine, Bupivacaine), opioids (Fentanyl, Alfentanil, Sufentanyl, meperidine) and hypnotics (Propofol, Etomidate, Ketamine) are known to lower the seizure threshold. The use of these agents needs careful titration in epileptic children.

Children may be unable to have their medication due to postoperative nausea and vomiting in the postoperative period. Most anticonvulsants, however, have a long elimination half-life of 24-36 hr, and if their levels are in the therapeutic range, a

24-hr period can elapse without significantly increasing the risk of seizures. However, parenteral medications may be needed post-procedure in some instances.

Congenital Bleeding Disorders [4]: Patients with Haemophilia A (deficiency of factor VIII), Haemophilia B (lack of factor IX), Von Willebrand Disease (deficient or abnormal plasma protein Von Willebrand Factor), Factor XI deficiency, *etc.* are at increased risk of significant bleeding from invasive dental procedures. Factor replacement therapy may be provided on a prophylactic basis 32ewto prevent bleeds or on-demand when a bleed occurs. Since the factor levels decline rapidly, the procedure should be performed within half-life duration for that factor which may be as short as 30 -60 min of administration of factor concentrate. The synthetic antidiuretic hormone desmopressin stimulates the release of endogenous FVIII and Vwf from the stores in patients with mild haemophilia and Vwd. DDAVP can be administered one-hour pre-procedure subcutaneously or intravenously. Antifibrinolytic agents like tranexamic acid (IV, oral and mouthwash) has been tried perioperatively to control bleeding with variable success.

## Pediatric Dental Treatment under Sedation/ Anesthesia during Covid-19 Pandemic [41 - 43]

Corona Virus pandemic & Covid-19 infection has posed innumerable challenges to humanity in recent times. Dental treatment in children under sedation/anaesthesia is one of them. Dentistry & sedation/anaesthesia involves close contact with the oral cavity, aerosol-generating drilling processes, positive pressure ventilation, intubation & extubation, coughing, gaging by patients *etc.* All these make it a 'high risk' from a covid infection transmission point of view for patients, doctors, and other health care workers alike. To prioritise & treat these children appropriately, evaluation and triage of these children are done by most units initially by video interviews (Table **7**).

**Table 7. Segregation of children to prioritise treatment during the COVID pandemic.**

| Triage status | Clinical criteria |
|---|---|
| Conservative management | Little/no pain/ can eat & sleep well, relieved with analgesics, the child doesn't have any other medical condition making him high risk, *e.g.*, cardiac anomalies, immune suppression *etc.* |
| Need for active review & possible intervention | Chronic infection, repeated use of antibiotics, cannot eat or sleep due to pain. |
| Urgent Intervention needed | Acute & fast-spreading infection, trismus, no relief with analgesics, affecting child & family in routine day to day activities. |

Those needing intervention are either treated on an official basis or admitted to the hospital; with or without sedation/ general anaesthesia as per the child's age & clinical condition. Usually, ASA I & II children (Table **8**) [44] are managed in an official basis. ASA III & above children will need to stay in hospital.

**Table 8. ASA physical status Classification system, Pediatric examples.**

| ASAClass | Pediatric Examples include but are not limited to |
|---|---|
| ASA I | A Child without systemic disease; Normal BMI percentile for Age |
| ASA II | A Child with mild systemic disease. *e.g.*, well-controlled epilepsy, Asthma & Congenital cardiac disease, Autism with Mild Limitations, Oncology in remission. |
| ASA III | A Child with severe systemic disease. *e.g.*, Uncontrolled Asthma, epilepsy and Congenital cardiac disease, Autism with strict limitations, Muscular Dystrophy, Difficult Airway, Morbid Obesity, Diabetes Insulin-dependent. |
| ASA IV | A Child with severe systemic disease that is a constant threat to life. *e.g.*, Sepsis, Shock, Disseminated Intravascular Coagulation, Severe Trauma, Congestive Cardiac Failure, Severe Respiratory Distress. |
| ASA V | A moribund Child is not expected to survive 24 hours with or without operation. |
| ASA VI | A Declared Braindead, whose organs are removed for donation. |
| ASA E | Emergency operation of any variety, 'E' preceded the number indicating the patient's physical status. |

Following precautions need to be taken while treating these children:

- The number of attendants accompanying the patient should be restricted to one caregiver per person and maintain social distancing (except for physical examination) and hand hygiene throughout.
- In addition to the standard pre-anaesthetic evaluation, all patients should be assessed for a potential COVID-19 infection.
- Universal precautions, including protection against aerosols, should be followed. These include the cap, goggles/visor, surgical mask, waterproof gown, gloves, and shoe covers. An N95 mask and double gloves should be used (Level 2 PPE).
- Premedication is highly recommended to avoid coughing, crying, and struggling children and reduce the risk of aerosolisation and droplet contamination. Intravenous (IV) induction *via* a cannula secured earlier is best. Sufficient time must be set aside for oral premedication and subsequent IV cannula placement. Nasal administration of premedication is not recommended because of the potential for high viral loads and the risk of coughing and sneezing.
- Till the child is taken on a dental chair for sedation/anaesthesia, Face mask covering nose and mouth to be kept on. The same mask may be used post-procedure with $O_2$ supplementation.

- IV induction is preferred, as inhalational induction increase exposure to respiratory droplets and aerosols. If inhalation sedation/induction becomes unavoidable, the lowest possible fresh gas flow should be used while maintaining a tight facemask seal. The double-layered mask is preferable to achieve adequate seal during $N_2O$: $O_2$ sedation with vacuum/ suction placed by the side of the mask.
- The head end of the patient should be covered during induction to minimise airborne contamination during airway instrumentation. An 'intubation box' (Fig. **30A**) made of clear plastic or acrylic sits over the patient's head and acts as a protective shield during AGP (aerosol-generating procedures). It has two Arm Holes to place hands to intubate with a standard Laryngoscope or Video Laryngoscope. The Arm Holes may be covered with a rubber seal to prevent tracking of Aerosols along with the hands. There are side holes to provide suction or any other help. The intubation box does help to minimise the exposure of Anaesthesiologists, dentists & Operating room personnel to Aerosol.
- If intubation is required, video laryngoscopy (preferably with disposable blades) is preferred, as the distance between the patient and the laryngoscopist is increased along with better first-pass intubation success.
- Use low flows, tight-fitting masks, rubber dams, extubation in deeper planes of sedation to prevent coughing from being undertaken to minimise contamination.
- 1st procedure in recovery area child may be placed in Intubation Box with $O_2$ provision till they are fully awake.

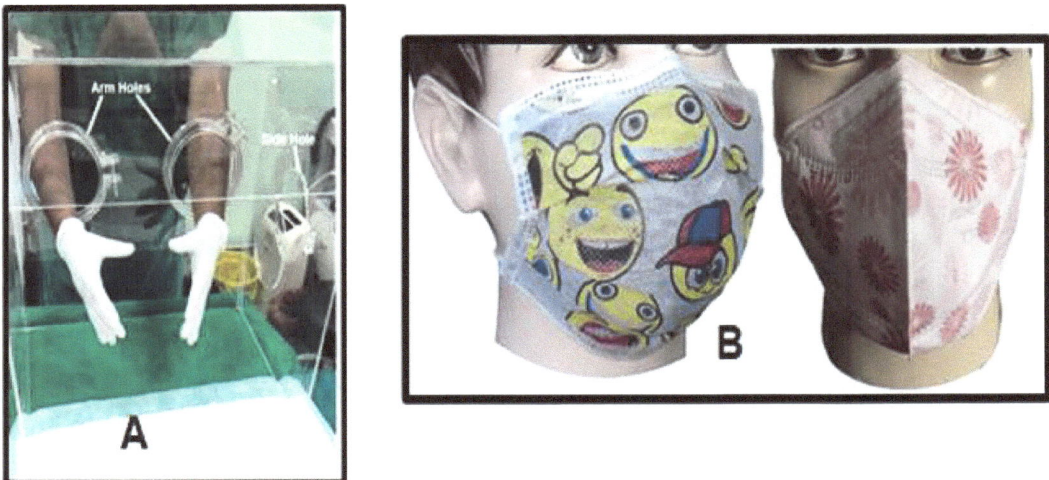

**Fig. (30).** A-Intubation box, B- Pediatric surgical & n95 mask.

## SUMMARY

Sedation & GA are behavioural control techniques increasingly used in paediatric dentistry. Advancements in knowledge, technology, monitoring concepts & understanding of paediatric anatomy, physiology & pharmacology, general anaesthesia & sedation have become safe practices in modern medicine. However, occasional adverse events are known to occur mainly in children with pre-existing medical conditions [3]. Careful selection of patient, the technique of anaesthesia, surgical skills & duration, competent anaesthesia provider, meticulous planning, abiding by safe protocols & education of parents provides the key for success.

## ACKNOWLEDGEMENTS

We sincerely acknowledge support from Ms. Pascalis from Porter Instrument Business Unit of Parker Hannifin for equipment photographs & Dr. Nandini Dave, senior paediatric Anaesthesia consultant from SRCC children's Hospital, Mumbai, India, for clinical photographs.

## REFERENCES

[1]     Acharya S. Chair-side general anaesthesia for pediatric dental patients-risky or risk-free. International Journal of PedodonticRehabilitation 2018; 3: 8-11.

[2]     Silva CC. Lavadoc, Areias C, *et al.* Conscious sedation vs general anaesthesia in pediatric dentistry- a review. Medical express (Sao Paulo, online) 2015; 2(1): M150104.

[3]     Bartella AK, Lechner C, Kamal M, Steegmann J, Hölzle F, Lethaus B. The safety of paediatric dentistry procedures under general anaesthesia. A five-year experience of a tertiary care center. Eur J Paediatr Dent 2018; 19(1): 44-8.
[PMID: 29569453]

[4]     Fernandes S. Deepa Suvarna, 'Anesthesia for pediatric dentistry.' 'Principles& Practice of Pediatric Anesthesia. Chapter 18 2016; 247-57.

[5]     Cote CJ, Wilson S. American Academy of Pediatrics & American Academy of Pediatric Dentistry. Guidelines for monitoring & management of Paediatric patients before, during and after sedation for Diagnostic and Therapeutic procedures. Pediatr Dent J 2019; 41(4): E26-52.

[6]     Nayak PA, Srikant N, Karuna YM, Baliga KN, Rao A. Parent's perception on general anaesthesia in paediatric dentistry: A questionnaire study. Indian J Public Health Res Dev 2019; 10(9): 235-41.
[http://dx.doi.org/10.5958/0976-5506.2019.02432.X]

[7]     Ramazani N. Different aspects of general anaesthesia in pediatric dentistry: A review. Iranian. Iran J Pediatr 2016; In Press: e2613.
[http://dx.doi.org/10.5812/ijp.2613] [PMID: 27307962]

[8]     Adewale L. Anaesthesia for paediatric dentistry. Contin Educ Anaesth Crit Care Pain 2012; 12(6): 288-94.
[http://dx.doi.org/10.1093/bjaceaccp/mks045]

[9]     Sharma A, Jayaprakash R. N Aravindha Babu *et al.* General anaesthesia in paediatric dentistry. Biomedical & Pharmacology Journal 2015; 8(Spl. Edn):. 189-94.

[10]    ain P, Sharma S, Sharma A, *et al.* Efficacy and safety of oral triclofos as a sedative for children undergoing sleep electroencephalogram: An observational study. J Ped Neurosci 2016; 11: 105-8.

[11] Wyne AH, Sheta SA, Al-Zahrani AM. Comparison of oral midazolam with a combination of oral midazolam and nitrous oxide-oxygen inhalation in the effectiveness of dental sedation for young children. J Indian Soc Pedod Prev Dent 2009; 27(1): 9-16.
[http://dx.doi.org/10.4103/0970-4388.50810] [PMID: 19414968]

[12] Corcuera-Flores JR, Silvestre-Rangil J, Cutando-Soriano A, López-Jiménez J. Current methods of sedation in dental patients - a systematic review of the literature. Med Oral Patol Oral Cir Bucal 2016; 21(5): 0.
[http://dx.doi.org/10.4317/medoral.20981] [PMID: 27475684]

[13] Samuel Oh. and Karl Kingsley, Efficacy of Ketamine in Pediatric Sedation Dentistry: A Systematic Review, Compendium: May. 2018; 39(5).

[14] Oyedepo, A Nasir, L O Abdur-Rahman, et al. Efficacy and safety of oral ketamine premedication in children undergoing day-case surgery. J West Afr Coll Surg 2016; 6(1): 1-15.

[15] Shapira J, Kupietzky A, Kadari A, Fuks AB, Holan G. Comparison of oral midazolam with and without hydroxyzine in the sedation of pediatric dental patients. Pediatr Dent 2004; 26(6): 492-6.
[PMID: 15646910]

[16] C. Fantacci1, G. C. Fabrizio1, P. Ferrara1, et al, Intranasal drug administration for procedural sedation in children admitted to pediatric Emergency Room, European Review for Medical and Pharmacological Sciences: 2018; 22: 217-22.

[17] Yuen VM, Hui TW, Irwin MG, Yao TJ, Wong GL, Yuen MK. ORIGINAL ARTICLE: Optimal timing for the administration of intranasal dexmedetomidine for premedication in children. Anaesthesia 2010; 65(9): 922-9.
[http://dx.doi.org/10.1111/j.1365-2044.2010.06453.x] [PMID: 20645951]

[18] Yuen VM, Hui TW, Irwin MG, Yuen MK. A comparison of intranasal dexmedetomidine and oral midazolam for premedication in pediatric anesthesia: a double-blinded randomized controlled trial. Anesth Analg 2008; 106(6): 1715-21.
[http://dx.doi.org/10.1213/ane.0b013e31816c8929] [PMID: 18499600]

[19] Zanaty OM, El Metainy SA. A comparative evaluation of nebulized dexmedetomidine, nebulized ketamine, and their combination as premedication for outpatient pediatric dental surgery. Anesth Analg 2015; 121(1): 167-71.
[http://dx.doi.org/10.1213/ANE.0000000000000728] [PMID: 25822924]

[20] Manoj M, Satya prakash MVS, Swaminathan S, Kamaladevi RK. Comparison of ease of administration of intranasal midazolam spray and oral midazolam syrup by parents as premedication to children undergoing elective surgery. J Anesth 2017; 31(3): 351-7.
[http://dx.doi.org/10.1007/s00540-017-2330-6] [PMID: 28271228]

[21] Mehran M, Tavassoli-Hojjati S, Ameli N, Zeinabadi MS. Effect of Intranasal Sedation Using Ketamine and Midazolam on Behavior of 3-6 Year-Old Uncooperative Children in Dental Office: A Clinical Trial. J Dent (Tehran) 2017; 14(1): 1-6.
[PMID: 28828011]

[22] Kyle R. Canton, Shawn Hendrikx, Gary Joubert, et al. Intranasal Ketamine for Procedural Sedation and Analgesia in Children: A Systematic Review: Pediatrics2018January, 141 (1 Meeting Abstract) 350

[23] H.S. Abdel-Ghaffar, S.M. Kamal, F.A. El Sherif, et al., Comparison of nebulised dexmedetomidine, ketamine, or midazolam for premedication in preschool children undergoing bone marrow biopsy, Paediatrics| 2018; 121(2): P445-452.

[24] Miller Textbook of Anesthesia. Miller Textbook of Anesthesia, 7th edition Flumezinil, Naloxone hydrochloride. pp. 736-811.

[25] Mason KP, Seth N. Future of paediatric sedation: towards a unified goal of improving practice. Br J Anaesth 2019; 122(5): 652-61.

[http://dx.doi.org/10.1016/j.bja.2019.01.025] [PMID: 30916013]

[26] Local Anaesthetic Toxicity Management Chi SI. Complications caused by nitrous oxide in dental sedation. J Dent Anesth Pain Med 2018; 18(2): 71-8.. https://www.asra.com/advisory-guidelines/articles/3/checklist-for-treatment-of-local-anesthetic-systemic-toxicity

[27] American Academy of pediatric dentistry. Use of local anaesthesia for pediatric dental patients. The Reference Manual of Pediatric Dentistry. Chicago, III, American academy of pediatric dentistry Portable Dental N2O systems. https://www.porterinstrument.com/breathing-circuits 2020; 318-23.

[28] Chi SI. Complications caused by nitrous oxide in dental sedation. J Dent Anesth Pain Med Porter Product catalogue https://wwwporterinstrumentcom/pdf/datasheets/Porter-Full-Products--nd-Accessories-Catalog-FM-1423pdf 2018; 18(2): 71-8.
[http://dx.doi.org/10.17245/jdapm.2018.18.2.71] [PMID: 29744381]

[29] Portable Dental N. https://www.porterinstrument.com/breathing-circuitsRamsay MA, Savege TM, Simpson BR. Controlled sedation with alphaxolone- alphadalone. Br Med J 1974; 2(5920): 656-9

[30] https://www.porterinstrument.com/pdf/datasheets/Porter-Full-Products-and-Accessories-Cata-og-FM-1423.pdf

[31] https://www.porterinstrument.com/dental-nitrous-applications

[32] Aboytes DB, Flores JR. Administration of Nitrous Oxide Analgesia, Use of this form of conscious sedation represents an effective alternative pain management strategy for dental procedures. Decisions in Dentistry: On Jan 9, 2018. https://decisionsindentistry.com/article/administration-nitrous-oxi-e-analgesia/

[33] American Academy of pediatric dentistry. Use of local anaesthesia for pediatric dental patients. The Reference Manual of Pediatric Dentistry. Chicago, III, American academy of pediatric dentistry: 2020, p. 318-23.

[34] Local Anaesthetic Toxicity Management.https://www.asra.com/advisory-guidelines/articles/3/checklist-for-treatment-of-local-anesthetic-systemic-toxicity.

[35] American Society of Anesthesiologists (ASA). Joint statement on pediatric dental sedation: 2021. https://www.asahq.org/advocacy-and-asapac/advocacy-topics/office-based-anesthesia-and-dental-anesthesia/joint-statement-pediatric-dental-sedation. Last assessed & revised on 20/01/2021

[36] Vutskits L, Davidson A. Miller's Anesthesia, 9thedition, Elsevier, 2019, 'Pediatric Anesthesia', Chapter 77, 2019; 2427-39.

[37] Standard ASA. and Guidelines, Statements, Distinguishing Monitored Anesthesia Care from Moderate Sedation Analgesia 2018.

[38] Johnson YJ, Nickerson M, Quezado ZMN. Case report: an unforeseen peril of parental presence during induction of anesthesia. Anesth Analg 2012; 115(6): 1371-2.

[39] Fakhruddin KS, Hisham EB, Gorduysus MO. Effectiveness of audiovisual distraction eyewear and computerized delivery of anesthesia during pulp therapy of primary molars in phobic child patients. Eur J Dent 2015; 9(4): 470-5.
[http://dx.doi.org/10.4103/1305-7456.172637] [PMID: 26929683]

[40] Nunna M, Dasaraju RK, Kamatham R, Mallineni SK, Nuvvula S. Comparative evaluation of virtual reality distraction and counter-stimulation on dental anxiety and pain perception in children. J Dent Anesth Pain Med 2019; 19(5): 277-88.

[41] Malhotra N, Joshi M, Datta R, Bajwa SS, Mehdiratta L. Indian society of anaesthesiologists (ISA national) advisory and position statement regarding COVID-19. Indian J Anaesth 2020; 64(4): 259-63.
[http://dx.doi.org/10.4103/ija.IJA_288_20] [PMID: 32362681]

[42] Matava CT, Kovatsis PG, Lee JK, *et al.* Pediatric Airway Management in COVID-19 Patients: Consensus Guidelines From the Society for Pediatric Anesthesia's Pediatric Difficult Intubation Collaborative and the Canadian Pediatric Anesthesia Society. Anesth Analg 2020; 131(1): 61-73.

[http://dx.doi.org/10.1213/ANE.0000000000004872]

[43]    Halla Z, Pathanjali K, Grainne Y, Helen R. COVID-19: implications for paediatric dental general anaesthetic services. Fac Dent J 2020; 11(3): 114-119.

[44]    ASA Physical Status Classification System, "https://www.asahq.org/standards-and-guidelines" Guidelines, Statements, Clinical Resources: December 13, 2020.

# CHAPTER 4

# Drugs Used in Pediatric Dentistry

**Abdulkadeer M. Jetpurwala[1], Shely P. Dedhia[1,\*]** and **Vidya Iyer[2]**

[1] *Department of Pediatric and Preventive Dentistry, Nair Hospital Dental College, Mumbai, India*

[2] *Ex Associate Professor, Department of Pediatric and Preventive Dentistry, CSI College of Dental Sciences, East Veli Street, Madurai, Tamilnadu, India*

**Abstract:** Children are in a state of delicate physiologic equilibrium and, unlike adults, are more susceptible to medications and their adverse effects. Medicines used for children should be carefully selected, and the minimum dose required should be administered. Possible adverse reaction in multidrug therapy is also essential. The pediatric dentist must also consider any other drug the child may be taking while prescribing drugs and understanding children's presenting signs and symptoms.

**Keywords:** Analgesics, Antibiotics, Antifungal, Antimicrobials, Non-steroidal anti-inflammatory drugs.

## INTRODUCTION

Children are more prone to infections because of their developing immune systems. The oral cavity is one such area where various bacterial, viral, and fungal infections are generally encountered, making using antimicrobials and analgesics mandatory. The oral cavity is also a zone of inflammatory responses from the gingival and periodontal tissues, and anti-inflammatory drugs are commonly prescribed for dental diseases.

Antimicrobials are substances that kill or suppress the growth or multiplication of microorganisms. Along with combating infections, managing pain is inherent to dental practice. Numerous analgesics are available, and the recent introduction of new agents provides even more options from which to choose while prescribing these drugs; it is essential and should be considered that children are not just "small adults." Children go through different stages of development, which variations in body weight, surface area, physiology, kidney function, liver,

\* **Corresponding author Shely P. Dedhia:** Department of Pediatric Dentistry, Nair Hospital Dental College, Mumbai, India; E-mail: jetabdulkadeer@yahoo.com

**Satyawan Damle, Ritesh Kalaskar & Dhanashree Sakhare (Eds.)**
**All rights reserved-© 2023 Bentham Science Publishers**

cognitive or immune function. This, in turn, influences the impact of drugs on the pharmacokinetic/ pharmacodynamics of their body.

Most children report to the dental office with the chief complaint of pain or swelling about the teeth or surrounding structures. The most typical cause of dental pain is an odontogenic infection caused by dental caries or trauma. In such emergencies, the primary emphasis should be given to pain relief and control of the underlying disease. Hence, a pedodontist/ dental professional needs to know the dosage and side effects of drugs used in different conditions [1].

## Calculation of Pediatric Dose [2]

The dose of drugs used in children varies from adults, primarily concerning age, metabolic activity, body surface area and excretory capacity of the child.

The appropriate dose of the drug for children can be calculated by the following formulae, depending on the child's age, weight, or body surface area, relating to the average adult dose.

Young's Rule

Dilling's Rule

Fried's Rule

Clarke's Rule

## According to the Body Surface Area

### *Non-Steroidal Anti-Inflammatory Drugs [3]*

Human beings have undoubtedly experienced pain since the beginning of time. From historic fossils to writings of ancient civilisations, evidence of pain and attempt at its relief has been noticed throughout history. Nonsteroidal anti-inflammatory drugs (NSAIDs) are commonly prescribed in dental practice to manage pain and swelling.

Nonsteroidal anti-inflammatory drugs are also called non-opioid analgesics. These drugs have some common actions, such as, Fig. (**1**).

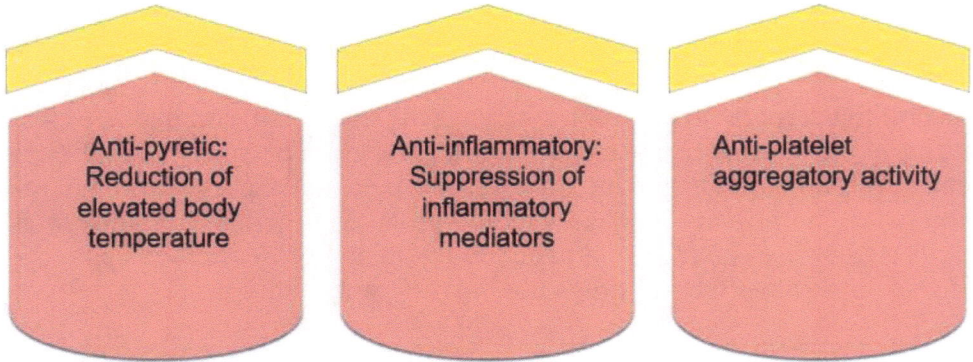

**Fig. (1).** Actions of nonsteroidal anti-inflammatory drugs.

## Analgesia: Pain Relief (Without Interfering with Opioid Receptors)

### *Classification*

Nonsteroidal anti-inflammatory drugs are classified according to their potential to cyclo-oxygenaseygenase (COX) enzyme during arachidonic acid metabolism (Table **1**) [4].

**Table 1. Classification of nonsteroidal anti-inflammatory drugs.**

| Type | Examples |
|---|---|
| **Nonselective COX inhibitors** | |
| Salicylates and their congeners | Acetyl salicylic acid (Aspirin), Salicylamide |
| Para amino phenol derivatives | Phenacetin, Paracetamol |
| Pyrazolone derivatives | Phenylbutazone, Oxyphenbutazone |
| Indoles and related drugs | Indomethacin, Sulindac |
| Aryl acetic acid derivatives | Diclofenac |
| Pyrrolo pyrrole derivatives | Ketorolac |
| Propionic acid derivatives | Ibuprofen, Ketoprofen |
| Anthralin acid derivatives | Flufenamic acid, Mefenamic acid |
| Oxicams | Piroxicam |
| **Preferential COX2 inhibitors** | Nimesulide, Meloxicam, Nabumetone |
| **Selective COX2 inhibitors** | Rofecoxib, Valdecoxib, Etoricoxib, Celecoxib |

## Mechanism of Action

### *Analgesic Action: (Fig. 2)*

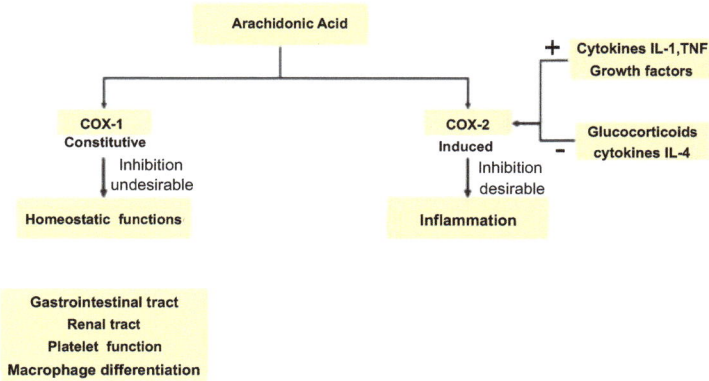

**Fig. (2).** Action of NSAIDs on arachidonic acid metabolism.

Although these drugs differ in their chemical structures, they have a similar mechanism of action.

Arachidonic acid is liberated from cell membranes converted to prostaglandins via the cyclo-oxygenase (COX 1 and 2) pathways during fever, pain and inflammation.

COX-1 activity is constitutively present in nearly all cell types at a constant level.

COX-2 activity is absent in most cells (except renal and neural cells) but can be induced by inflammation.

Increased prostaglandin production leads to:

Increased permeability of blood vessels.

Hyperalgesia is associated with inflammation.

The release of prostaglandins in the central nervous system lowers the threshold of the significant pain circuits.

Headache and vascular pain.

NSAIDs inhibit cyclo-oxygenase (COX1 and COX2) enzymes and block the synthesis of prostaglandins, thereby producing beneficial therapeutic effects.

## *Anti-pyretic Action:*

The maintenance of average body temperature is a physiologic phenomenon. Adults' usual body temperature range is 36.1-37.2°C (97-99°F). Body temperature is slightly higher in infants. Suppose the core temperature increases by a few degrees, psychosomatic changes such as confusion, delirium, and febrile convulsions can occur. When body temperature is elevated, the hypothalamic thermal regulation centre is set at a higher temperature, regulating the body temperature according to the new setting. It includes peripheral vasoconstriction, which decreases heat loss.

NSAIDs reset the hypothalamic thermal regulation centre to a lower temperature and cause sweating which helps in reducing the body temperature.

Paracetamol should be used as a first-line antipyretic in children. Other NSAIDs should be used only if the patient does not respond to paracetamol.

## General Properties of NSAIDs:

The available properties of NSAIDs are as under (Fig. 3).

Weakly acidic compounds with ionization constants ranging from 3.0 to 5.0

Varying degrees of lipid solubility and almost completely absorbed orally.

Highly protein bound, having a small volume of distribution.

Metabolized in the liver and mostly excreted in the urine.

**Fig. (3).** General properties of NSAIDs.

Commonly used NSAIDs in pediatric dental practice have been discussed below:

I) Nonselective COX inhibitors:

1. Salicylates and their congeners:

Salicylates are esters or salts of salicylic acid, e.g., methyl salicylate, sodium salicylate and acetylsalicylic acid (aspirin).

They have analgesic, antipyretic, anti-inflammatory, and anti-platelet aggregatory action.

## Adverse Effects

Aspirin should be avoided in infants and children below 12 years of age unless specifically indicated, such as juvenile rheumatoid arthritis. Serious and often fatal complications like Reye's syndrome have been associated with aspirin administration in children. Reye's Syndrome may occur after a few days of viral infection, especially varicella and influenza virus, in children below 12. There is anicteric liver dysfunction due to hepatic mitochondrial injury and metabolic encephalopathy.

They cause peptic ulcers and gastrointestinal bleeding. They also have uricosuric properties.

## Dosage

The usual adult dose for aspirin varies according to its use. The analgesia and amount antipyrine amount in divided doses are 30-65 mg/kg/day.

## *Paracetamol [5]:*

Paracetamol has analgesic and antipyretic actions, but it has weak anti-inflammatory activity. It is an analgesic/antipyretic choice when salicylates or other NSAIDs are contraindicated, e.g., asthmatic patients, peptic ulcer patients and children. Paracetamol cannot inhibit cyclo-oxygenase enzymes in the presence of peroxides present at the site of inflammation. Peroxides are not present in the brain. This explains its poor anti-inflammatory but good antipyretic properties. It is indicated in management mild to moderate pain and fever (Fig. **4**). It is available as tablets, suspensions, suppositories, and injections.

| 1 | Fever due to infection or inflammation or pulpal procedure etc. |
| 2 | Pain due to trauma or odontogenic infections |
| 3 | Headache, musculoskeletal pain |

Fig. (4). Indications of Paracetamol.

## Dosage

The pediatric dose is determined according to the age of the patient. The recommended dose is being 10-15 mg/kg/day to be repeated 4-6 hours (Table **2**).

Table 2. Age-adjusted Dosage.

| 3months- 1 year | 60-120 mg |
|---|---|
| 1 – 5 years | 120-250 mg |
| 6 -12 years | 250-500 mg |

The common adverse effects due to paracetamol have been summarized in Table **3**.

Table 3. Adverse effects.

| Hypersensitivity |
|---|
| Renal or hepatic impairment |

## *Diclofenac [5]:*

Diclofenac has potent anti-inflammatory, analgesic, and antipyretic actions. Diclofenac is available as a sodium or potassium salt. The sodium salt is enteric coated to ensure optimum bioavailability. This leads to some delay in the onset of action. The potassium salt is absorbed rapidly, and the beginning of the movement is faster. They are available in the form of tablets, syrups, and injections.

## Dosage

The dose for children over one year is 2-3 mg/kg/day in divided doses.

## Indications:

It is commonly indicated for inflammatory degenerative chronic disease, musculoskeletal diseases, and acute dental pain.

## Side effects

It may cause perforation of existing gastric ulcers, gastrointestinal bleeding, and blood dyscrasias.

## *Ibuprofen [5]:*

It has anti-inflammatory, analgesic, and antipyretic effects. The analgesic effect is independent of anti-inflammatory activity and has central and peripheral products. Temperature is reduced in febrile patients. Ibuprofen is a potent inhibitor of cyclo-oxygenase and prostaglandin synthesis. The indication of ibuprofen is given in Table **4**. Ibuprofen prevents formation of thromboxane A by platelets. The adverse effects of ibuprofen are shown in Figure 5. It is available as tablets, capsules, and suspensions.

**Table 4. Indications.**

| Musculoskeletal Pain |
| --- |
| Inflammatory and Degenerative Arthritis |
| Dental Pain |

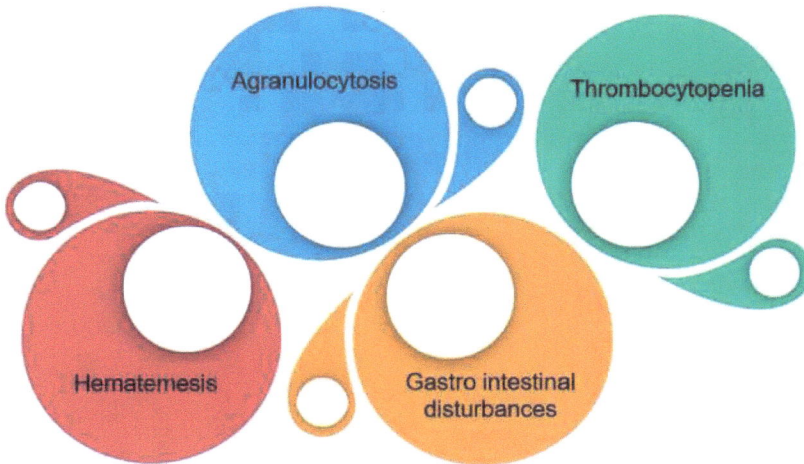

**Fig. (5).** Common adverse effects of Ibuprofen.

## Dosage

The recommended dose for analgesic/antipyretic effect is 5-10 mg/kg every 4-6 hours. It should not be given to children less than 7 kgs.

Ibuprofen is often used alone or in combination with paracetamol.

### *Preferential COX 2 inhibitors:*

### *Meloxicam*

Meloxicam is a new derivative of the oxicam group developed to treat rheumatoid arthritis and osteoarthritis. It has a greater selective inhibitory action against COX 2, responsible for its nonsteroidal anti-inflammatory effects like antipyretic and analgesic actions. Hence, this drug has less chances of inducing gastrointestinal adverse effects [6, 7].

### *Mefenemic Acid*

It is an anthranilic acid derivative used to treat mild to moderate pain. It is commonly used to manage myalgia, arthritis, post-operative pain, and toothache. It is a non-selective COX inhibitor and prevents the formation of prostaglandins. It has good antipyretic action as well.

Dosage: It is prescribed as 20 mg/kg/day in three divided doses.

Adverse effects: Headache, vomiting, gastrointestinal disturbances, and skin rashes are commonly seen side effects.

**Ketorolac:** ketorolac is used for short term management of moderate to severe pain for short duration treatment up to seven days. It can be administered orally as well as sublingually. It functions as a carboxylic acid derivative to non-selectively block prostaglandin synthesis.

Dosage: the recommended dosage is 0.5mg/kg every eight hours.

Adverse effects: Nausea, vomiting, gastrointestinal symptoms, itching and dryness of mouth are commonly seen. Severe side effects include toxic epidermal necrosis (TEN) and Steven's Johnson syndrome.

There is no rule selecting analgesics in the management of pain in pediatric dentistry. The dental surgeon should consider the child's age, weight, general physical and medical condition, degree of pain the child experienced, and selectman most the analgesic with minor side effects (Table 5).

**Table 5. Commonly Prescribed analgesics and Dosages.**

| Drugs | Adult Dose | Pediatric Dose | Route of Administration | Available Forms | Side Effects | Contraindications |
|---|---|---|---|---|---|---|
| Paracetamol | 0.5-1 gm every 4-6 hrs Maximum dose 4g/day | Paracetamol | 0.5-1 gm every 4-6 hrs Maximum dose 4g/day | Paracetamol | 0.5-1 gm every 4-6 hrs Maximum dose 4g/day | Paracetamol |
| Diclofenac sodium | 75-150 mg/day in 2-4 divided doses, Maximum dose - 150mg/day | 2-3mg/Kg/day in 2-4 divided doses | Oral/ Parenteral | Tab/Inj | Perforation of gastric ulcer, Gastrointestinal bleeding, Blood dyscrasias | Active peptic ulcer |
| Ibuprofen | 400-600mg/dose every 6-8 hrs Maximum dose 2400mg/day | 5-10mg/Kg every 6-8hrs | Oral | Tab | Haematemesis, Agragranulocytosis, GI disturbances, Thrombocytopenia | Avoided in peptic ulcer patients |

## *Antimicrobial Drugs [8]*

Antimicrobial therapy has an essential role in managing odontogenic infections, as it can shorten the period of illness and minimise the associated risks. Depending on their source, these drugs can be divided as:

Antibiotics

Antimicrobials

## *Antibiotics*

They are chemical substances synthesised by various species of micro-organisms. They produce suppression of growth or destruction of other microorganisms.

## *Antimicrobials*

They are synthetically derived agents which act against microbes by killing the organisms or suppressing their growth.

These terms are often used interchangeably.

## The Following Factors Must Be Considered Before Deciding to Administer Antibiotics in Pediatric Dentistry

In the case of acute infection, the use of antibiotics is based on the degree of disease, rate of progression and systemic manifestations.

Antibiotics are rarely recommended to treat mild trauma, though in cases involving important soft tissue or dentoalveolar lesions, antibiotic prophylaxis against infection is advisable.

Healthy children requiring the extraction of a single deciduous tooth with an abscess, or endodontic treatment of a permanent tooth, may be operated upon without antibiotic treatment.

In contrast, immunocompromised children, or patients with cardiac problems, require antibiotic prophylaxis [9].

Before any dental treatment of children with some syndrome, medical problem, or any other unfamiliar disorder, it is advisable to consult the pediatrician/family physician.

The antimicrobial medicines' doses are subject to mean inhibitory concentrations (MIC) and mean bactericidal concentrations (MBC). These are especially important to understand the drug's effect on the micro-organism.

The choice of antimicrobial drugs is also based on two methods.

**Empirical therapy:** the antimicrobial chosen is based on clinical knowledge about the condition and commonly associated bacteria with the lesion observed.

**Antibiotic Sensitivity:** the antimicrobial is chosen after culturing the micro-organism and assessing the same sensitivity towards different agents.

**General Principles When Prescribing Antibiotics for Commonly Occurring Conditions [8]**

- **Oral Wound Management**

Factors related to hosting risk and type of wound must be evaluated when determining the risk for infection and subsequent need for antibiotics. Facial lacerations may require topical antibiotic agents. Intraoral lacerations that appear to have been contaminated by extrinsic bacteria, open fractures, and joint injury have an increased risk of infection and should be covered with antibiotics.

- **Pulpitis/apical Periodontitis/draining Sinus Tract/localised Intra-oral Swelling**

Bacteria can access the pulpal tissue through caries, exposed pulp or dentinal tubules, cracks into the dentin, and defective restorations. If a child presents with acute symptoms of pulpitis, treatment (i.e., pulpotomy, pulpectomy, or extraction) should be rendered. Antibiotic therapy usually is not indicated if the dental infection is contained within the pulpal tissue or the immediately surrounding tissue.

## • Acute Facial Swelling of Dental Origin

A child presenting with a facial swelling secondary to a dental infection should receive immediate dental attention. Depending on clinical findings, treatment may consist of treating or extracting the tooth/teeth in question with antibiotic coverage or prescribing antibiotics for several days to contain the spread of infection and then treating the involved tooth/teeth. Intravenous antibiotic therapy and referral for medical management may be indicated.

## Pediatric Periodontal Diseases

In pediatric periodontal diseases (*e.g.*, Neutropenias, Papillon-LeFevre syndrome, Leukocyte adhesion deficiency), the immune system cannot control the growth of periodontal pathogens; In some cases, treatment may involve antibiotic therapy.

## Viral Diseases

Conditions, such as acute primary herpetic gingivostomatitis should not be treated with antibiotic therapy unless strong evidence indicates a secondary bacterial infection.

## *Classification of Antimicrobial/Antibiotic Agents [10]:*

The classification of antimicrobial agents is based on their spectrum, mechanism of action and efficacy against specific microorganisms (Table **6**).

Table 6. Classification of antimicrobial/ antibiotic agents.

| Classification | Examples |
|---|---|
| Depending on the spectrum of action<br>Broad-spectrum antibiotics<br>Narrow spectrum antibiotics<br>Gram-positive bacteria<br>Gram-negative bacteria | Tetracycline, Chloramphenicol<br>Penicillin's Erythromycin, Vancomycin, Lincomycin etc.<br>Streptomycin, Gentamicin, Kanamycin |
| Depending on the mechanism of action<br>Interference with the cell wall synthesis<br>Damaging the cell membrane function<br>Inhibition of bacterial protein synthesis<br>Interference with bacterial DNA<br>Interference with bacterial metabolism | Penicillin, Cephalosporins, Vancomycin, Cycloserine<br>Polymyxin, Colistatin, Nystatin<br>Tetracycline, Chloramphenicol, Macrolides (Erythromycin),<br>Aminoglycosides (Streptomycin), Lincomycin<br>Fluoroquinolones, Metronidazole, Acyclovir, Rifampicin<br>Sulfonamide, Ethambutol, Pyrimethamine |

*(Table 6) cont.....*

| Classification | Examples |
|---|---|
| Depending on the efficacy against specific microorganism<br>Antibacterial agents<br>Antifungal agents<br>Antiprotozoal agents<br>Antiviral agents<br>Antihelminthic agents | Penicillin, Erythromycin, Streptomycin, Tetracycline, Chloramphenicol etc.<br>Nystatin, Griseofulvin, Amphotericin<br>Paromomycin<br>Idoxuridine, Acyclovir, Zidovudine<br>Mebendazole, Niclosamide |

## Penicillin [11]:

They were initially obtained from Penicillium notatum, but the current source is Penicillium chrysogenum. The basic structure of penicillin consists of a thiazolidine ring fused with a beta-lactam ring resulting in 6-amino-penicillanic acid (6 APA).narrow-spectrum spectrum antibiotics suitable for odontogenic infections, as shown in Table (7).

**Table 7. Classification of Penicillin.**

| Classification | Examples |
|---|---|
| Natural Penicillin's<br>SemiSynthetic penicillin<br>Acid-resistant penicillin<br>Penicillinase resistant penicillin<br>Acid labile<br>Acid-resistant<br>c) Extended-spectrum penicillin<br>Aminopenicillins<br>Carboxypenicillins<br>Ureidopenicillins | Penicillin G. (Benzyl Penicillin) Procaine benzylpenicillin, Benzathine penicillin I.P.<br>Potassium phenoxymethylpenicillin (Penicillin V) Potassium phenoxy ethyl penicillin (Phenethicillin)<br>Methicillin, Cloxacillin, Nafcillin<br>Flucloxacillin<br>Ampicillin, Amoxycillin<br>Carbenecillin, Ticarcillin<br>Piperacillin |

## Beta-lactamase Inhibitors

Many microorganisms have developed resistance against penicillin by the production of beta-lactamase enzyme. When given along with penicillin, certain drugs inhibit the bacterial beta-lactamase enzyme and improve the drug's efficacy, *e.g.*, Clavulanic acid sulbactam.

## Antimicrobial Spectrum:

Penicillin is effective mainly against gram-positive and gram-negative cocci and gram-positive bacilli, Streptococci, Staphylococci, Gonocooci, Pneumococci, Meningococci, *Corynebacterium diphtheriae*, Clostridium, Bacteroides, *Treponema pallidum, etc.*

## Mechanism of Action:

Penicillins are bactericidal drugs effective against rapidly multiplying organisms. They act by inhibiting the synthesis of cell wall mucopeptide (peptidoglycans).

## Preparations and Doses:

I. Natural penicillin:

Benzyl penicillin (Penicillin G) available as an injectable form containing 5,00,000 units/ml. Tablets 50,000 to 5,00,000 units (600 mg = 1 million units).

## Dosage

The recommended dose depends on the age of the child.

Neonates- 50mg/kg/day in 2 divided doses

Infants and children- 100mg/kg/day in four divided doses.

Rapid urinary excretion of benzylpenicillin necessitates its parenteral administration every 4 or 6 hours causing considerable inconvenience to the patient. To overcome this, repository preppreparatio actions are relatively insoluble (Table 8). They slowly release benzylpenicillin, thus producing a relatively slow but prolonged antibiotic concentration in blood.

**Table 8. Repository penicillin preparations.**

| Procaine Benzylpenicillin |
|---|
| Fortified rocaine benzylpenicillin |
| Benzathine penicillin |

## Semi-synthetic Penicillin

Semi-synthetic preparations overcome the drawbacks of benzylpenicillin. Organic radicals replace the natural side chains of 6-aminopenicillanic acid. However, it has flaws like inactivation by gastric acid, short duration of action, narrow spectrum of activity, the possibility of anaphylaxis, *etc.*

## Acid-resistant Penicillin

Potassium phenoxy methyl penicillin (Penicillin V)

Potassium phenoxy ethyl penicillin.

They are relatively resistant to inactivation by gastric acid. Hence, they can be given orally.

## Dosage

The child's age determines the dose of potassium phenoxymethylpenicillin.

6-12 years- 250 mg

1-5 years - 125 mg

< 1 year - 62.5 mg to be given in 4 divided doses (1 mg = 1600 units).

## Penicillinase Resistant Penicillin

They are effective against penicillinase producing microorganisms.

Cloxacillin: 0.5 to 1 gm/day in 3-4 divided doses (adult dose)

50 to 100 mg/kg/day in 4 to 6 divided doses.

Methicillin

Nafcillin (I.M.)

## Extended Spectrum Penicillin

Aminopenicillins

Carboxypenicillins

Ureidopencillins

Extended-spectrum penicillin has the following characteristics:

Active against anaerobes.

Most useful in infections caused by *P. aeruginosa* and other gram-negative organisms.

Act synergistically with aminoglycoside antibiotics.

Less active against gram-positive organisms compared to penicillin G.

# Ampicillin

It is more effective against harmful gram-negative bacteria but less sensitive than benzylpenicillin.

## Antimicrobial Spectrum

*H. influenzae, Strep. viridans, Proteus mirabilis, Neisseria gonorrhoea, Salmonella, E. coli, Shigella, Aerobacter* (certain strains), *Enterococci.*

Ampicillin is inactivated by penicillinase, and hence it is ineffective against staphylococci resistant to benzylpenicillin. They are water-soluble, acid-resistant and practical on oral administration.

## Dosage

The recommended dose for children under 13 years is

Orally: 50-100 mg/kg/day

Parenterally: 25-50 mg/kg/day given in divided doses.

## Adverse Effects

It includes nausea, vomiting, maculopapular skin rashes, while diarrhoea is common with oral ampicillin.

## Amoxycillin

It is semisynthetic penicillin with a broad-spectrum antibacterial activity like that of ampicillin. It is the most used antibiotic for odontogenic infections. They are available as capsules, dispersible tablets, suspensions, and injections.

## Advantages

The advantages of amoxicillin over ampicillin are given in Table **9**.

Table 9. Advantages of amoxicillin.

| Blood levels on oral administration of similar oral doses are twice that of ampicillin. |
| --- |
| The incidence of skin rashes and diarrhoea is less than ampicillin. |
| It is less protein-bound, hence faster urinary excretion. |

## Dosage

Children less than 12 years- 20-40 mg/kg/day in 3 divided doses.

## Cephalosporins [12]:

They are derived from *Cephalosporium acremonium*. They have a dithiazolidine ring fused with a beta-lactam ring to form 7-amino-cephalosporins acid (7 ACA).

## Antimicrobial Spectrum

Possess a wide range of activity against gram-positive and gram-negative bacteria.

Gram-positive organisms: Beta hemolytic streptococci, staphylococci, Pneumococci, *C. diphtheriae*.

Gram-negative organisms: *E-coli, Proteus mirabilis, K. pneumonia, N. gonorrhoea* and *Paracolobacterium species*.

The newer derivatives are effective against *Pseudomonas aeruginosa,* Enterobacter, Cephalosporins act by inhibiting bacterial cell wall synthesis like penicillin and are bactericidal.

## Classification

Cephalosporins are divided into generations according to their introduction in clinical practice (Table **10**).

Table 10. Classification of Cephalosporins.

| Classification | Example |
|---|---|
| First Generation | Cephalexin, Cefadroxil |
| Second Generation | Cefaclor, Cefuroxime |
| Third Generation | Ceftazidime, Cefixime, Cefdinir |
| Fourth Generation | Cefepime, Cefpirome |

First-generation cephalosporins are primarily effective against gram-positive and some gram-negative bacteria.

Second-generation cephalosporins have a more comprehensive range of action against gram-negative bacilli, less activity against gram-positive cocci and are ineffective against anaerobes pseudomonas.

Third-generation cephalosporins have poor activity against gram-positive cocci but are more active against gram-negative bacilli and variable action against Pseudomonas.

Fourth-generation cephalosporins are resistant to beta-lactamases and can penetrate the blood-brain barrier.

Cephalosporins are chemically like the penicillin group of drugs. They are also vulnerable to bacteria that produce a β-lactamase enzyme, and they may be used in conjunction with clavulanic acid.

## Fluoroquinolones [13]:

## Ciprofolxacin

Ciprofloxacin is a synthetic chemotherapeutic antibiotic of the fluoroquinolone drug class. It is a second-generation fluoroquinolone antibacterial. It kills bacteria by interfering with the enzymes that cause DNA to rewind after being copied, stopping the synthesis of DNA and protein.

## Antimicrobial Spectrum

Gram-positive: methicillin-susceptible *Staphylococcus aureus* (MSSA), *Streptococcus pneumoniae*.

Gram-negative: *Enterobacteriaceae, H. influenzae,* other *Haemophilus* spp., *N. gonorrhoea, N. meningitides, M. catarrhalis, P. aeruginosa, S. maltophilia*

Atypical: *Legionella pneumophilia*

## Adverse Reaction

CNS: headache, insomnia, dizziness; hallucinations, depression, psychotic reactions (rare)

Connective tissue: tendon injury

Renal: interstitial nephritis

Cardiovascular: arrhythmia

Ciprofloxacin is considered contraindicated within the pediatric population, pregnancy, nursing mothers, and patients with epilepsy or other seizure disorders. It has been reported to have cartilage depression in children and should be avoided.

**Dosage:** 25mg/Kg/day divided in 2 doses (12 hrs each).

## Ofloxacin

Ofloxacin is a quinolone group antibiotic that inhibits the bacterial topoisomerase and DNA gyrase enzymes. It has a broad-spectrum antibiotic effective against both gram-positive and gram-negative bacteria

Antibacterial spectrum:

*Staphylococcus aureus, Strep pneumonia, Strep pyogenes, Enterobacter aerogenes, E. Coli, H Influenzae, Klebsiella gonorrhoea*

Adverse reaction:

Usually well-tolerated, it may cause nausea, vomiting, tendonitis, and cardiotoxicity.

Contraindications

Pregnancy, lactating mothers, seizure disorders and psychiatric problems. Should be used with caution in children

Dosage:

Child under 30kg, the dose should be 15 – 20 mg/kg/day in two divided doses.

## Nitroimidazoles [14]

## Metronidazole

It is a nitro-imidazole derivative. Although metronidazole is effective against penicillin-resistant anaerobic gram-negative bacilli, it only has moderate activity against microaerophilic gram-positive cocci. In severe infections, metronidazole is best used with penicillin to ensure coverage against aerobic gram-positive bacteria. The development of resistance to this agent by common odontogenic pathogens is rare. Metronidazole has excellent anaerobic gram-negative activity and a low degree of toxicity, which is beneficial for treating odontogenic infections.

## Antimicrobial Spectrum

Anaerobic microorganisms.

Nonsporing, anaerobic, gram-negative bacilli such as Bacteroides.

Trichomonas infection

Lacks activity against aerobic bacteria.

## Mechanism of Action

Interacts with the bacterial DNA with a lethal effect (bactericidal).

## Preparation and Dosage

They are available as tablets, suspensions, and injectable forms.

The recommended pediatric dose is 30 - 50 mg/kg/day orally in 3-4 divided doses.

## Therapeutic Uses

Metronidazole is effective against infections caused due to non-sporing gram-negative anaerobes (Bacteroides). It is also used for acute odontogenic diseases such as ulcerative gingivitis (Vincent's stomatitis).

The adverse effects of metronidazole are given in Table **11**.

**Table 11. Adverse Effects of Metronidazole.**

| **Nausea, Anorexia, Abdominal Discomfort** |
|---|
| Metallic taste in the mouth |
| Headache, dizziness |
| Stomatitis, cystitis |
| Peripheral neuropathy, rarely epileptic seizures |
| Mild blood dyscrasias like prolymphocytic leucopenia |
| Possible carcinogenic and mutagenic effects in animals |

## Ornidazole

It is a synthetic nitroimidazole derivative with an antimicrobial spectrum like metronidazoles. However, it is tolerated better. It has abroad antimicrobial range and is also effective in protozoal and anaerobic infections.

## Antimicrobial Spectrum

The antimicrobial spectrum is like metronidazole

**Mechanism of Action**

Disrupts the DNA replication and transcription process

**Dosage**

It is generally available as a combination drug along with ofloxacin

Available as tablets and suspension

It is administered at 10-25 mg/kg/day in two divided doses

**Therapeutic Uses**

Anaerobic infections

Amoebiasis

Trichomoniasis

Giardiasis

**Adverse Reactions**

Headache

Nausea and vomiting

Skin rashes

**Macrolide Antibiotics [15]:**

They have a lactone ring in their chemical structure. The commonly used drugs in this group are:

Erythromycin

Roxithromycin

Azithromycin

Clarithromycin

These drugs inhibit protein synthesis by binding to the 50s ribosome.

# Erythromycin

It is the most effective drug of all macrolide antibiotics. It is obtained from Streptomyces erythreus (fungus). Depending on the serum concentration, they show bacteriostatic or bactericidal effects.

## Antibacterial Spectrum

Gram-positive cocci including Streptococci, Staphylococci, Pneumococci, Neisseria and some strains of Influenza, C. diphtheriae, Mycoplasma etc. The gastric juice partially destroys them; hence, it must be administered in the form of enteric-coated tablets; this also minimises gastric upset associated with these drugs. Erythromycin esters like erythromycin stearate, estolate and ethyl succinate are better tolerated orally.

## Dosage

The erythromycin dose is 30-50 mg/kg/day in 4 divided doses.

The macrolide antibiotics should not be considered first-line therapy to treat odontogenic infections. They should be reserved for patients with a penicillin allergy or against penicillin-resistant organisms. Newer macrolides like azithromycin, clarithromycin, and roxithromycin have a similar antimicrobial spectrum as erythromycin but are more resistant to acid hydrolysis. They also act against *H. influenzae, M. catarrhalis, T. gondii* and *M. avium* complex.

## Other Related Antimicrobials include

Lincomycin

Clindamycin

Vancomycin

Bacitracin

## Clindamycin

Clindamycin has excellent activity against gram-positive organisms, including anaerobes and beta-lactamase-producing strains. Low drug concentrations are bacteriostatic, but bactericidal activity is achieved clinically with the usual recommended doses. Because of its broad spectrum of coverage and excellent clinical efficacy, coupled with the increase in penicillin-resistant microorganisms, clindamycin is widely used to treat odontogenic infections.

## Dosage

In children less than 1 month 15-20 mg/kg/day, in older children, 20-40 mg/kg/day are given in 3-4 divided doses.

## Tetracyclines [16]:

Tetracyclines are of limited use in pediatric dentistry. Although they are active against a range of gram-positive and gram-negative aerobic and anaerobic bacteria, their usefulness has been greatly diminished due to widespread resistance.

Doxycycline and Minocycline possess better anaerobic activity than tetracycline, but neither of these agents should be considered as first-line therapy for odontogenic infections.

## Dosage

It is given in 20-40 mg/kg/day in 2-4 divided doses.

## Adverse effects

Gastrointestinal disturbances are common with tetracyclines, and hypersensitivity reactions such as skin rashes and drug-induced fever can occur. The use of tetracyclines in children under 13 is contraindicated due to the risk of permanent discolouration of teeth and interference with bone development.

The enteral route of administration of the tetracycline group of drugs has declined in dentistry. Doxycycline has been used to soak the tooth in managing avulsion of teeth when the extraoral dry time of the tooth has been prolonged. At the same time, minocycline has been used as an intra-canal medicament as part of the triple antibiotic paste (Ciprofloxacin, Metronidazole and Minocycline).

## Antifungal Agents [17]:

The fungal infection may be a primary disease or may occur secondarily to antibiotic therapy, malignancy, diabetes mellitus and corticosteroid therapy.

## Classification

The classification of antifungal agents has been shown in Table **12**.

**Table 12. Classification of antifungal agents.**

| Type | Examples |
|---|---|
| Antibiotics<br>Polyenes<br>Heterocyclic | Nystatin, Hamycin, Natamycin |
| Antimetabolites | Flucytosine |
| Azoles<br>Imidazoles<br>Topical<br>Systemic<br>b) Triazoles Systemic<br>Other topical agents | Clotrimazole, Miconazole, Ketoconazole<br>Fluconazole, Itraconazole, Allylamine, Terbinafine<br>Benzoic acid, Quinidochlor |

## Nystatin

It is obtained from *Streptomyces noursei.*

## Antifungal Spectrum

Candida, Histoplasma, Blastomycoses, Trichophyton and Microsporum audouini. On parenteral administration, it produces toxic effects (*e.g.*, nephrotoxicity); hence its use is restricted to treating localized infections caused by Candida.

## Mechanism of Action

Nystatin acts by interfering with vital cellular mechanisms such as respiration, glucose utilisation, *etc.*

## Preparation and Dose

Nystatin suspension contains 1, 00,000 units/ml; oral topical application is usually made 3 times a day.

Children less than one year 1, 00,000 units eight hourly.

1 to 6 year 2, 00,000 units 8 hourly.

Above 6 yrs-5, 00,000 units 8 hourly.

## Adverse Reaction

Local application - mild adverse effects.

Orally administered- nausea, vomiting and diarrhoea.

Parenterally administered nephrotoxicity.

## Antiviral Drugs

## Acyclovir [18]:

It is an antiviral medication which works on the principle of decreasing the production of viral DNA. It is used primarily in the treatment of herpes simplex infection. It is used in children with the severe signs of acute herpetic gingivostomatitis, chickenpox and shingles.

## Preparations and Dosage

It is available in syrups, tablets and drops and topical application for pediatric use. It is used in 20 mg/kg per dose at six-hour intervals.

## Adverse Effects

Commonly seen side effects include nausea, vomiting, and diarrhoea. In the topical application there is localised itching or eczema.

A summary of the commonly prescribed antibiotics and their doses, route of administration, side effects and contraindications has been given in Table **13**.

**Table 13. Commonly prescribed antibiotics for Oro dental infections.**

| Drugs | Adult Dose | Pediatric Dose | Route of Administration | Available Forms | Side Effects | Contraindications |
|---|---|---|---|---|---|---|
| Amoxicillin | 250-500mg 3 times/day | 20-40mg/Kg/ day in 3 doses | Oral/ Parenteral | Tab/Cap/ Dry syrup/Inj | Pseudomembranous colitis, leucopenia, Anemia. | Hypersensitivity |
| Cefixime | 200mg Two times a day for 7-10days | 8mg/Kg/day in 2 divided doses | Oral | Tab/Cap/ Syrup | Pseudomembranous colitis, Thrombocytopenia | Hypersensitivity |
| Amoxicillin + Clavulanic acid | 200-600mg every 12 hrs | 20-40mg/Kg/ day in 3 doses | Oral/Parenteral | Capsule/ Dry syrup/Inj | Candida, anaphylactic reaction, Superinfection | Allergy |
| Ciprofloxacin | 200mg 2 times a day for 7 -10 days | 25mg/Kg/day divided into 2 doses (12 hrs each). To be avoided in children below 18 yrs. | Oral /parental/ Topical | Tab/Inj/ Drops | Tremor, Confusion, Convulsions, Phototoxicity | Avoid exposure to strong sunlight. |
| Cefadroxil | 0.5-1g O D or B I D | 30mg/Kg/ day in 2 doses | Oral | Tab/Cap/ syrup/Suspension | Angioedema, Candida, anaphylactic reaction, superinfection | hypersensitivity |

*(Table 13) cont.....*

| Drugs | Adult Dose | Pediatric Dose | Route of Administration | Available Forms | Side Effects | Contraindications |
|-------|-----------|----------------|------------------------|-----------------|--------------|-------------------|
| Erythromycin | 250-500mg (stearate or estolate salts) or 400mg ethyl succinate salt every 6 hrs. | 30 to 50 mg /Kg/ day in divided doses every 6hrs | Oral | Tab/Cap/ Dry syrup/Susp | Ototoxicity, Neurotoxicity, Hepatotoxicityagranulocytosis | Hypersensitivity, Porphyria, Hepatic impairment |
| Metronidazole | 250-750mg every 8 hrs, not to exceed 4g in 24 hrs | 30-50 mg/Kg/day in 3 divided doses for 5-10 day | Oral/ Parenteral/ Rectal | Tab/ Susp/ Inj/ Suppo | Metallic taste, Glossitis, Stomatitis, Ataxia, Hepatitis | Hypersensitivity |
| Ornidazole | 500mg twice daily for five days | 10mg/ Kg every 12 hrs | Oral/ Parenteral | Tab/Inj/Susp | Temporary loss of consciousness, Taste disturbances Vertigo, | Hypersensitivity |

## Contraindications and Adverse Effects

The contraindications and adverse effects of drugs commonly used in pediatric dentistry have been shown in Table **14**.

**Table 14. Contraindications and adverse effects of drugs commonly used in dentistry.**

| Drug | Contraindication | Adverse reaction |
|------|------------------|------------------|
| NSAIDs | Asthma | Bronchospasm |
| Aspirin | Allergy to aspirin Bleeding disorders Children under 12 years Diabetes mellitus G-6PD deficiency Liver disease | Anaphylaxis Gastric bleeding Reye's syndrome Interferes with blood sugar Control Hemolysis Bleeding tendency |
| Paracetamol | Liver disease | Hepatotoxicity |
| Penicillin | Allergy | Anaphylaxis |
| Ampicillin/ Amoxycillin | Allergy to penicillin Chronic lymphoblastic leukemia | Anaphylaxis Rash |
| Cephalosporin | Allergy to penicillin | Anaphylaxis |
| Erythromycin Estolate | Liver disease | Hepatotoxicity |
| Tetracycline | Children under 12 yrs. | Staining of teeth |
| Metronidazole | Blood dyscrasias, CNS disease, Liver disease | Leucopenia, Neuropathy Hepatotoxicity |

## TOPICAL DRUGS USED IN PEDIATRIC DENTISTRY

**Topical Antimicrobial Oral Rinse -** Chlorhexidine gluconate 0.12% oral rinse

**Dose and Directions**: Rinse with 15 ml for 30 secs and expectorate. Use twice a day after breakfast and dinner.

**Pediatric Significance**: Because of the tooth staining properties of chlorhexidine gluconate oral rinse, applying the medication with a cotton-tipped applicator and placing it on the ulcer helps to minimise its side effect.

Minor irritation and mucosal sloughing have been noted with use in children.

A pharmacist can compound this oral rinse without alcohol, but it needs to be formulated at a 0.2% concentration to have a comparable antimicrobial effect. Most flavouring agents destroy the antimicrobial effect of chlorhexidine and the foaming agents in toothpaste. All foamy residue from toothbrushing should be rinsed away before using this agent. Although commonly used, clinical effectiveness and safety have not been established in children younger than age 18 [19].

**Topical Anti-inflammatory Paste - Amlexanox Oral Paste 5%**

**Directions:** Apply to the ulcers after meals and before bed until healed.

**Pediatric Significance**: This agent has been shown to increase the healing rate and pain relief by about one day.

Children should be instructed to wash their hands after use to prevent irritation, especially from the accidental rubbing of the eyes. A burning sensation may occur after applying this paste that children may not well accept.

The clinical effectiveness and safety have not been established in children younger than age 18, but the paste is probably safe and offers a reasonable alternative to topical steroids [20].

**Topical Steroid Medications [21]**

Triamcinolone acetonide

**Directions:** Coat the lesion with a thin film after each meal and bedtime. Do not eat or drink for 30 mins after application. Use until the ulcer is no longer painful.

**Pediatric Significance**: Topical steroids for intraoral use are not generally recommended for children younger than the age of 2 years. These medications should not be used for more than seven days to decrease the potential risk of adrenocortical insufficiency unless the child is being supervised adequately for this complication.

Oropharyngeal candidiasis is another side effect that some children develop with steroid use.

The gel formulations may sting on application and tend to separate and harden when mixed with the occlusive oral pastes.

**Topical Mouth Rinses – Dexamethasone 0.5mg/5 ml.**

Betamethasone syrup 0.6mg/5ml

**Directions:** Rinse with one teaspoon (5ml) for 2 mins 4 times a day, after meals and before bedtime. Do not eat and drink for 30 mins after use.

**Pediatric Significance**: Liquid steroids, used as oral rinses, is indicated when there are multiple and widespread lesions or when a direct topical application to individual ulcers is complex because of location.

The alcohol content varies from 5% for Dexamethasone to less than 1% for Betamethasone syrup. Dexamethasone is sweetened with glycerin and saccharin.

Rinsing with these liquid steroids is not indicated for children who cannot cooperate or expectorate.

**Systemic Corticosteriods - Prednisone, 5 mg., 10 mg., 20 mg. Tablets**

**Directions**: 20 – 60 mg every morning for 5 to 10 days.

**Pediatric Significance**: Systematic steroids should be prescribed in consultation with a physician and limited to short-burst therapy to decrease the risk of adrenocortical suppression. A maintenance phase should be instituted, including topical steroids when frequent recurrences.

The maximum dosage is 60 mg./d for the shortest duration, not to exceed ten days.

Some children experience insomnia, headache, irritability and candidal infections. Prednisone oral solution one mg./mL with 5% alcohol is also available for children who cannot swallow tablet.

Patients who are taking or have undergone corticosteroid therapy should be given special consideration during dental management as corticosteroids can lead to suppression of hypothalamic-pituitary-adrenal axis and may lead to precipitation of adrenal crisis under a stressful situation.

## Topical Benzydamine Mouthwashes

It is used to relieve pain, discomfort, and inflammation of the mouth, gums, and throat. It provides relief from pain and swelling and aids in speeding up the healing process. It is a non-steroidal anti-inflammatory drug used at a dose is 0.15%. it is helpful in oral ulcers, gingivitis, and gag reflex patients [22].

## Drug Interactions [23]

When more than one drug is prescribed to a child, the possibility of drug interaction exists. This may lead to further complications. Some everyday drug interactions have been listed in Table **15**.

**Table 15. Drug Interactions.**

| Drug | Interaction | Effect |
|---|---|---|
| Aspirin ulcer | Corticosteroids, Oral anticoagulants Oral hypoglycemics | Peptic ulcer Increases anticoagulant effect Increased hypoglycemic effect |
| Paracetamol | Anticonvulsants, Carbamazepine | Hepatotoxicity Hepatotoxicity |
| Erythromycin | Carbamazepine Theophylline | Toxicity Toxicity |
| Metronidazole | Anticoagulants | Increases anticoagulant effect |
| Tetracycline | Iron supplements Anticoagulants | Reduced serum tetracycline Increases anticoagulant effect |

## CONCLUSION

In today's world of advancement, clinicians are advised to take maximum precautions as far as the methodology of proper infection control is concerned. Antibiotics or antimicrobials should not be prescribed routinely unless indicated, as these drugs can lose their efficacy due to the development of resistant strains of micro-organisms. When prescribing these drugs, the potential of adverse drug reactions and drug interactions should always be considered.

## REFERENCES

[1]     Paudel KR, Sah NK, Jaiswal AK. Prevalence of pharmacotherapy in the department of paediatric dentistry. Kathmandu Univ Med J 2010; 8(30): 190-4. [KUMJ].
        [PMID: 21209533]

[2]  Elias GP, Antoniali C, Mariano RC. Comparative study of rules employed for calculation of pediatric drug dosage. J Appl Oral Sci 2005; 13(2): 114-9.
[http://dx.doi.org/10.1590/S1678-77572005000200004] [PMID: 20924533]

[3]  Phero JC, Becker D. Rational use of analgesic combinations. Dent Clin North Am 2002; 46(4): 691-705.
[http://dx.doi.org/10.1016/S0011-8532(02)00022-8] [PMID: 12436825]

[4]  Spink M, Bahn S, Glickman R. Clinical implications of cyclo-oxygenase–2 inhibitors for acute dental pain management. J Am Dent Assoc 2005; 136(10): 1439-48.
[http://dx.doi.org/10.14219/jada.archive.2005.0059] [PMID: 16255470]

[5]  Gazal G, Al-Samadani KH. Comparison of paracetamol, ibuprofen, and diclofenac potassium for pain relief following dental extractions and deep cavity preparations. Saudi Med J 2017; 38(3): 284-91.
[http://dx.doi.org/10.15537/smj.2017.3.16023] [PMID: 28251224]

[6]  Tate AR, Acs G. Dental postoperative pain management in children. Dent Clin North Am 2002; 46(4): 707-17.
[http://dx.doi.org/10.1016/S0011-8532(02)00028-9] [PMID: 12436826]

[7]  Pain management in infants, children, adolescents, and individuals with special health care needs The Reference Manual of Pediatric Dentistry. Chicago, Ill.: American Academy of Pediatric Dentistry 2020; pp. 362-70.

[8]  Use of antibiotic therapy for pediatric dental patients The Reference Manual of Pediatric Dentistry. Chicago, Ill.: American Academy of Pediatric Dentistry 2020; pp. 443-6.

[9]  Palma Aguirre JA, Rodríguez Palomares C. [Indications and contraindications for analgesics and antibiotics in pediatric dentistry]. Pract Odontol 1989; 10(1): 11-12, 14, 16 passim.
[PMID: 2696955]

[10]  Ullah H, Ali S. Classification of Anti☐Bacterial Agents and Their Functions. 2016.
[http://dx.doi.org/10.5772/intechopen.68695]

[11]  Miller EL. The penicillins: a review and update. J Midwifery Womens Health 2002; 47(6): 426-34.
[http://dx.doi.org/10.1016/S1526-9523(02)00330-6] [PMID: 12484664]

[12]  Harrison CJ, Bratcher D. Cephalosporins. Pediatr Rev 2008; 29(8): 264-73.
[http://dx.doi.org/10.1542/pir.29.8.264] [PMID: 18676578]

[13]  Jackson MA, Schutze GE. AAP Committee on Infectious diseases. The Use of systemic and topical fluoroquinolones. Pediatrics 2022; 138(5); e20162706.
[http://dx.doi.org/10.1542/peds.2016-2706] [PMID: 27940800]

[14]  Sivakumar N, Anupam S, Kumar MS. Prescription of metronidazole in pediatric dentistry – an evidence-based approach. J Clin Diagn Res 2018; 12(12): ZE08-11.
[http://dx.doi.org/10.7860/JCDR/2018/37544.12349]

[15]  Klein JO. History of macrolide use in pediatrics. Pediatr Infect Dis J 1997; 16(4): 427-31.
[http://dx.doi.org/10.1097/00006454-199704000-00025] [PMID: 9109154]

[16]  Zeichner SL. Tetracycline Update. Pediatr Rev 1998; 19(1): 32.
[http://dx.doi.org/10.1542/pir.19.1.32] [PMID: 9439167]

[17]  Antifungal agents for common paediatric infections. Can J Infect Dis Med Microbiol 2008; 19(1): 15-8.
[http://dx.doi.org/10.1155/2008/186345] [PMID: 19145261]

[18]  James SH, Whitley RJ. Treatment of herpes simplex virus infections in pediatric patients: current status and future needs. Clin Pharmacol Ther 2010; 88(5): 720-4.
[http://dx.doi.org/10.1038/clpt.2010.192] [PMID: 20881952]

[19]  Fiorillo L. Chlorhexidine Gel Use in the Oral District: A Systematic Review. Gels 2019; 5(2): 31.

[http://dx.doi.org/10.3390/gels5020031] [PMID: 31212600]

[20]    Singh A, Hasan AA, Umarji HR. Evaluation of the efficacy of topical Amlexanox oral paste and Rebamipide tablets in managing Recurrent Aphthous Ulcers. Int J Curr Res 2018; 10(07): 71105-711.

[21]    Kiran MS, Vidya S, Aswal G, Kumar V, Rai V. Systemic and topical steroids in the management of oral mucosal lesions. J Pharm Bioallied Sci 2017; 9(5) (Suppl. 1): 1.
[http://dx.doi.org/10.4103/jpbs.JPBS_91_17] [PMID: 29284925]

[22]    Goswami D, Jain G, Mohod M, Baidya DK, Bhutia O, Roychoudhury A. Randomized controlled trial to compare oral analgesic requirements and patient satisfaction in using oral non-steroidal anti-inflammatory drugs versus benzydamine hydrochloride oral rinses after mandibular third molar extraction: a pilot study. J Dent Anesth Pain Med 2018; 18(1): 19-25.
[http://dx.doi.org/10.17245/jdapm.2018.18.1.19] [PMID: 29556555]

[23]    Flint SR, O'Sullivan C, Arthur N. An update of adverse drug reactions of relevance to general dental practice. J Ir Dent Assoc 2000; 46(2): 67-70.
[PMID: 11326529]

**CHAPTER 5**

# Management of Children with Systemic Diseases

**Bahman Seraj[1,*], Gholam Hossein Ramezani[2], Razieh Jabbarian[3], Mona Sohrabi[3] and Alireza Mirzaei[4]**

[1] *Department of Pediatric Dentistry, Dental Faculty, Tehran University of Medical Science, Tehran, Iran*

[2] *Department of Pediatric Dentistry, Dental Faculty, Islamic Azad University of Medical Science, Tehran, Iran*

[3] *Department of Pediatric Dentistry, Qazvin University of Medical Sciences, Qazvin, Iran*

[4] *RWTH Aachen University, 52062 Aachen, Germany*

**Abstract:** Significant oral problems are associated with many medical disorders. Close cooperation and consultation between the dentist and the child's physician are essential to render optimum medical care. Prevention of oral disease is the primary consideration for these children. Medically compromised children can be challenging to treat and affect dental care [30]. To treat medically compromised patients safely, it is essential to Obtain a relevant and thorough medical history and understand the possible implications of the illness on dental treatment and the potential importance of the condition on treatment planning and the caries risk associated with the medical condition. With advances in medical treatment, significantly more children survive longer with more complex medical needs, and these children will present to the general dentist for dental treatment.

**Keywords:** Children, Compromised Patient, Dental Management, Emergency, Medical Disorders, Systematic Diseases.

## INTRODUCTION

Medically compromised patients are individuals with any physical, develop-mental, mental, sensory, behavioural, cognitive, or emotional disability. Their effective participation in society can be limited due to individual disorder and environmental barriers. These patients are at risk for tooth decay and other oral diseases due to various factors such as compromised immunity, financial obstacles for parents, difficulty in maintaining oral health due to sensory or motor disorders and aversion to dental treatment (Figs. **1** & **2**). Oral diseases are among the most prevalent ailments among these disabled children worldwide, and dental

\* **Corresponding author Bahman Seraj:** Department of Pediatric Dentistry, Dental Faculty, Tehran University of Medical Science, Tehran, Iran; E-mail: erajbah@as tums.ac.ir

**Satyawan Damle, Ritesh Kalaskar & Dhanashree Sakhare (Eds.)**

care is the greatest unattended health need of these disabled. Therefore, these patients have a low oral health-related quality of life (OHRQoL). The psychological reactions associated with a disability affects the disabled, parents, caregivers, and family members. Lack of awareness of the parents of these children about the importance of oral health, health care system, stress and unique concerns of their parents, and limited financial resources available are the reasons for delays in the assessment and treatment of oral health of these children. For this reason, in many cases, home care is so neglected that they require extensive dental treatment. Therefore, raising parental awareness is a critical issue. The role of a dental professional is also vital in the rehabilitation of these patients in the social environment. This specialist should be fully aware of these patients' systemic, extraoral and intraoral signs and symptoms and how to treat them but should also be aware of multidisciplinary areas so that, if necessary, these patients can be treated after consultation with other specialists.

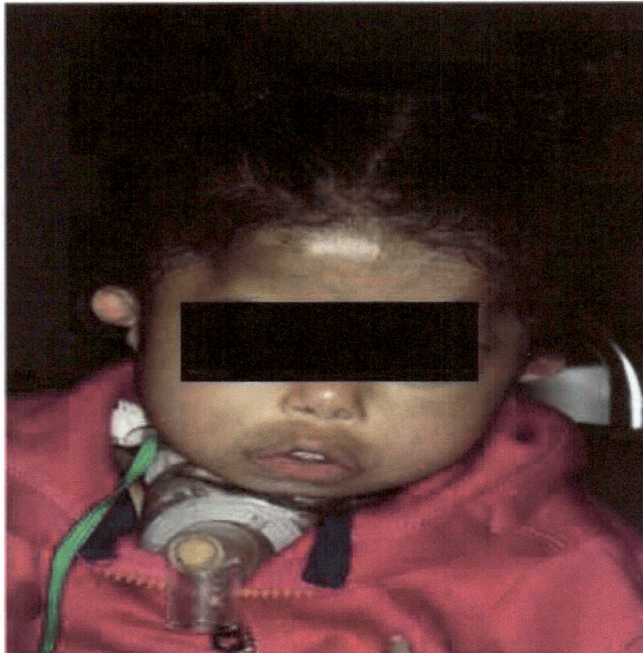

**Fig. (1).** A South African Child of mixed ancestry heritage, aged four years with CHARGE syndrome.

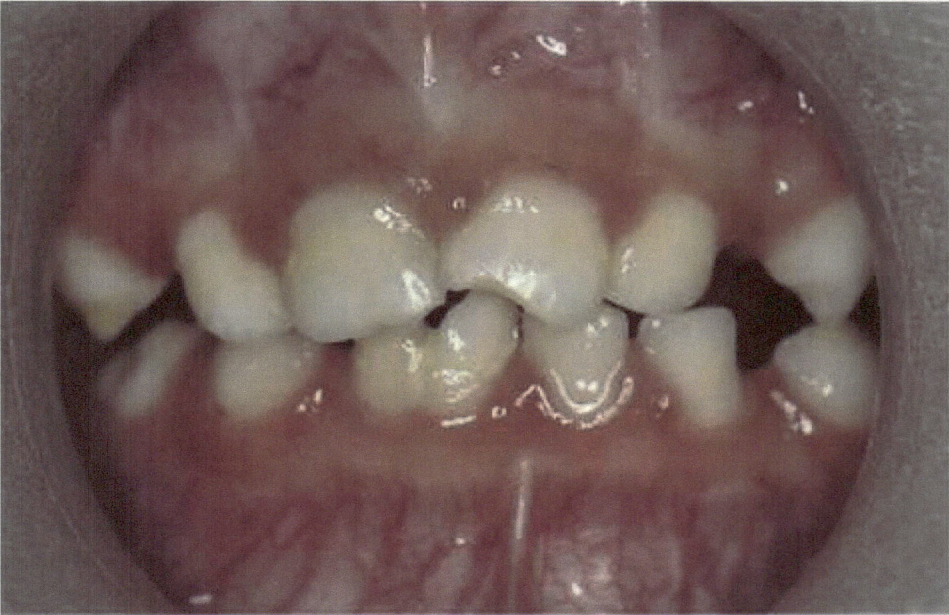

**Fig. (2).** Plaque accumulation and mild to moderate gingival hyperplasia are evident. The incisal edge of her anterior incisor was chipped, and there was a fusion of her 81 and 82.

**1) Respiratory system**

                **1-1**) Asthma

                **1-2**) Bronchopulmonary dysplasia

                **1-3**) Cystic fibrosis

**2) Cardiovascular system**

                **2-1**) congenital heart disease

                **2-2**) Acquired heart disease

**3) Circulatory system**

                **3-1**) Hemophilia A

                **3-2**) VonWillbrand Disease

                **3-3**) Sickle cell anaemia

**4) Immune system**

                **4**-1) AIDS

                **4-2**) Leukemia

                **4-3**) Hematopoietic stem cell transplantation

**5) Gastrointestinal system**

                **5-1**) Crohn's disease

                **5-2**) Celiac disease

## 6) Kidney system

**6-1**) Chronic renal failure
**6-2**) End-stage renal failure

## Asthma

Asthma has been defined as a chronic inflammatory disorder of the airways. Globally, death rates from asthma in children range from 0 to 0.7 per 100,000 people, and most of all, these deaths are preventable. Childhood asthma misses many school days and may deprive children of academic achievement and social interaction [1]. The etiology is poorly understood, but it is a complex disorder involving immunological, infectious, biochemical, genetic, and psychological factors. Asthma episodes are caused by oedema of the mucous membranes, increased mucus secretion, and smooth muscle spasms, which block the airflow to the lungs and cause wheezing, coughing, breathlessness and chest tightness.

Asthma can demonstrate a broad spectrum of oral and dental manifestations affecting both the hard and soft tissues of the mouth. The most observed are higher caries prevalence, oral candidiasis, periodontal diseases, dental erosion, Ulcerations, xerostomia and Halitosis.

The prevalence of caries is higher in patients with asthma. According to a meta-analysis, the rate of stimulated and non-stimulated saliva flow in asthma patients is significantly reduced. Salivary buffer capacity and salivary pH were reduced considerably in asthma patients only when saliva was unstimulated.

Medications taken by these patients are also effective in the caries process. Some dry powder inhalers consist of sugar (lactose monohydrate). Also, 30 minutes after taking beta-2 agonist inhalers, the pH of saliva and plaque will be less than the critical value of 5.5 and the saliva flow rate is also reduced [2].

Children with bronchial asthma should receive special dental preventive attention as presented with a greater risk for oral and dental diseases than healthy children. During the dental treatment of these patients, every effort should be made to avoid acute attacks. Patients should continue to take their medications until they see a dentist. Patients taking bronchodilators should receive a dose before the appointment. To reduce the anxiety of these patients, behavioural control methods, nitrous oxide-oxygen sedative, hydroxyzine hydrochloride, and diazepam, can be used. The use of barbiturates, narcotics and aspirin compounds is contraindicated in these patients.

If the patient shows signs of respiratory distress and wheezing during dental work, place the patient in an upright or semi-upright position and use the albuterol bronchodilator spray. If the condition does not improve, 100% oxygen can be used. Finally, if the condition persists, it is recommended to use epinephrine (0.01 mg/kg with a maximum initial dose of 0.3 mg) intramuscularly and get medical help [3, 4].

## Bronchopulmonary Dysplasia

Bronchopulmonary dysplasia is a chronic lung disease with a higher prevalence in premature infants. The condition occurs following respiratory distress syndrome, requiring prolonged ventilation with a high oxygen concentration during infancy, leading to bronchial ulceration, necrosis with plugging of bronchiolar lumina, and inflammatory cells. Pathologic changes compromise further lung development: Airway resistance increases due to inflammation and bronchiolar fibrosis, leading to hypoxemia and putting these children in need of an oxygen supply until lung function and size improves [4].

Some children develop right ventricular hypertrophy (cor pulmonale) and may require diuretic therapy to prevent congestive heart failure [4].

Dental care for children with bronchopulmonary dysplasia requires more chair time than usual. Spending a long time of life in the hospital makes these children exhibit significant oral defensiveness. Consultation with a pulmonologist is necessary, and any elective dental care should be postponed until the condition is controlled [4].

If there is a need for continuous oxygen delivery, the appointments must be short with frequent breaks to prevent the development of pulmonary vasoconstriction. Additional oral hygiene is necessary when these children eat regular small meals to maintain the proper caloric intake [4].

## Cystic fibrosis

Cystic fibrosis is the most common lethal genetic disorder [4]. It is an autosomal recessive condition that affects many exocrine and mucus-secreting glands [5]. The abnormal CF transmembrane conductance regulator (CFTR) gene has been located on the long arm of the chromosome [3, 7]. The defective gene causes abnormal water and electrolyte (sodium and chloride) transport across the epithelial cell. Eventually, it creates the appearance of "salty skin", which is the hallmark of the disease [3, 4]. The condition involves multiple systems of the gastrointestinal tract (pancreas), respiratory tract and other endocrine glands, such as the salivary glands and sweat glands. The clinical manifestations of this disease are variable and include chronic productive cough, recurrent chest infections, halitosis, chest deformity, xerostomia, clubbing of the fingers and toes [5, 6].

Lung disease progresses and leads to shortness of breath. Most patients die of pneumonia and respiratory failure [4]. Antibiotics, pancreatic enzyme alternatives, physiotherapy, high protein and high-calorie diet and exercise are used to treat these patients [3, 4]. The use of tetracycline antibiotics may be unavoidable due to long periods of antibiotic use and drug resistance [5].

The incidence of dental caries in these patients is low due to long-term use of antibiotics, pancreatic enzyme replacements and increased salivary buffering capacity. Delayed tooth development, enamel opacities, discolouration due to tetracycline (Fig. **3**), calculus, open bite, mouth breathing, and malocclusion are seen in these patients [4, 6].

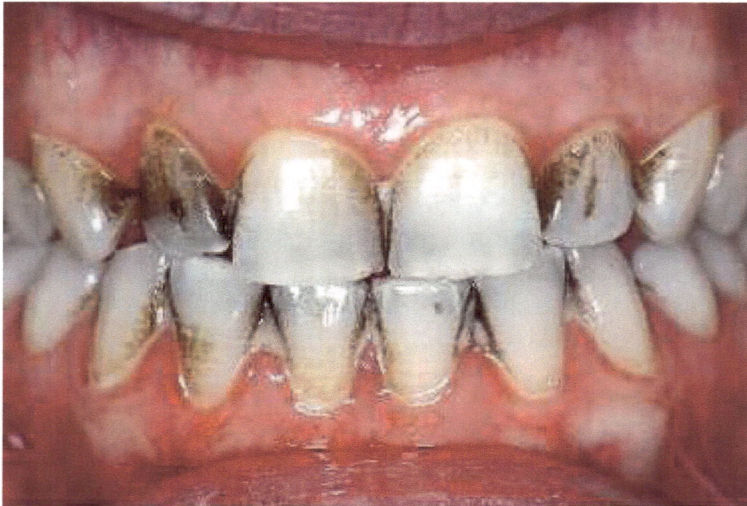

**Fig. (3).**  Black discolouration of teeth following the utilization of the carbapenem antibiotic meropenem.

The dentist should consider the patient's preference when working with these patients and place the patient in a more upright position. Be sure to consult with the patient's physician regarding the use of sedation, general anaesthesia, and nitrous oxide [3, 4]. The dentist should ask about the use of bisphosphonates in patients with osteoporosis and osteopenia and consider the necessary considerations. Several patients with cystic fibrosis should not be present in the office at the same time to prevent cross-infection with *Pseudomonas aeruginosa*, which is the most common pathogen involved in the respiratory system in these patients [3]. A significant percentage of these children may have liver involvement and defects in the clotting process, which should be considered to control bleeding following surgical procedures [6].

## Congenital Heart Disease

Congenital Heart Disease (CHD), the largest group of pediatric cardiovascular diseases, involves 8-10 cases per 1000 live births. Different chromosomal abnormalities such as Down syndrome (trisomy 21) and Turner syndrome (45, X chromosome) are associated with heart disease, but these represent fewer than 5% of the total [7]. The aetiology of CHD is obscure in most cases. Still, some known risk factors include maternal rubella, diabetes, alcoholism, irradiation and drugs such as thalidomide, phenytoin sodium and warfarin sodium.

Following are the eight most common congenital heart diseases which account for over 80% of the total: ventricular septal defects, patent ductus arteriosus, tetralogy of Fallot, transposition of the great vessels, atrial septal defects, pulmonary stenosis, coarctation of the aorta and aortic stenosis [4, 7].

Congenital heart disease can be classified into acyanotic (shunt or stenotic) and cyanotic lesions depending on clinical presentation. The cyanotic group of conditions is characterised by right to left shunting of blood within the heart, presenting as cyanosis, hypoxemia, clubbing of fingers, dyspnea on exertion, and paroxysmal dyspneic attack and heart murmur. Examples of such defects are the tetralogy of Fallot, transposition of the great vessels, pulmonary stenosis, and tricuspid atresia [4, 7, 8].

acyanotic congenital heart disease presents minimal or no cyanosis and is commonly divided into two major groups. The first group consists of defects that cause left-to-right shunting of blood within the heart. This group includes ventricular and atrial septal defects. The second major group of defects are stenotic and cause obstruction (*e.g.*, aortic stenosis and coarctation of the aorta) [4, 7, 8].

## Acquired Heart Disease

### *Rheumatic Fever*

Acute rheumatic fever (ARF) is a multisystem disease occurring some weeks after an untreated Group A streptococcus (GAS) infection of the throat or skin in genetically susceptible individuals. ARF may occur at all ages but usually between 5 and 15 years. Factors such as malnutrition, limited access to health care, crowded and unsanitary living conditions increase the spread of group A streptococcus and consequently the prevalence of ARF [6]. Major and minor clinical manifestations of ARF include carditis, arthritis, chorea, erythema marginatum, subcutaneous nodules, arthralgia and fever [9]. Rheumatic heart disease (RHD) is caused by recurrent ARF episodes and involves permanent damage to the heart valves [4]. Individuals with RHD are at increased risk of complications of valvular disease, including heart failure, arrhythmias, atrial fibrillation, stroke, thromboembolism, infective endocarditis and premature death [9]. Strategies to combat the disease include primary prophylaxis of penicillin following strep A diagnosis or secondary prevention for patients with ARF or RHD [10]. According to WHO guidelines, secondary prophylaxis should be continued for at least five years after the last ARF episode or until the age of 18 (whichever is longer) and for a more extended period in cases of carditis or RHD [9]. In 2013, the World Heart Federation (WHF) stated to achieve a 25 per cent reduction in premature deaths from ARF and RHD in people under 25 by 2025 [10].

## Infective Endocarditis Prophylaxis

Transient bacteremia, which occurs following specific dental procedures, can act as an initiating factor for developing infective endocarditis in susceptible patients. All dental procedures that involve manipulation of gingival tissue or the periapical region of teeth or perforation of the oral mucosa in cases listed below require antibiotic prophylaxis according to Table 1 [4]:

**Table 1. IE antibiotic prophylaxis regimen for dental procedures.**

| Situation | Agents[&] | Adults | Children |
|---|---|---|---|
| *Oral* | Ampicillin | 2 g | 50 mg/kg |
| *Unable to take oral medication* | Ampicillin OR Cefazolin or ceftriaxone | 2 g IM or IV 1 g IM or IV | 50 mg/kg IM or IV 50 mg/kg IM or IV |
| *Allergic to penicillins or ampicillin—oral* | Cephalexin *† OR Clindamycin OR Azithromycin or clarithromycin | 2 g 600 mg 500 mg | 50 mg/kg 20 mg/kg 15 mg/kg |
| *Allergic to penicillin or ampicillin and unable to take oral medication* | Cefazolin or ceftriaxone† OR Clindamycin | 1g IM or IV 600 mg IM or IV | 50 mg/kg IM or IV 20 mg/kg IM or IV |

IM, intramuscular; IV, intravenous. [&] Regimen: single dose 30 to 60 minutes before the procedure. *Other first- or second-generation oral cephalosporin in equivalent adult or pediatric dosage. †Cephalosporins should not be used in individuals with a history of anaphylaxis, angioedema, or urticaria with penicillin or ampicillin [4].

- Prosthetic cardiac valve or prosthetic material used for cardiac valve repair
- Previous infective endocarditis
- Unrepaired cyanotic CHD, including palliative shunts and conduits
- Completely repaired congenital heart defect with prosthetic material or device,

whether placed by surgery or by catheter intervention, during the first six months after the procedure

• Repaired CHD with residual defects at the site or adjacent to the area of a prosthetic patch or prosthetic device (which inhibits endothelialisation)

• Cardiac transplantation recipients who develop cardiac valvulopathy [4].

## Dental Management

The most critical issue in planning dental care for these children is the prevention of dental diseases. Physicians should refer them for a dental evaluation and regular clinical and radiographic monitoring as soon as they are diagnosed. A preventive program including oral health advice, diet counselling, fluoride therapy, and fissure sealant is necessary for these patients [6]. Active dental disease should be treated before heart surgery. The dentist should consult the patient's cardiologist about details of the patient's condition, medications, and dental treatment plan. Due to the risk of infection and endocarditis in these patients, pulp therapy of deciduous teeth with a poor prognosis is not recommended. It is replaced by the extraction and placement of a fixed space maintainer. Endodontic treatment of permanent teeth is unimpeded if the case selection is valid and the ideal treatment is performed [4].

Suppose the patient suffers from multiple carious teeth. To negate the risk of infective endocarditis with further operative procedures, it is preferable to complete the treatment under general anaesthesia in one appointment. Although a routine dental environment is also possible, there is a need to prescribe alternative antibiotics or wait for a month between charges to reduce bacterial resistance [7].

## Hemophilia A

Hemophilia A is inherited as an X-linked recessive disorder resulting in a deficiency of plasma factor VIII coagulant activity. It accounts for about 85% of all haemophilia patients, more common in men, and according to factor VIII, plasma level classifies as severe (<1%), moderate (1% to 5%) and mild (6% to 40%). In unusual bleeding, the laboratory test presents average platelet count, bleeding time, thrombin time, and prothrombin time, but a prolonged activated partial thromboplastin time [3, 7].

Muscle and joint haemorrhages which are debilitating sometimes, besides easy bruising and prolonged hemorrhage after trauma or surgery, are clinical hallmarks of the disease. A treatment approach serves prophylactic therapies to prevent joint disease and haemorrhage accidents. This approach acts more successful on knee joints; although preventive measures, the ankle joints are the first to be affected. Intramuscular hematomas can compress vital structures and cause nerve paralysis and vascular or airway obstruction. Factor VIII replacement therapy should be used in cases of major surgery and life-threatening bleeding. Today, prophylactic use of clotting factor concentrates is the primary treatment approach of severe haemophilia A. In mild and moderate cases of haemophilia A, Vasopressin (desmopressin) can be used. It increases the plasma levels of factor VIII and von Willebrand factor (vWF) and peaks in 20 to 60 minutes with a duration of 4 hours. Unfortunately, 15% of patients develop antibodies against factor VIII [3, 11].

## Von Willebrand Disease

Abnormal Von Willebrand factor in quantity or quality results in Von Willebrand disease (vWD). The disease encompasses type 1 and types 3 (mild to moderate and severe quantitative deficiencies of vWF, respectively) and type 2 (qualitative defects of vWF). The most common clinical manifestations include epistaxis and gingival and gastrointestinal bleeding, which desmopressin can adequately control. Supportive therapy with antifibrinolytic agents (tranexamic acid) is also essential in vWD [3, 12].

## *Case Report*

An 8.10-year-old boy without a history of significant bleeding events presented with his parents to the Pediatric Dentistry Postgraduate Clinic complaining of lack of eruption of both permanent upper central incisors. The parents manifested an excellent general health status of their son and no reported previous significant bleeding episodes (e.g., from gingiva during tooth brushing), medical disorders (particularly bleeding diathesis), or exposure to surgical interventions. On the oral examination, both incisors were palpable and covered with fibrous gingival tissue, not associated with previous bleeding (Fig. **4**).

Signed informed consent was obtained from the parents before the treatment. It was decided to perform a vestibular squared incision over the gingiva with flap apical reposition to expose the incisal third of both incisor crowns. The surgical procedure was carried out under local anaesthesia, employing a water-irrigated laser hand-piece system (Waterlase YSGG®, Biolase Technology, Inc., Irving, CA, USA) and sutures in both sides of the flap (Fig. **5**). The patient was discharged without apparent local or systemic complications and postoperative hygiene/diet instructions [26].

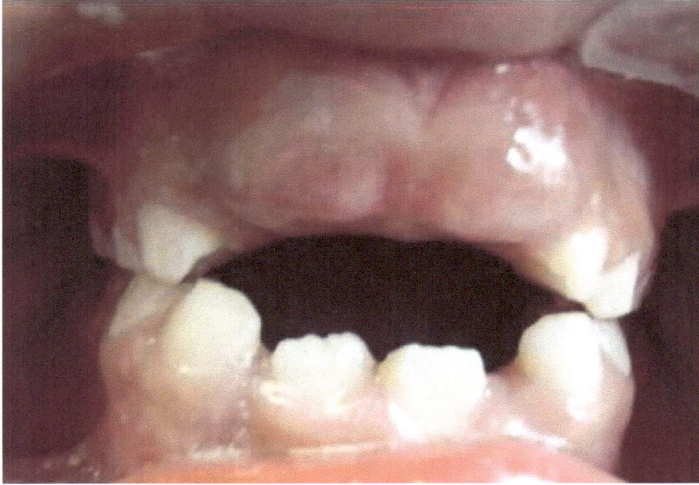

**Fig. (4).** Initial frontal view.

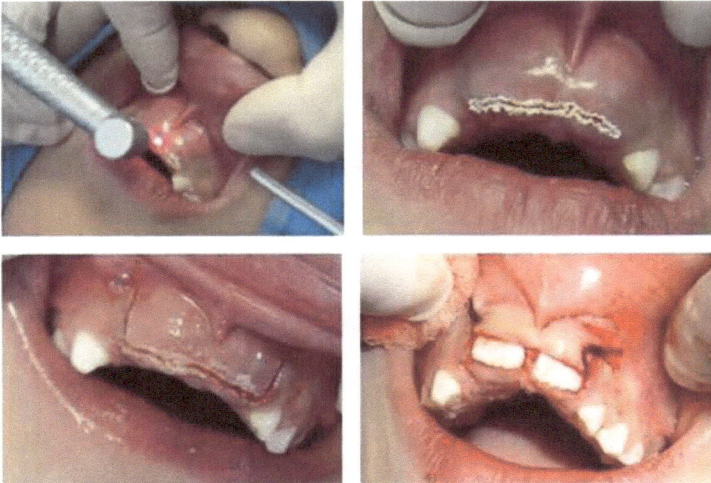

**Fig. (5).** Surgical procedure stages.

Three days later, the patient returned to the clinic exhibiting profuse gingival bleeding, difficult to control with external pressure application using wet gauze (Fig. **6**). After consulting with the Pediatric Hematologist, routine laboratory blood tests for blood clotting times were carried out because there was no history of spontaneous bleeding or other hemorrhagic events. The results were within the normal limits, except for the aPTT, slightly lower. Then, the wound was resutured and covered with Gelfoam with a surgical splint. The patient was closely monitored in an ambulatory approach. After two days, the bleeding persisted (Fig. **7**), and the child looked pale and weak. New laboratory-specific tests were performed, including quantification of factors VIII and IX and Von Willebrand. The clot factor VIII manifested a deficit of 6% regarding the average plasmatic level; according to this information, the child was diagnosed with mild haemophilia A. To control the bleeding, the patient was intravenously infused with tranexamic acid (250 mg), vitamin K (5 mg), and normal saline for 8-hours; after this time, the bleeding was finally stopped patient was discharged. Close control visits were programmed. Ten days after the event at the final examination, the child did not show additional unusual bleeding episodes (**Fig 8**) or other oral/systemic complications.

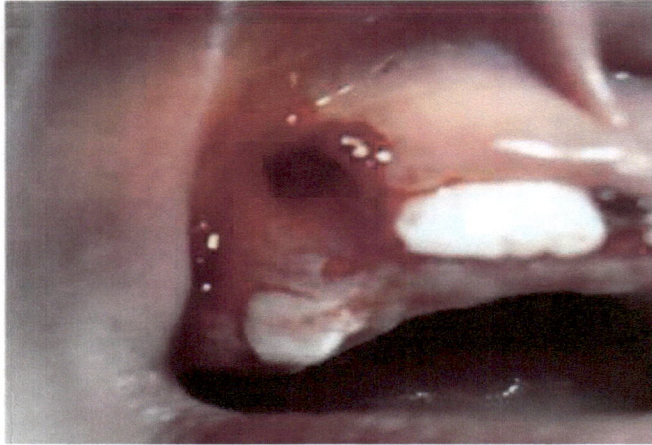

**Fig. (6).** 3-day postoperative view. The suitable suture was removed. The wound was resutured.

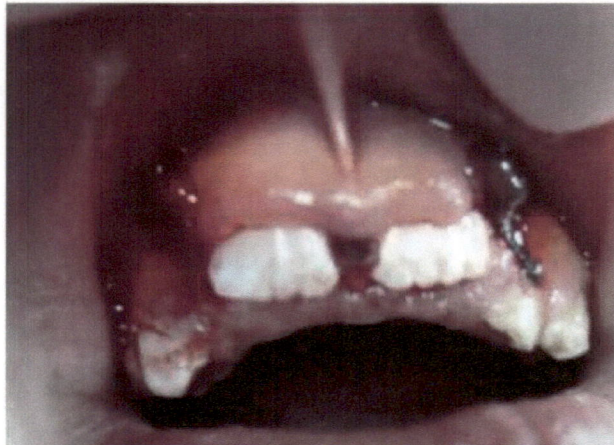

**Fig. (7).** 2 days later. The new suture was also retired and then resutured. Pharmacological treatment was initiated intravenously.

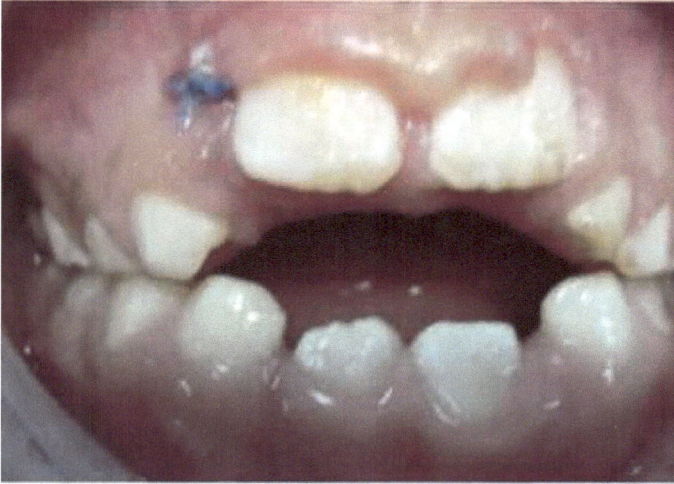

**Fig. (8).**  Final view after 8 hours of treatment. Bleeding was finally controlled.

## Dental Treatment Consideration

A comprehensive consultation with the haematologist is necessary to determine the hemostatic condition of the patient and restore the system to avoid bleeding during invasive procedures. Supragingival scaling in mild and moderate haemophilia cases does not require any treatment. However, in the case of subgingival scaling, pretreatment should be discussed with the haematologist. The risk of block and specific infiltration anaesthesia in mild to moderate diseases are low but should not be performed in severe hemophilias until the hemostatic problem is corrected; because they carry high risk and can cause deep hematoma and potential airway obstruction. If pulpotomies, pulpectomies, and root canal therapy do not extend beyond the apex, it can be done without significant bleeding. The surgical technique should be atraumatic and primary closure should be obtained to protect the blood clot. Orthodontic treatment is not a contraindication, but wires with sharp edges and placement of bands require special attention.

In moderate to severe haemophilia cases, oral surgery requires an infusion of factor VIII concentrate before treatment. Local hemostatics (pressure, sutures, gelatin sponge, cellulose materials, thrombin, microfibrillar collagen, fibrin glue, etc.) and oral antifibrinolytics (tranexamic acid mouthwash) help achieve hemostasis. Vasopressin, ε-aminocaproic acid, and tranexamic acid can also be used systemically after dental extractions [3, 12, 13].

## Sickle Cell Anaemia

Sickle cell anaemia (SCA) is the most common genetic blood disorder. Transmission of the disease is autosomal recessive. Sickle cell anaemia is the homozygous state in which the sickle gene is inherited from both parents. Sickle cell disease (SCD) is when a person inherits two mutated globin genes, at least one of which is always a sickle mutation.

Sickle haemoglobin (HbS) is produced by replacing glutamic acid with valine in the sixth amino acid of beta-globin and condition of hypoxia [4]. The lifespan of a sickle-shaped globule is reduced to 12 to 17 days, and its haemoglobin level is reduced from the average level of 12-18 g/dl to 6-9 gr/dl [3]. These sickle-shaped cells are easily destroyed (haemolysis). They can also adhere to the lining of the blood vessels, thus blocking tiny blood vessels (vaso occlusion) and leading to pain and necrosis. Vaso-occlusion can lead to a sickle cell crisis. Affected children may be pale, tired, weak, and breathless. They may complain of painful joints and swelling of the hands and feet [6]. Painful crises are triggered by stress, fever, infection, hypoxia, hypothermia, dehydration, and hypotension [3, 4].

Other problems in these patients include acute complications such as stroke, priapism, acute chest syndrome, splenic sequestration and chronic complications such as cardiovascular problems, pulmonary hypertension, renal function impairment, retinal and conjunctival damage, osteomyelitis, osteoporosis [3, 14]. Spleen function is impaired in many patients, resulting in decreased immunoglobulin production, anaemia, thrombocytopenia, and reticulocytosis [3, 4]. In this disease, infection is the leading cause of death in children under three years. Respiratory tract infections and septicemia are the most common infections in these patients. In these patients, for prophylaxis against pneumococcal infection, the antibiotic penicillin V potassium 125 mg is given twice a day from the age of two months, and the dose is doubled at the age of 3. It should be continued until the age of 5 [3]. The gold standard of treatment for pain control in times of crisis is analgesic opioid derivatives [15]. Hydroxyurea, an oral chemotherapeutic drug, is currently the only licensed treatment for SCD. It is used as a therapy to prevent complications of SCD, including pain, stroke, acute chest syndrome, decreased organ function, hospital admissions and the need for transfusions by raising fetal haemoglobin, improving nitric oxide metabolism, reducing red cell-endothelial interaction [14].

Radiographic findings include generalised radiolucency, coarse trabecular pattern, pronounced lamina dura, dentin hypomineralisation, interglobular dentin in the periapical region, calcifications in the pulp chamber, and hypercementosis. There is a high incidence of malocclusions in patients with SCD (bimaxillary protrusion with flared incisors, increased overjet and diastemas). Vasoocclusive episodes in the jawbones or dental pulp cause tissue infarction and cause toothache or facial pain in the absence of pathological symptoms. These episodes in the mental foramen area can also cause lower lip paraesthesia. The prevalence of caries in children with this disease is down due to antibiotics [3, 4].

A complete medical history should be provided for the dental treatment of these patients. Treatment sessions should be short and stress-free. Ask the patient about the use of bisphosphonates. In non-crisis times, all dental procedures can be performed in the office. A complete blood cell count test should be performed if hydroxyurea is used. Do not use respiratory suppressants for sedation. Because inadequate oxygenation can trigger a crisis, treatment under general anaesthesia should be avoided as much as possible [3, 4, 6]. For treatment under general anaesthesia, consult a haematologist and anesthesiologist. Patients with a haemoglobin level of less than seven g/dl and a hematocrit of less than 20% may need a blood transfusion. Restorative and pulpotomy treatments are preferable to tooth extraction. In the case of necrotic teeth that need pulpectomy, extraction is recommended if the success of the treatment is low and there is a possibility of recurrence of the infection [3, 4].

## AIDS

The first experience of human immunodeficiency virus (HIV) infection may be an influenza-like illness that is even asymptomatic. The patient then enters a latent phase, during which the patient remains asymptomatic. Eventually, the disease will enter the third stage of acquired immune deficiency syndrome (AIDS) when the number of CD4 T cells reaches less than 200/ml [5]. HIV is mainly transmitted through unprotected sex, infected blood transfusions, infected needles, and from mother to child during pregnancy, delivery, or breastfeeding [4].

Oral candidiasis is still the most common oral manifestation in these patients, including those undergoing antiretroviral therapy (ART) [16]. Oral ulcers in these patients are caused by recurrent viral infections, including herpes simplex virus (HSV), human papillomavirus (HPV), varicella-zoster virus (VZV), and cytomegalovirus [4].

The most common lesions in children with HIV infection include candidosis (pseudomembranous, erythematous, angular cheilitis), linear gingival erythema [27] (Figs. **9** & **10**), herpes simplex infection, parotid enlargement and recurrent aphthous ulcers. Oral candidiasis may be a predictor of recurrent oropharyngeal candidiasis [5]. Chronic candidiasis can signify a poor prognosis and a rapid decline in immune function. Swelling and inflammation of the salivary glands, especially the parotid gland, are seen in these patients, resulting in xerostomia [4].

Xerostomia also provides the conditions for oral candidiasis and dental caries [5]. In these patients, aphthous ulcers, especially of the significant type with erythematous margins [4].

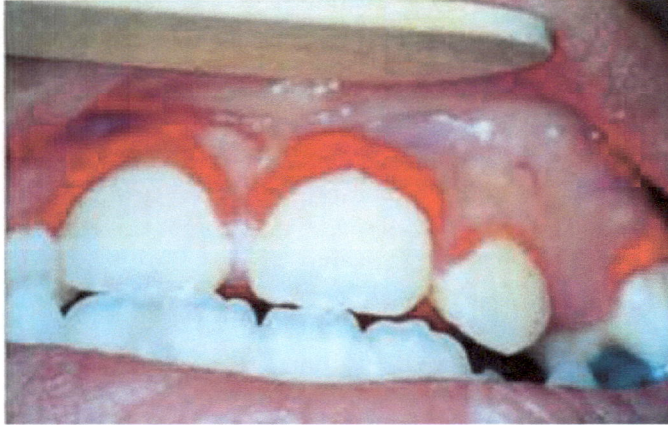

**Fig. (9).** Linear Gingival Erythema in an 8yeras (HIV) Old female. Note the absence of inflammatory swelling female.

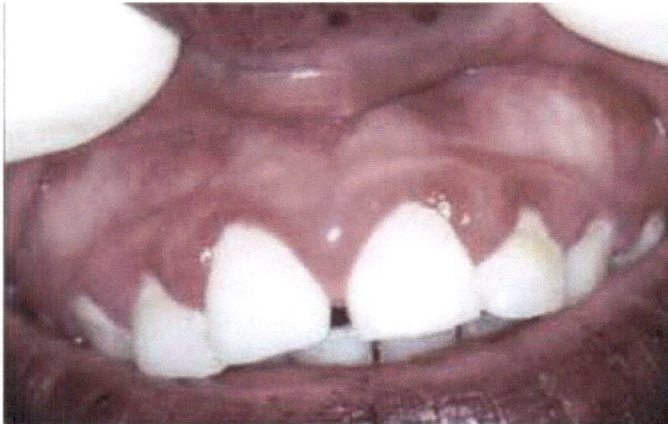

**Fig. (10).** Conventional gingivitis in 17 years old the gingiva is swollen because of inflammation.

Less common lesions in children with HIV infection include periodontal disease, seborrheic dermatitis (perioral), viral infections (cytomegalovirus, human papillomavirus, varicella-zoster virus, molluscum contagiosum) and xerostomia [5]. Progressive and premature periodontitis, which may be the first sign of HIV infection in adults, does not respond well to routine periodontal treatments and requires aggressive curettage treatment with chlorhexidine digluconate mouthwash [4].

Lesions strongly associated with HIV infection but rare in children include neoplasms (Kaposi's sarcoma and non-Hodgkin's lymphoma), hairy leukoplakia, and tuberculosis ulcers [5]. Kaposi's sarcoma, the most common malignancy in HIV patients, is associated with the human herpesvirus (HHV-8) and is mainly sexually transmitted [4]. The most common sites are the hard palate and maxillary gingivae, which appear as red, blue, or purple macules that turn into papules, nodules, or sores [5]. Lymphoma is rare in these patients, and non-Hodgkin's lymphoma usually occurs. The first manifestations may be painless swelling in the maxillary gingivae and throat. The average survival time after diagnosis is approximately six months [4]. Oral hair leukoplakia (OHL) is the second most common HIV-related oral mucosal lesion in adults and is rare in children. This lesion is a predictor of disease progression and usually affects the lateral margins of the tongue [5].

According to systematic reviews, the prevalence of oral lesions includes angular cheilitis, erythematous candidiasis, oral herpes, pseudomembranous candidiasis, Kaposi sarcoma, and oral hairy leukoplakia in HIV-positive patients is lower for those on highly active antiretroviral therapy (HAART). Still, oral mucosal hyperpigmentation was higher in patients on HAART [17].

The average risk of HIV infection following only one accidental needle stick is 0.3%. Assuming that all dental patients may be infected, full implementation of health and prevention protocols is essential [4].

## Leukemia

Leukaemia is the most common childhood cancer and the second leading cause of death after accidents, resulting from replacing platelets, leukocytes, and red blood cells with malignant leukocytes. Acute lymphocytic leukaemia (ALL) is the cause of about 80% of childhood cancer, and with advances in diagnosis and treatment, the survival rate of all affected children is about 85%. The peak incidence is four years old [3, 4]. According to meta-analysis studies, maternal smoking before, during, or after pregnancy was not associated with childhood ALL, although paternal smoking was associated with a significantly increased risk of youth ALL during pregnancy [18].

The most common signs and symptoms of the disease, which are found in more than 50% of children, include hepatomegaly, splenomegaly, pallor, fever and bruising. Other symptoms seen in a third to a half of children include recurrent infections, fatigue, limb pain, hepatosplenomegaly, bruising/petechiae, lymphadenopathy, bleeding tendency and rash. The most common bone lesion in these patients is generalised osteoporosis due to enlargement of bone marrow spaces with the proliferation of leukemic cells, which causes bone pain [3, 4].

More common intraoral findings include lymphadenopathy, petechiae and ecchymosis of mucous, gingival bleeding, gingival hypertrophy, mucosal pallor and non-specific ulcerations. Other manifestations in these patients are toothache, jaw pain, numbness of the chin and lips, cerebral palsy and loose teeth due to the pressure of leukocyte infiltration on nerves and blood vessels. Radiographic findings are loss of lamina dura, widening of the periodontal ligament space, destruction of cancellous bone and alteration in the crypts of developing teeth (position and morphology) (Figs. **11** & **12**) [3, 4, 28].

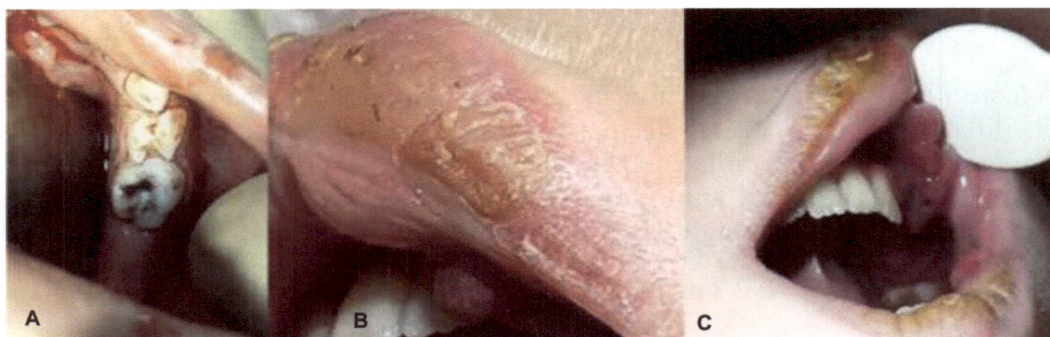

**Fig. (11).** (**A**) Caries in the lower primary molars, intraoral bleeding, and gingival enlargement/hyperplasia. (**B**) Cracked lips and gingival enlargement. (**C**) Cracked lips, gingival enlargement/hyperplasia, and buccal bleeding.

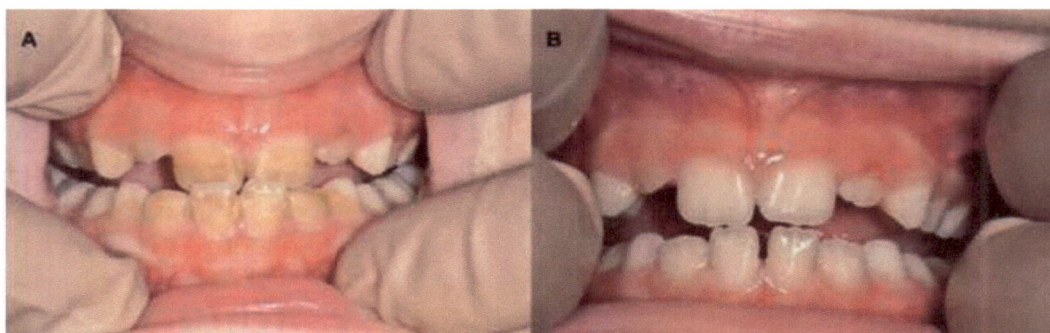

**Fig. (12).** (**A**) Enamel discolouration and presence of calculus stone. (**B**) Picture showing an intraoral view of the patient shown in **Fig 12A** after removing the discolouration and calculus stone in a few sessions of scaling and polishing.

Treatment of ALL consists of 4 steps. 1. Remission-induction: A combination of anti-leukaemia drugs is used during the four weeks. 2. Central nervous system (CNS) prophylaxis: This prophylactic treatment is prescribed to protect the nervous system from leukemic cells due to the lack of chemotherapy drugs passing through the blood-brain barrier. At this stage, cranial irradiation or intrathecal injection of a chemotherapeutic agent is performed. 3. Consolidation/intensification: This step intensifies leukaemia treatment and kills any remaining leukemic cells. 4. Maintenance: in this phase, the growth of cancer cells is suppressed by administering methotrexate and 6-mercaptopurine. This phase continues for two years for girls and three years for boys [3, 4]. Chemotherapy causes side effects such as taste dysfunction, xerostomia, mucositis, opportunistic infections, decreased salivary immunoglobulins IgA and IgG, Spontaneous oral bleeding and teeth with short, thin, tapered roots, or hypo mineralised or hypomature enamel. Radiotherapy causes side effects such as xerostomia, mucositis, incomplete jaws and facial skeleton development, decreased growth hormone and thyroid-stimulating hormone, and atrophy of the soft tissue microdontia enamel hypoplasia, incomplete calcification of teeth and arrested root development [8].

Before any dental treatment, the dentist should consult a pediatric haematologist or oncologist and determine the best time for treatment. At least one month before initiation of leukaemia treatment, all children should be evaluated by a dentist [4, 8]. Impacted teeth, root tip, nonrestorable teeth, teeth with acute or chronic infection and mobile teeth should be extracted ideally two weeks before the initiation of cancer treatment [3]. Pulpotomy and pulpectomy should not be performed on primary teeth. Any local stimuli such as orthodontic appliances and space maintainers should be removed, especially if the patient has poor oral health [4, 8].

Patients undergoing cancer treatment suffer from xerostomia and mucositis due to the side effects of chemotherapy and radiotherapy. Therefore, it is recommended that the child rinse his mouth several times a day with cold water or normal saline [8]. Brush your teeth with a soft toothbrush after each meal. Sponge and foam toothbrushes are not recommended due to their ineffectiveness. Brushing should be stopped when the platelet count is lower than $20,000/mm^3$ or when the absolute neutrophil count (ANC) is less than $500/mm^3$. In these conditions, moist gauze is recommended [3, 8]. Chlorhexidine mouthwash is recommended for patients with periodontal problems. Fluoride supplements are recommended for patients to control the caries process caused by xerostomia and sucrose-containing drugs [3]. Candidiasis is common in these patients due to a suppressed immune system, and nystatin is recommended for treatment [4]. Toothaches in the absence of pathological symptoms need serious investigation. These pains may be due to the infiltration of leukemic cells into the blood vessels of the dental pulp and obstruction of blood supply to the pulp (liquefaction necrosis) or a side effect of chemotherapy drugs, such as vincristine and vinblastine [3, 4] (Fig. **13**).

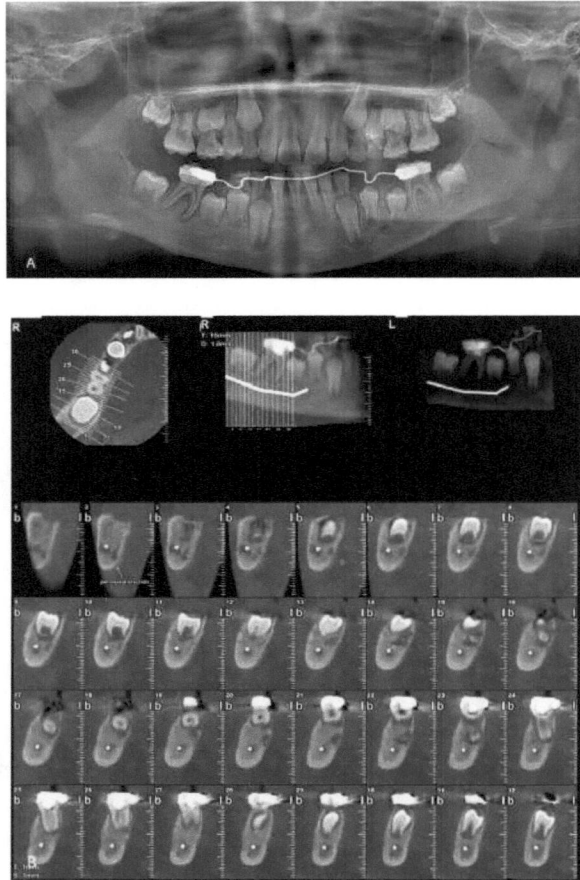

Fig. (13). **A**, Panoramic view of a 10-year-old child with necrosis and dental abscess in the lower correct six teeth area. The tooth was covered with a lingual arch that was caries-free on all surfaces after removing the space maintainer. **B**, On the patient's CBCT view, multiple lesions were seen in the apical area and periosteal reactions. After malignancy was suspected, the leukaemia was finally confirmed by a blood test.

The patient's blood cell count decreases one week after the treatment cycle and increases after two to three weeks. Therefore, blood cell counts return to normal between chemotherapy cycles and are a good time for dental treatment. It is best to have a complete blood and platelet count before starting dental treatment [3].

Dental treatment should only be performed if the absolute neutrophil count (ANC) has improved and exceeds $1,000/mm^3$ and if the platelet count (at least $50,000/mm^3$) and function are adequate. Dental surgical procedures and administration of local anaesthetic blocks should be avoided during periods of thrombocytopenia [4, 8]. If the platelet count is 40,000-75,000/mm3, platelet transfusions are required before and 24 hours after dental treatment [3]. Root canal therapy for permanent teeth is not recommended during periods of immunosuppression. Pulp therapy should be performed at least one week before cancer treatment if the tooth is symptomatic. If this is not possible, the tooth should be extracted, and antibiotics should be administered for a week. Tooth extraction in patients due to the risk of osteonecrosis should be done very atraumatic and careful [3].

According to the guideline presented in a review study for antibiotic prophylaxis in cancers, prophylaxis is recommended in children with relapsed ALL receiving intensive chemotherapy expected to result in severe neutropenia (ANC <500/μL) for at least seven days. Antibiotic prophylaxis is not recommended routinely for children receiving induction chemotherapy for newly diagnosed ALL. Antibacterial prophylaxis should not be used in children whose treatment is not expected to result in severe neutropenia. If systemic antibacterial prophylaxis is planned, levofloxacin is the preferred agent and should be limited to the scheduled period of severe neutropenia (ANC <500/μL) [19].

## Hematopoietic Stem Cell Transplantation

Replacement of bone marrow during Hematopoietic stem cell transplantation (HSCT) is a treatment approach for patients with hematologic disorders, congenital immunodeficiencies, lipidoses, and inborn errors of metabolism, as well as for marrow support to allow the administration of higher doses of chemotherapy and radiotherapy in patients with solid tumours [3]. This approach has also been effective as a rescue therapy for leukaemia patients [4].

Each phase of Hematopoietic stem cell transplantation (HSCT) is associated with specific considerations [20]:

### *Phase I: Preconditioning*

Oral manifestations of the underlying disease and recent cancer treatment impact oral complications of the patient. These might include oral infections, gingival leukemic infiltrates bleeding, ulceration and temporomandibular dysfunction [20].

There are two significant differences between dental and oral care for pediatric cancer and HSCT: 1) Receiving cytotoxic therapies in just a few days before the transplant, and 2) Prolonged duration of immunosuppression following the transplant [20].

All dental treatments should be completed before induction of immunosuppression. Elective dentistry will need to be postponed until immunological recovery, at least 100 days following HSCT, or longer if chronic GVHD or other complications are present [20].

### Phase II: Conditioning Neutropenic Phase

From the hospital admission until 30 days post-HSCT, this phase involves different conditioning regimens and supportive medical therapies. Oral complications are typically severe and high prevalent, including mucositis, xerostomia, oral pain, bleeding, opportunistic infections, taste dysfunction, neurotoxicity (including dental pain, muscle tremors), and temporomandibular dysfunction (including jaw pain, headache, joint pain) [20].

Oral mucositis usually begins seven to 10 days after initiation of conditioning, and symptoms continue approximately two weeks after the end of the training [20].

Dental procedures usually are not allowed in this phase due to the patient's severe immunosuppression. Consultation is necessary for the need of emergency treatment [20].

### Phase III: Engraftment to Hematopoietic Recovery

Three to four weeks after transplantation, both intensity and severity of complications decrease. Oral fungal infections and herpes simplex virus infections are most notable. Attention to xerostomia and oral GVHD manifestations is of utmost importance. Haemorrhage, neurotoxicity, temporomandibular dysfunction, and granulomas/papillomas sometimes are observed [20].

Oral hygiene should be optimised, and a cariogenic diet should be avoided. HSCT patients are susceptible to intraoral thermal stimuli between two- and four months post-transplant, which resolves spontaneously within a few months. Topical application of neutral fluoride or desensitising toothpaste helps reduce the symptoms [20].

### Phase IV: Immune Reconstitution/Recovery from Systemic Toxicity

After day 100 post-HCT, chronic toxicity of the conditioning regimen causes oral complications, including salivary dysfunction, craniofacial growth abnormalities, late viral infections, oral chronic GVHD, and oral squamous cell carcinoma [20].

Xerostomia and relapse-related oral lesions may be observed. Invasive dental treatment should be avoided in patients with profound impairment of immune function [20].

## *Phase V: Long-Term Survival*

Craniofacial, skeletal, and dental developmental issues are some of the complications faced by cancer survivors and usually develop among children who were less than six years of age at the time of their cancer therapy. Long term effects of cancer therapy may include tooth agenesis, microdontia, crown disturbances (size, shape, enamel hypoplasia, pulp chamber anomalies), root disturbances (early apical closure, blunting, changes in condition or length), reduced mandibular length, and reduced alveolar process height. Patients may also experience permanent salivary gland hypofunction/dysfunction or xerostomia [20].

## Crohn's Disease

Inflammatory bowel disease (IBD) is a recurring inflammatory disorder involving the intestines. Crohn's disease and ulcerative colitis are two main types, with the former affecting the large intestine, small intestine, or both and the latter involving the colon and rectum [3]. Clinical symptoms include abdominal pain, diarrhoea, rectal blood loss, decreased appetite, weight loss, fever and growth failure in children. The patient experiences episodes of exacerbations interspersed with remission intervals [21].

Oral manifestations of Crohn's disease include aphthous ulcers, lip and buccal mucosa swelling or cobblestoning, mucogingivitis, angular cheilitis and chronic granulomatous lesions (Figs. **14** & **15**) [29]. Up to 40% of children may have one or more of these symptoms [3].

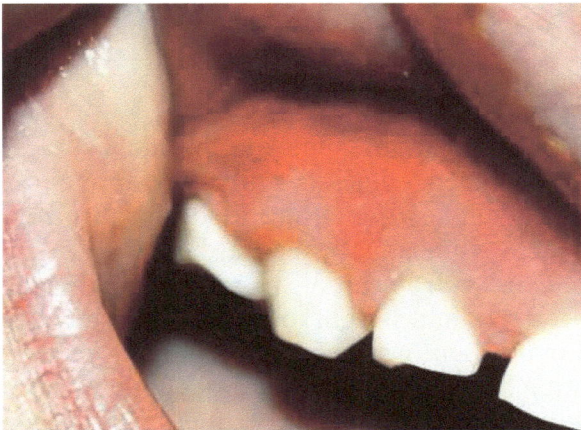

**Fig. (14).** Mild mucosal erythema of the right anterior maxillary gingiva.

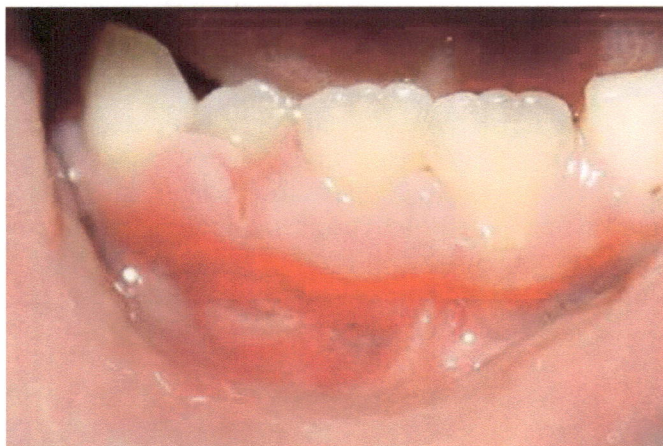

**Fig. (15).** Nodular swellings of the interdental papillae between the right permanent mandibular central and lateral incisors and primary canine. Ulceration of the free gingival margin between the incisors is seen. Also noted is linear ulceration with hyperplastic margins involving the alveolar mucosa.

Orofacial granulomatosis sometimes precedes the onset of ulcerative colitis by 1–2 years [7]. Oral lesions are usually asymptomatic and self-limiting but may be a marker of disease severity [3]. Control of gastrointestinal disease is the first and most crucial step in treating oral lesions [21]. If the patient experiences discomfort due to oral lesions, cinnamon- and benzoate-rich diet should be avoided, and topical agents such as lidocaine and topical steroids such as triamcinolone 0.1% or beclomethasone can be used [3, 21]. Lip swelling and deep linear ulcerations can be treated with topical tacrolimus (0.5 mg/kg) and intralesional steroid injections [21]. Severe and persistent symptoms may require immunosuppressors, *e.g.*, Thalidomide [3].

**Celiac Disease**

Celiac disease is a systemic, autoimmune and chronic disorder in individuals with genetic susceptibility to gluten. Gluten is a mixture of proteins found in wheat, rye and barley. These patients suffer from food malabsorption and nutritional deficiencies due to minor intestinal mucosa damage. Therefore, children with gastrointestinal problems such as chronic diarrhoea, abdominal pain and bloating, unexplained malabsorption and weight loss should be screened for celiac disease [3]. Extraintestinal manifestations such as iron deficiency anaemia, osteoporosis, herpetiform dermatitis, diabetes mellitus, reproductive disorder, cardiovascular diseases, ataxia and neurological disorders (tingling, pain and numbness due to nerve damage) are also seen in these patients. A gluten-free diet improves the symptoms of neuropathy and ataxia [3, 22].

Diagnosis is clinical, supported by haematology, biochemistry and small bowel biopsy. A gluten-free diet and replacement of any iron or vitamin deficiency are essential [5]. These patients are at risk of consuming too much fat and insufficient fibre, iron, vitamin D, and calcium. The most beneficial naturally gluten-free foods are green vegetables, legumes, fish and meat, rich in iron and folic acid. Pseudo-cereals (amaranth, quinoa, buckwheat, and other grains) are a good source of carbohydrates, dietary fibre, vitamins, and polyunsaturated fatty acids, a relatively good source of protein that is better in quality and quantity than wheat [23].

Oral manifestations include aphthae, dry mouth sensation, glossitis, angular stomatitis and dental enamel defects [3, 5]. According to existing studies, the incidence of caries is lower in these patients due to special diets, which needs further investigation [3] (Fig. **16**).

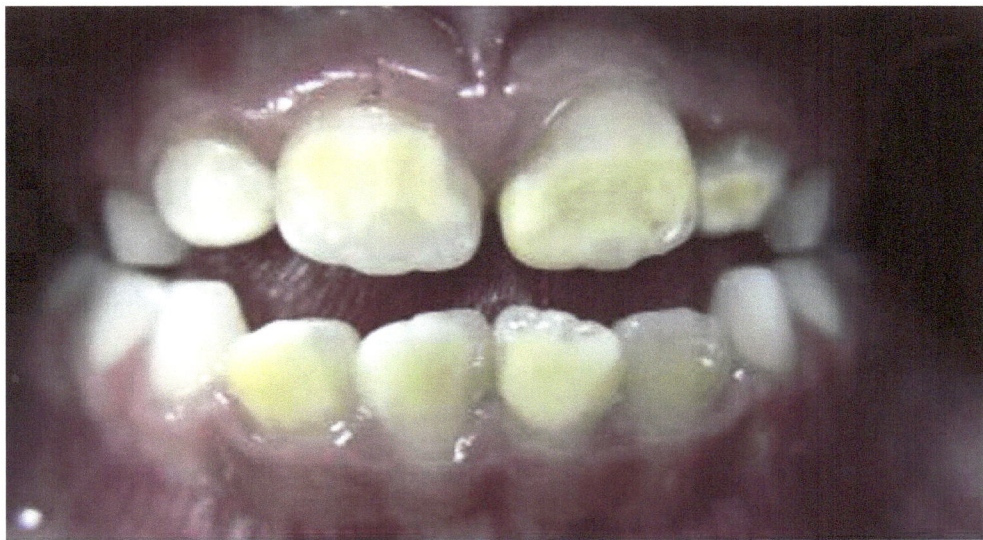

**Fig. (16).** Grade I (Aine classification) dental enamel defects in an 8-year-old boy with celiac disease.

## Chronic Renal Failure

Chronic renal failure (CRF) is a progressive disease characterised by the gradual destruction of nephrons. Subsequently, kidney function reduces, and the glomerular filtration rate (GFR) falls while serum levels of urea rise [24]. The most common chronic conditions affecting the kidneys are Ureteric reflux, Obstructive uropathy, Glomerulosclerosis, Medullary cystic disease, Systemic lupus erythematosus, Cystinosis [7].

Children suffering from CRF at a young age show growth retardation and a delay in the development of the dentition. An early effect is enamel hypoplasia due to enamel development and mineralisation [24].

Anaemia due to decreased erythropoietin output, decreased erythrocyte production, and reduction of erythrocyte life due to hypertension causes parlour of the oral mucosa. Hematoma's formations, tendency to bruise and increased bleeding time, chronic marginal gingivitis, uremic gingivostomatitis resembling candidiasis is also seen [24, 25].

Calcium absorption is decreased due to the production inhibition of vitamin D metabolites. Consequently, partial or complete loss of lamina dura, loss of trabeculation, ground glass appearance, metastatic calcifications and large bony giant cell lesion is seen in hard tissues [25].

As the preferred diet is a protein-reduced supplemented with calories, intake of softened food can lead to excessive calculus formation. Despite this, caries experience is not higher than usual, which may be due to increased concentration of urea in saliva and, consequently, a more increased saliva pH [25].

**End-Stage Renal Disease**

End-Stage Renal Disease (ESRD) is characterised by diminished endocrine and metabolic functions of the kidney with subsequent retention and accumulation of toxic metabolites. Blood pressure increases due to fluid overload and the production of vasoactive hormones via the renin-angiotensin system, increasing the risk of developing congestive heart failure [7, 25].

No special consideration is necessary for the patients with renal disease receiving conservative medical treatment unless avoiding nephrotoxic drugs (such as tetracyclines or aminoglycosides) and monitor blood pressure during the procedures due to frequent hypertension [24].

However, for hemodialysis patients, consultation with the nephrologist is necessary to know about the patient's condition, medications under usage and comorbidities such as diabetes. Most important of all is the decision about antibiotic prophylaxis. Because of the controversies about antibiotics, an antibiotic prophylaxis indication should be evaluated individually.

The anticoagulant effect of heparin increases bleeding time, so dental treatment with risk of bleeding should be postponed to non-dialysis day [24].

Local anaesthetics can be safely used because they have hepatic elimination. Paracetamol remains the best choice for pain management. Other anti-inflammatory drugs such as ibuprofen or naproxen could cause hypertension and worsen the bleeding tendency. Aspirin is contraindicated because it increases platelet dysfunction, the risk of gastric bleeding and contributes to the deterioration of renal function. Finally, a reduction of compliance should be expected as poor quality of life and depression have been associated with hemodialysis [8, 24].

## CONCLUSION

A child suffering from a systemic disease is different from a healthy child in that an average child can play, take part in day-to-day activities, attend school regularly and remain a centre of love and affection for parents and relatives. A child with systemic diseases is sick, physically and emotionally unstable and usually uncooperative. Hence, there is a heavy burden on the family members. It has been observed that children with systemic diseases exhibit more dental and oral health problems compared to normal healthy children of their age. Enamel disturbances and related disorders are frequently seen in children with endocrinal disorders and malabsorption syndromes. The role of prevention must never be underestimated for these children. Appropriate dietary counselling and oral hygiene measures must be adapted to their specific needs. Finally, the children and their families may often be neglected or isolated by society; hence a dentist's role as a sympathetic, understanding counselor must never be overlooked.

## CONSENT FOR PUBLICATION

Not applicable.

## CONFLICT OF INTEREST

The authors declare no conflict of interest, financial or otherwise.

## ACKNOWLEDGEMENT

Declared none.

## REFERENCES

[1]    Serebrisky D, Wiznia A. Pediatric asthma: a global epidemic. Ann Glob Health 2019; 85(1): 6.
       [http://dx.doi.org/10.5334/aogh.2416] [PMID: 30741507]

[2]    Sharma S, Gaur P, Gupta S, Kant S. Impact of asthma on oral health: A review. Int J Recent Sci Res
       2018; 9(5): 26512-4.

[3]    Nowak A, Christensen JR, Mabry TR, Townsend JA, Wells MH. Pediatric dentistry: Infancy through
       adolescence Elsevier Philadelphia: 2018.

[4]    Dean JA, Avery DR, McDonald RE. McDonald and Avery Dentistry for the child and adolescent
       Elsevier Imprint: Mosby: 2016.

[5] Scully C, Welbury R, Flaitz C, Almeida OP. Colour atlas of orofacial health and disease in children and adolescents: diagnosis and management Taylor & Francis Group; London: CRC Press. 2001.

[6] Welbury R, Duggal MS, Hosey MT. Paediatric dentistry. Fifth Edition (Oxford, 2018; online edn, Oxford Academic, 12 Nov. 2020).
[http://dx.doi.org/10.1093/oso/9780198789277.001.0001]

[7] Cameron AC, Widmer RP. Handbook of Pediatric Dentistry E-Book Elsevier Imprint: Mosby: 2013.

[8] Badrinatheswar GV. Pedodontics: practice and management Jaypee Brothers Medical Publishers. 2010.

[9] Kevat PM, Reeves BM, Ruben AR, Gunnarsson R. Adherence to Secondary Prophylaxis for Acute Rheumatic Fever and Rheumatic Heart Disease: A Systematic Review. Curr Cardiol Rev 2017; 13(2): 155-66.
[PMID: 28093988]

[10] Abrams J, Watkins DA, Abdullahi LH, Zühlke LJ, Engel ME. Integrating the Prevention and Control of Rheumatic Heart Disease into Country Health Systems: A Systematic Review and Meta-Analysis. Glob Heart 2020; 15(1): 62.
[http://dx.doi.org/10.5334/gh.874] [PMID: 33150127]

[11] Srivastava A, Brewer AK, Mauser-Bunschoten EP, *et al.* Guidelines for the management of hemophilia. Haemophilia 2013; 19(1): e1-e47.
[http://dx.doi.org/10.1111/j.1365-2516.2012.02909.x] [PMID: 22776238]

[12] Gupta A, Epstein JB, Cabay RJ. Bleeding disorders of importance in dental care and related patient management. J Can Dent Assoc 2007; 73(1): 77-83.
[PMID: 17295950]

[13] Shastry SP, Kaul R, Baroudi K, Umar D, Hemophilia A. Hemophilia A: Dental considerations and management. J Int Soc Prev Community Dent 2014; 4(3) (Suppl. 3): S147-52.
[PMID: 25625071]

[14] Nevitt SJ, Jones AP, Howard J. Hydroxyurea (hydroxycarbamide) for sickle cell disease. Cochrane Database Syst Rev 2017; 4(4): CD002202.
[PMID: 28426137.]

[15] Saramba MI, Shakya S, Zhao D. Analgesic management of uncomplicated acute sickle-cell pain crisis in pediatrics: a systematic review and meta-analysis. J Pediatr (Rio J) 2020; 96(2): 142-58.
[http://dx.doi.org/10.1016/j.jped.2019.05.004] [PMID: 31351033]

[16] El Howati A, Tappuni A. Systematic review of the changing pattern of the oral manifestations of HIV. J Investig Clin Dent 2018; 9(4): e12351.
[http://dx.doi.org/10.1111/jicd.12351.] [PMID: 30019446.]

[17] de Almeida VL, Lima IFP, Ziegelmann PK, Paranhos LR, de Matos FR. Impact of highly active antiretroviral therapy on the prevalence of oral lesions in HIV-positive patients: a systematic review and meta-analysis. Int J Oral Maxillofac Surg 2017; 46(11): 1497-504.
[http://dx.doi.org/10.1016/j.ijom.2017.06.008] [PMID: 28684301]

[18] Chunxia D, Meifang W, Jianhua Z, *et al.* Tobacco smoke exposure and the risk of childhood acute lymphoblastic leukemia and acute myeloid leukemia. Medicine (Baltimore) 2019; 98(28): e16454.
[http://dx.doi.org/10.1097/MD.0000000000016454] [PMID: 31305478]

[19] Lehrnbecher T, Fisher BT, Phillips B, *et al.* Guideline for antibacterial prophylaxis administration in pediatric cancer and hematopoietic stem cell transplantation. Clin Infect Dis 2020; 71(1): 226-36.
[http://dx.doi.org/10.1093/cid/ciz1082] [PMID: 31676904]

[20] Guideline on dental management of pediatric patients receiving chemotherapy, hematopoietic cell transplantation, and/or radiation. Pediatr Dent 2013; 35(5): E185-93.
[PMID: 24290549]

[21]    Tan CXW, Brand HS, de Boer NKH, Forouzanfar T. Gastrointestinal diseases and their oro-dental manifestations: Part 1: Crohn's disease. Br Dent J 2016; 221(12): 794-9.
[http://dx.doi.org/10.1038/sj.bdj.2016.954] [PMID: 27982000]

[22]    Mearns E, Taylor A, Thomas Craig K, *et al.* Neurological manifestations of neuropathy and ataxia in celiac disease: a systematic review. Nutrients 2019; 11(2): 380.
[http://dx.doi.org/10.3390/nu11020380] [PMID: 30759885]

[23]    Nardo GD, Villa MP, Conti L, *et al.* Nutritional deficiencies in children with celiac disease resulting from a gluten-free diet: A systematic review. Nutrients 2019; 11(7): 1588.
[http://dx.doi.org/10.3390/nu11071588] [PMID: 31337023]

[24]    Costantinides F, Castronovo G, Vettori E, *et al.* Dental Care for Patients with End-Stage Renal Disease and Undergoing Hemodialysis. Int J Dent 2018; 2018: 1-8.
[http://dx.doi.org/10.1155/2018/9610892] [PMID: 30538746]

[25]    Koch G, Poulsen S. Pediatric dentistry: a clinical approach. Wiley-Blackwel. 2017.

[26]    Ricardo Martínez-Rider. Arturo Garrocho-Rangel, Raúl Márquez-Preciado, María Victoria Bolaños-Carmona,et al. Socorro Islas-Ruiz,Amaury Pozos-Guillén, Dental Management of a Child with Incidentally Detected Hemophilia: Report of a Clinical Case. Case Rep Dent 2017; 2017: 7429738.

[27]    Barasch A, Safford MM, Catalanotto FA, Fine DH, Katz RV. Oral soft tissue manifestations in HIV-positive vs. HIV negative children from an inner-city population: A two-year observational study. Pediatr Dent 2000; 22(3): 215-20.

[28]    Cammarata-Scalisi F, Girardi K, Strocchio L, et al. Oral Manifestations and Complications in Childhood Acute Myeloid Leukemia. Cancers (Basel) 2020; 12(6): 1634.

[29]    Woo VL. Oral Manifestations of Crohn's Disease: A Case Report and Review of the Literature. Case Rep Dent 2015; 2015: 830472.

[30]    Cooley RO, Sobel RS. Dental treatment considerations for the medically compromised child. Pediatr Clin North Am 1982; 29(3): 613-29.
[http://dx.doi.org/10.1016/S0031-3955(16)34183-9] [PMID: 6211651]

# CHAPTER 6

# Management of Special Children

**Bhavna H. Dave**[1,*] and **Pratik B. Kariya**[1]

*¹ Department of Pediatric and Preventive Dentistry, K.M. Shah Dental College and Hospital, Sumandeep Vidyapeeth Deemed to Be University, Vadodara, Gujarat, India*

**Abstract:** Patients with a spread of medical conditions, some unknown to them, ask for dental treatment. Usually, this can often be mixed with the intake of a posh variety of medicines. Dental management aims to produce safe and effective treatment while not causative a medical crisis. Consequently, dental treatment might be changed to keep with the patient's medical constraints, and occasionally, MD consultation can be required. Information of the medical standing of patients obtained through correct medical history-taking is key to safe patient management. The health profile of a country's population is additionally relevant for the supply of oral health care. However, there's a scarceness of data regarding the medical standing of patients seen. This chapter throws lightweight on the consecutive management of dental patients with medical emergencies with this read.

**Keywords:** Blood Coagulation Disorders, Children, Dental Management, Diabetes Complications, Drug Hypersensitivity, Emergency Treatment, Medical Emergencies, Metabolic Disease, Myocardial Ischemia Therapy.

## INTRODUCTION

Individuals with special health care needs are at greater risk for oral diseases throughout their lifetime. Oral diseases are of significant concern due to their direct and devastating impact on the health and quality of life of those with specific systemic health problems. Such individuals have unique needs and require oral health care of a special nature. Familiarity with the patient's medical history is essential. It decreases the risk of aggravating a medical condition while rendering dental care [1].

---

\* **Corresponding author Bhavna H. Dave:** Department of Pediatric and Preventive Dentistry, K.M. Shah Dental College and Hospital, Sumandeep Vidyapeeth Deemed to Be University, Vadodara, Gujarat, India; E-mail: bhavnadave1964@gmail.com

**Satyawan Damle, Ritesh Kalaskar & Dhanashree Sakhare (Eds.)**
**All rights reserved-© 2023 Bentham Science Publishers**

## Pre- Appointment Preparation (Table-1)

a. Acquiring a thorough health history

b. Understand the significance of the disease that the patient may endorse.

c. Consult with the child's primary care physician

d. History of medications

e. History of allergies

## Assessment of the Medically Compromised Patient

**Table 1. Assessment of the medically compromised patient.**

| Complete Health History | Assessment and management tools |
|---|---|
| • Date of Last Physical Examination.<br>• Name, Address and Contact number of Specialists.<br>• List of Medical conditions being treated.<br>• List of medications.<br>• Allergies and Medical emergencies experienced.<br>• Hospitalizations. | • Complete blood count (CBC) with Plat. Count and white blood cells (WBC diff).<br>• Prothrombin time (PT)/ international normalised ratio (INR).<br>• Partial thromboplastin time (PTT); BT.<br>• Liver function tests (LFTs)<br>• Hepatic Serology, Serum Creatinine.<br>• Fasting blood sugar test (FBS).<br>• Postprandial glucose test PP and glycated haemoglobin (HbA1C).<br>• CD4 count and Viral Load. |

Note: At each visit, the history should be consulted and updated. Caries- risk assessment should be performed periodically [2].

## Various Medical Conditions

• Cardiovascular diseases
• Pulmonary diseases
• Hematological disorders
• Endocrine disorders
• Hepatological Diseases
• Neurological disorders
• Immunological disorders

## Management of Patients with Cardiovascular Diseases

Management implications in oral health care depend mainly on intervention and cardiovascular risk (Table **2**). The anxiety and pain associated with dental care can cause enhanced sympathetic activity and adrenaline (epinephrine) release, increasing the heat load and the risk of angina or arrhythmias.

**Table 2. Grading of hypertension and dental management considerations.**

| American Society of Anesthesiologists (ASA) grading of hypertension and dental management considerations | | | |
|---|---|---|---|
| Blood pressure (mmHg) (Systolic, diastolic) | ASA Grade | Hypertension Stage | Dental aspects |
| <140, <90 | I | – | Routine dental care Recheck BP before Starting regular dental Care. |
| 140–159, 90–99 | II | 1 | |
| 160–179, 95–109 | III | 2 | Recheck BP and seek medical advice before Routine dental care Restrict use of adrenaline (epinephrine) Conscious sedation may Help |
| >180, >110 | Iv | 3 | Recheck BP after 5 min Quiet rest medical advice before Dental care Only emergency care Until BP controlled Avoid vasoconstrictors |

Before any procedure, it is crucial to note down the vital (Fig. **1**). The constant monitoring of the vitals is necessary. Various modalities to be followed, especially for dental management, are there for different cardiac conditions (Table **3**).

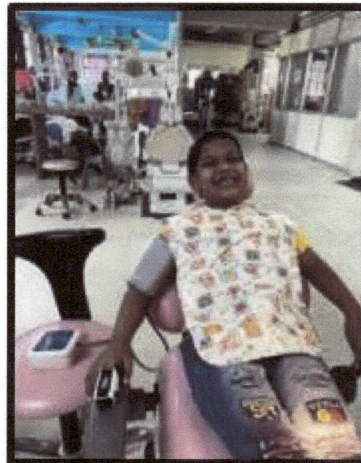

**Fig. (1).** Recording Vitals before the dental procedure for a patient with congenital heart disease.

## Management of Patients with Endocrinology Diseases

The endocrine system is widespread and consists of glands that exert their effects through chemicals (hormones) secreted into the blood circulation. Hormones are chemical messengers of various types, which usually act at some distance from their source and can be classified according to their main function [3]. This section covers the management of endocrine disorders (Table **4**) (Figs **2** & **3**).

**Table 3. Dental management of patients with cardiac conditions.**

| Cardiac condition | Feature | Dental management | Emergency management |
|---|---|---|---|
| **Hypertension** | High blood pressure >140 mmHg systolic pressure, >90 mmHg diastolic pressure | Proper and regular medications to be taken even for the day of dental treatment. Blood pressure to be recorded. Preferably morning appointment. Either anxiolytic agents (5-10 mg diazepam the night before and 1-2 hours before the appointment) or consideration of sedation with nitrous oxide in an anxious patient. Vasoconstrictor use should be limited, not to exceed 0.04 mg of adrenaline. | Conservative treatment for an emergency dental visit with the use of analgesics and antibiotics (NSAIDs not prescribed for more than five days) |
| **Heart failure** | The incapacity of the heart to function correctly, pumping insufficient blood towards the tissue and leading to fluid accumulation within the lungs, liver, and peripheral tissues | Position- semi-supine to avoid orthostatic hypotension Aspirin should not be prescribed. Vasoconstrictor dose to be limited to two anaesthetic capsules when the patient is under digitalis agents (digoxin, methyldigoxin) | Patient seated with the legs lowered, with nasal oxygen at 4-6 litres/ minute. Sublingual nitroglycerin tablets (0.4-0.8mg) every 5-10 minutes if blood pressure is maintained |
| **Cardiac arrhythmias** | Abnormality in rate, regularity, or site of origin of the cardiac impulse | Anxiolytics- to reduce stress and anxiety. Caution while using electrical devices (if pacemakers are present) | Arrhythmia during the dental procedure- cease the practice and assess vitals. Sublingual nitrates are to be administered in the event of chest pain. The patient should be placed in the Trendelenburg position with vagal manoeuvring. |

(Table 3) cont.....

| Cardiac condition | Feature | Dental management | Emergency management |
|---|---|---|---|
| **Infective endocarditis** | Usually develops in individuals with underlying structural cardiac defects who develop bacteremia with organisms likely to cause endocarditis. | Antimicrobial prophylaxis should be administered for procedures associated with significant bleeding. | - |
| **Ischemic heart disease** | Characterised by a reduction (partial or total) in coronary blood flow. | In dental practice- a minimum safety period of 6 months has been established before any oral surgical procedure can be carried out. The patient should bring nitrates if used on each visit. For anxious patients- premedication can be administered to lessen anxiety and stress. Position- most comfortable (semi-supine) and should get up carefully to avoid orthostatic hypotension. | Patient under antiplatelet medication- excessive local bleeding is to be controlled. |
| **Cardiac pacemakers and implantable cardioverter-defibrillators** | ICD – a small battery-powered electrical impulse generator implanted in patients susceptible to sudden cardiac death due to ventricular fibrillation and ventricular tachycardia. | Before any therapeutic service- a cardiologist should be consulted. Electrical cords should not be placed over the patient's chest. A lead apron should be used while taking an x-ray. Hand scaling is preferred over ultrasonic. | Symptoms such as difficulty breathing, light-headedness, dizziness, change in pulse rate, prolonged hiccoughing, swelling in chest and arm, and chest pain indicate pacemaker malfunction. Under such conditions, the cardiologist should be consulted immediately. |

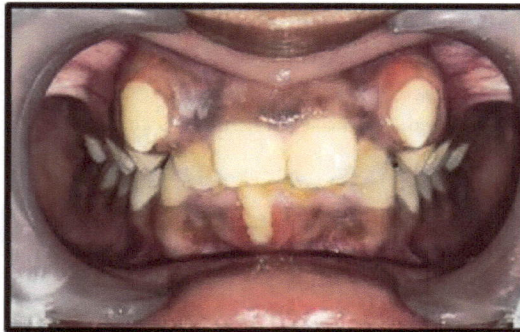

**Fig. (2).** Patient with type I Diabetes Mellites having swollen and bleeding gums.

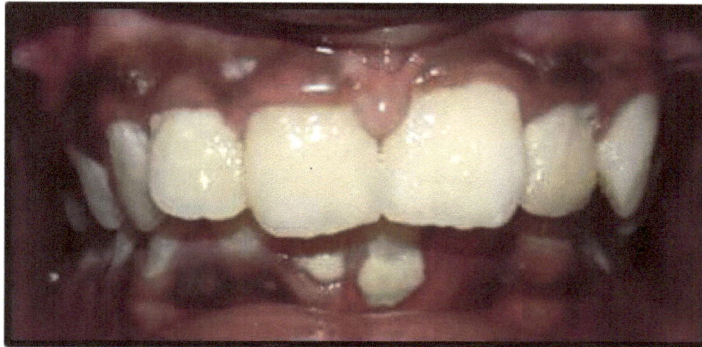

**Fig. (3).** Swollen gums in Juvenile diabetes.

## Dental Management of Patients with Hematological Diseases

**Hematologic Diseases** are disorders that primarily affect the blood & blood-forming organs. Hematologic diseases include rare genetic disorders, anaemia, HIV, sickle cell disease & complications from chemotherapy or transfusions (Fig. 4) (Table 5).

**Table 4. Dental Management of patients with an endocrine disorder.**

| Condition | Feature | Dental management |
|---|---|---|
| **Diabetes insipidus** | Swollen and inflamed gums Hypercalcemia, hypokalemia, renal disease, or drugs such as lithium). More commonly, it is because of reduced ADH secretion–cranial diabetes insipidus, which is caused by head injuries (when it may be temporary), a tumour (usually craniopharyngioma), infiltration, or infiltration vascular disease in the region of the hypothalamus or pituitary, or it may be idiopathic. | • Local anaesthesia (LA) is the most satisfactory means of pain control. <br> • Conscious sedation (CS) may be needed to control anxiety. <br> • This disorder usually does not complicate dentistry except for dryness of the mouth. <br> • Carbamazepine used in treating trigeminal neuralgia may have an additive effect with other drugs used to treat diabetes insipidus. <br> • Transient diabetes insipidus can be a complication of head injury, but a head injury can also cause the opposite effect–excessive ADH levels. |

*(Table 4) cont.....*

| Condition | Feature | Dental management |
|---|---|---|
| **Growth hormone excess: gigantism and acromegaly** | In gigantism, all the organs, soft tissues, and skeleton enlarge, leading to excessively tall stature, thickening of the soft tissues with a prominence of the supraorbital ridge, coarse oily skin, thick spade-like finger sand deepening of the voice.<br>Only those bones with growth potential, particularly the mandible, can enlarge in acromegaly. There is a thickening of the soft tissues, and the hands become large and spade-like [4]. | • Local analgesia is suitable.<br>• If necessary, conscious Sedation may be given provided the airway is clear.<br>• GA may be hazardous.<br>• Dental management may be complicated by:<br>• blindness, diabetes mellitus, hypertension, cardiomyopathy, arrhythmias, hypopituitarism, kyphosis, and other deformities affect respiration, making GA hazardous.<br>• The glottic opening may be narrowed, and the cords' mobility reduced.<br>• A goitre may further embarrass the airway<br>• Mandibular enlargement leads to prognathism (class III malocclusion) with the spacing of the teeth and thickening of all soft tissues, but most conspicuously of the face.<br>• Orthognathic Surgery may be needed and fatal if you have followed such Surgery in the past because of airway obstruction.<br>• The paranasal airs in use are enlarged, and the skull thickened [1]. |

*(Table 4) cont.....*

| Condition | Feature | Dental management |
|-----------|---------|-------------------|
| **Diabetes mellitus** | **Acute**<br>Thirst<br>Polyuria and polydipsia<br>Weight loss and weakness<br>Lethargy<br>Confusion/aggression/<br>behavioural changes<br>Abdominal pain<br>Nausea and vomiting<br>Ketoacidosis<br>Dehydration<br>renal failure<br>Coma<br>**Chronic**<br>Thirst<br>Polyuria and polydipsia<br>Weight loss and weakness<br>Lethargy<br>Irritability<br>recurrent skin, oral and genital<br>Visual deterioration<br>paresthesia (hands and<br>feet) | • Optimum control would aim to keep blood glucose levels at 4–7 mmol/L before meals (pre-prandial) and at no higher than10 mmol/L 2 hours after meals (postprandial), and HbA1c (long-term glucose level) at 7% or less.<br>• Weight should be reduced, and physical activity stepped up.<br>• Diet may help diabetic control; recommendations are to:<br>• Eat more starches, such as bread, cereal, and starchy vegetables. Eat five portions of fruits and vegetables every day.<br>• Soluble fibre, found mainly in fruits, vegetables, and some seeds, is beneficial as they help slow down or reduce the intestinal absorption of glucose.<br>• Legumes, such as cooked kidney beans, are among the highest soluble-fibre foods.<br>• Other fibre-containing foods, such as carrots, also positively level blood glucose.<br>• Eat fewer sugars and sweets.<br>• The 'Greenspan syndrome' (diabetes, lichen planus, and hypertension) may result from purely coincidental associations of common disorders probably related to drug use.<br>• Poorly controlled diabetics (whether type 1or2) should also be referred for improved blood glucose control before performing the non-emergency treatment [3]. |

*(Table 4) cont.....*

| Condition | Feature | Dental management |
|---|---|---|
| **Hypothyroidism** | • Hypothyroidism is often unrecognized.<br>• With raised TSH but normal T4 levels, subclinical hypothyroidism may be found in up to 10% of postmenopausal females.<br>• Hypothyroidism may cause symptoms like weight gain, lassitude, dry skin, myxedema, loss of hair, cardiac failure, ischemic heart disease, bradycardia, anaemia, neurological or psychiatric changes, hypotonia, cerebellar signs of ataxia, tremor, dysmetria, polyneuropathy, cranial nerve deficits, entrapment neuropathy (*e.g.*, Carpal tunnel syndrome), myopathic weakness, dementia, apathy, mental dullness, irritability, and sleepiness. | • The main danger is the precipitation of myxedema coma using sedatives (including diazepam or midazolam), opioid analgesics (including codeine), or tranquillizers.<br>• These should therefore be either avoided or given in a low dose.<br>• LA is satisfactory for pain control.<br>• Conscious Sedation can be carried out with nitrous oxide and oxygen.<br>• Diazepam or midazolam may precipitate coma.<br>• GA may be complicated because of possible ischemic heart disease and the danger of coma, and the respiratory centre is also hypersensitive to drugs such as opioids or sedatives.<br>• GA, if unavoidable, should be delayed if possible until thyroxine has been started.<br>• Associated problems may include hypoadrenocorticism, anaemia, hypotension, diminished cardiac output, and bradycardia.<br>• Occasional associations include hypopituitarism and other autoimmune disorders such as Sjogren syndrome.<br>• Povidone-iodine and similar compounds are best avoided [1]. |

*(Table 4) cont.....*

| Condition | Feature | Dental management |
|---|---|---|
| **Hyperthyroidism** | • Hyperthyroidism may cause exophthalmos, eyelid lag, and eyelid retraction. In addition, it mimics the effects of adrenaline (epinephrine) and can cause anorexia, vomiting or diarrhoea, weight loss, anxiety, tremor, sweating, and heat intolerance. Cardiac disturbances, particularly in older patients, include tachycardia, arrhythmias (especially atrial fibrillation), or cardiac failure.<br>• Thyrotoxic periodic paralysis comprises mild to severe weakness attacks, during which low serum potassium levels.<br>• Myasthenia gravis may occasionally be associated. | • Patients with sympathetic overactivity in untreated hyperthyroidism can be anxious and irritable and may faint.<br>• LA is the primary means of pain control; any risk of adrenaline (epinephrine) exacerbating sympathetic overactivity is only theoretical, and prilocaine with felypressin is not known to be safer than lidocaine.<br>• Conscious sedation is frequently desirable to control excessive anxiety.<br>• Benzodiazepines may potentiate antithyroid drugs; therefore, nitrous oxide, which is more rapidly controllable, is probably safer.<br>• Povidone-iodine and similar compounds are best avoided.<br>• Carbimazole occasionally causes agranulocytosis, which may cause oral or oropharyngeal ulceration. |
| **Hypoparathyroidism** | • Low plasma calcium leads to muscle irritability and tetany,<br>• Carpopedal spasms (Trousseau's sign; contracture of the hand and fingers (main accoucheur– obstetrician's hand) on occluding the arm with a cuff).<br>• numbness and tingling of arms and legs; and even laryngeal stridor | • There may be facial paresthesia and facial twitching caused by tetany (Chvostek's sign).<br>• Idiopathic (congenital) hypoparathyroidism may present the following features- enamel hypoplasia, shortened roots with osteodentine formation, delayed eruption, and sometimes chronic mucocutaneous candidiasis. |

(Table 4) cont.....

| Condition | Feature | Dental management |
|---|---|---|
| **Hyperparathyroidism** | • The main features include hypercalcemia and renal disease (most patients have renal calcifications),<br>• skeletal disease (bone pain, pathological fractures, giant cell tumours, bone rarefaction),<br>• peptic ulceration,<br>• pancreatitis,<br>• hypertension<br>• arrhythmias.<br>• Therefore, the expression 'stones, bones and abdominal groans' sometimes applies. | • Giant cell lesions of hyperparathyroidism (brown tumours) are rare. Histologically they are indistinguishable from central giant cell granulomas of the jaws.<br>• The parathyroid function should be investigated if found, particularly in a middle-aged patient or with renal failure.<br>• LA is the primary means of pain control, especially if hypertension and arrhythmias are present.<br>• CS is preferably carried out with nitrous oxide and oxygen.<br>• GA may be challenging because of cardiovascular complications and sensitivity to muscle relaxants.<br>• Dental treatment in patients with hyperparathyroidism may be complicated by renal disease, peptic ulceration, bone fragility, or pluriglandular disease. |

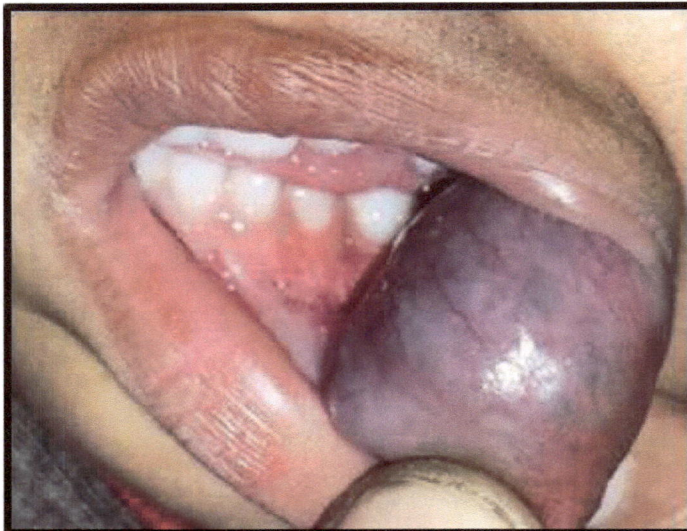

**Fig. (4).** Strawberry gums of an anaemic patient.

**Table 5. Shows dental management of bleeding disorders.**

| Condition | Feature | Dental management |
|---|---|---|
| Haemophilia A | • Hemophilia A is an X-linked disorder resulting from a deficiency in blood clotting factor VIII, a vital component of the coagulation cascade.<br>• Hemophilia is characterized by excessive bleeding, particularly after trauma and sometimes spontaneously.<br>• Hemorrhage appears to stop immediately after the injury (due to normal vascular and platelet hemostatic responses), but intractable oozing with rapid blood loss soon follows. (Fig. **5**)<br>• Hemorrhage is dangerous either because of acute blood loss or bleeding into tissues, particularly the brain, larynx, pharynx, joints, and muscles. | • Many of the coagulation defects present a hazard to Surgery and LA<br>• Injections, but in general, the teeth erupt and exfoliate without problems,<br>• Non-invasive dental care is safe. Close cooperation is needed between<br>• The physician and dentist to plan safe, comprehensive dental care.<br>• Antifibrinolytic agents include tranexamic acid (Cyklokapron)<br>• Desmopressin (DDAVP)<br>• Factor VIII must be replaced to a level adequate to ensure hemostasis<br>• If bleeding starts or is expected. The following tests are typically required:<br>■ Complete blood count, APTT, PT, factor VIII assay [5]<br>■ Specific factor VIII antibody test<br>■ Hepatitis B, hepatitis C, HIV tests<br>■ Liver function tests<br>■ Blood grouping and cross-matching in case of emergency when Surgery is contemplated. |

*(Table 5) cont.....*

| Condition | Feature | Dental management |
|---|---|---|
| Platelet disorders | Factors consider in haemophilia management<br>* Aggravation of bleeding by drugs<br>* Anxiety<br>* Dental neglect necessitating frequent dental extractions<br>* chronic pain<br>* Factor V inhibitors<br>* Hazards of anaesthesia, nasal intubation, and intramuscular injections<br>* Hepatitis and liver disease<br>* HIV infection<br>* trauma, Surgery, and subsequent bleeding | • Antiplatelet agents may be safely withdrawn seven days before surgery when prescribed for primary prevention. Still, any decision to stop antiplatelet therapy used for secondary prevention must balance the risk of thrombosis and ischemia against bleeding.<br>• No evidence continuing antiplatelet monotherapy causes major bleeding problems like dental extractions during or after minor surgery.<br>• Patients are more at risk of permanent disability or death from thromboembolic episodes if they stop antiplatelet medications before a surgical procedure. Therefore, advice from a specialist should be sought before withholding treatment, or the patient may need to be referred to a hospital setting for the course.<br>• Dentoalveolar surgical procedures likely to be carried out in primary care will be classified as minor, *e.g.*, simple extraction of up to three teeth, gingival Surgery, crown and bridge procedures, dental scaling, and the surgical removal of teeth.<br>• When more than three teeth need to be extracted, multiple visits will be required, by quadrants, or singly at separate visits.<br>• Scaling and gingival Surgery should initially be restricted to a limited area to assess whether bleeding is problematic [6]. |

*(Table 5) cont.....*

| Condition | Feature | Dental management |
|---|---|---|
| Bleeding disorders | • Initial indications of a haemostatic defect may start with standard bleeding features like epistaxis and gingival bleeding, swollen gums, and may occur after wounds and Surgery. Defects in haemostasis may include platelet activation and function abnormalities, contact activation or clotting proteins, or may signal excess antithrombin function. The more common causes of a bleeding tendency include:<br>• Aspirin (one tablet impairs platelet function for almost one week, but this rarely causes significant postoperative haemorrhage), NSAIDs, and other antiplatelet drugs<br>• Warfarin (the most common anticoagulant, which interferes with clotting factor production via vitamin K blockage)<br>• Von Willebrand disease is the most common inherited bleeding disorder.<br>• Acquired bleeding tendencies, such as:<br>• Bone marrow disease<br>• Immune disorders<br>• Liver disease<br>• Renal disease. | • Prolonged postoperative bleeding is defined if any of the following appertains:<br>•Bleeding continues for 12 hours.<br>•Bleeding causes the patient to return for attention.<br>•Bleeding causes an extensive hematoma/ecchymosis.<br>•The patient needs a transfusion.<br>• Saliva contains fibrinolytic agents that may aggravate the situation.<br>• In most cases, the cause is local. Bleeding can be managed using simple local haemostatic measures such as applying pressure on the wound with sterile pads (moistened with water, normal saline, or 5% tranexamic acid solution), using absorbable oxidised cellulose sponges, or suturing, as well as giving postoperative instructions verbally and in writing [7]. |

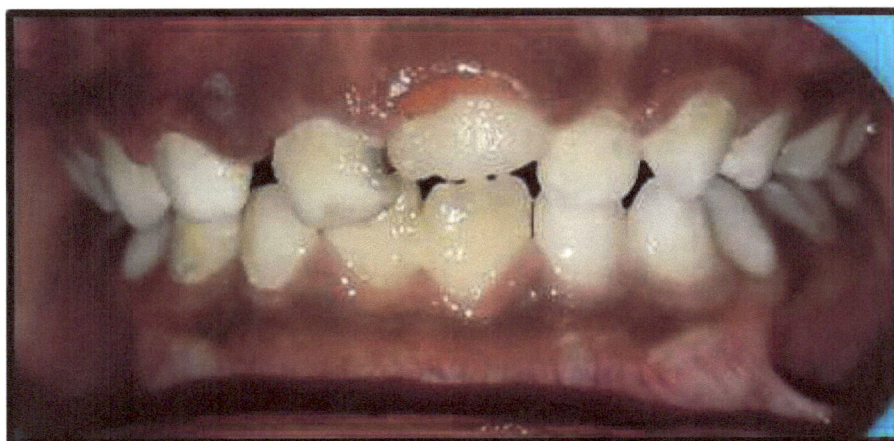

**Fig. (5).** Vascular hemangioma.

The following section deals with a list of platelet disorders (Table **6**).

**Table 6. Dental management of patients with Platelet disorders.**

| Condition | Feature | Dental management |
|---|---|---|
| **Anaemia** | • Typically, none in the early stage's general lassitude <br> • Cutaneous <br> pallor <br> brittle nails <br> koilonychia (spoon-shaped nails – iron deficiency) <br> • Oral sore mouth ulceration angular stomatitis glossitis burning mouth symptoms <br> • Cardiorespiratory <br> • Dyspnea <br> tachycardia <br> congestive cardiac failure <br> murmurs <br> palpitations <br> angina pectoris <br> • Blood picture shows morphological changes of the red cell (4) | • LA is satisfactory for pain control. <br> • CS can be given if full oxygenation is possible. <br> • A sore, physically regular tongue can develop before the Hb falls below the lower limit of normal. <br> • Atrophic glossitis – soreness of the tongue with depapillation or colour change – is the best-known effect of severe anaemia. <br> • The Paterson–Brown-Kelly (Plummer–Vinson) syndrome of glossitis and dysphagia with hypochromic (iron-deficiency) anaemia is uncommon. <br> • Candidiasis can be aggravated or precipitated by anaemia. <br> • Angular stomatitis is a well-known sign of iron deficiency anaemia but affects only a minority. <br> • Occasionally, adequate treatment of anaemia alone, without antifungal therapy, relieves the infection. <br> • Most patients with chronic mucocutaneous candidiasis are iron-deficient, particularly the familial and diffuse types. Treatment with iron appears to improve the response to antifungal therapy. <br> • Aphthous-like ulceration is sometimes associated with iron deficiency, which, if remedied, can sometimes bring about a cure. <br> • Staining the teeth with iron can be prevented in children by using sodium iron as the iron source, as it is also sugar-free and more palatable than ferrous sulphate. <br> • Some iron preparations can cause tooth erosion, as can chewable vitamin C [5]. |
| **Leukaemia's** | • The main types of leukaemia are: <br> • acute lymphocytic leukaemia (ALL) – accounts for 65% of childhood acute leukaemia but affects both children and adults <br> • chronic lymphocytic leukaemia (CLL) – is twice as common as chronic myelocytic leukaemia and is an adult disorder affecting older people <br> • acute myelocytic leukaemia (AML) – the most common acute leukaemia in adults <br> • chronic myelocytic leukaemia (CML) – most common in adults. | Orofacial manifestations include mucositis, ulcers, or gingival swelling and bleeding. <br> Bleeding tendencies and susceptibility to infection can often complicate dental management. <br> Septicaemias may spread from oral infections in these patients, as in other immunocompromised persons. <br> Cytotoxic drugs are potentially hazardous to staff, who should only handle them wearing medical gloves and protective eyewear should dispose of waste and sharps carefully. They should not handle it at all during pregnancy [8] (Table **7**). |

**Table 7. Synopsis of principles of oral health care in leukaemia.**

| Pre-chemotherapy | During induction chemotherapy | During remission | Long-term |
|---|---|---|---|
| **Assessment** | Continuation of preventive | Continuation of preventive | Continuation of preventive |
| **Treatment planning** | Oral health care | Oral health care | Oral health care |
| **Removal of unsavable teeth** | Antifungal prophylaxis (*e.g.*, Nystatin) | - | Monitoring of craniofacial and |
| **Treatment of caries** | Antiviral prophylaxis (*e.g.*, Acyclovir) | - | Dental development |
| **Dietary advice** | Dietary advice | Dietary advice | Dietary advice |
| **Initiation of fluoride prophylaxis** | Initiation of fluoride prophylaxis | Initiation of fluoride prophylaxis | Initiation of fluoride prophylaxis |
| **Oral hygiene advice** | Oral hygiene advice | Oral hygiene advice | Oral hygiene advice |
| **Initiation of chlorhexidine prophylaxis** | Initiation of chlorhexidine prophylaxis | Initiation of chlorhexidine prophylaxis | Initiation of chlorhexidine prophylaxis |

## Dental Management of Patients with Haematological Diseases

Life is impossible without the liver. The liver (hepar) consists of hepatocytes, organised for optimal contact with sinusoids (blood vessels) and bile ducts. It breaks down sugar, proteins, and fats, stores nutrients, produces bile, metabolises the drug, and removes toxins from the blood. Bile drains to the gallbladder and the small intestine via the bile duct. It is intimately associated with the head of the pancreas, swelling of which may cause biliary obstruction and jaundice [9]. This section covers Dental Management of Hepatological Condition (Table **8**).

## Dental Management of Patients with Respiratory Disorders: (Table 9)

- Infections of the respiratory tract can occur in:
  - The upper respiratory tract
  - The lower respiratory tract
  - Both.
- Organisms capable of infecting respiratory structures include bacteria, viruses & fungi.
- Viruses such as rhinovirus and parainfluenza virus cause the majority of upper respiratory tract infections
- Depending on the organism and extent of infection, the symptoms can range from mild to severe and even life-threatening.

**Table 8. Dental management in a patient with Hepatological condition.**

| Condition | Feature | Dental management |
|---|---|---|
| **Hepatitis** | • They include fatigue, nausea, vomiting, abdominal pain or discomfort, loss of appetite, low-grade fever, jaundice, and itching.<br>• Recovery is usually uneventful.<br>• Blood and faces become non-infective during or shortly after the acute illness.<br>• There is no evidence of either a carrier state or progression to chronic liver disease.<br>• About 15% have relapses over a 6–9-month period, but the mortality is less than 0.1%. | • There is a bleeding tendency if the platelet count is low or if the prothrombin time (and INR) is prolonged.<br>• Patients with average platelet counts and regular prothrombin times (INR) can undergo dental intervention safely.<br>• As little as 0.0000001 ml of HBsAg-positive serum can transmit hepatitis B.<br>• The main danger is from needle stick injuries; some 25% may transmit HBV infection.<br>• There is a higher risk for oral surgeons, periodontologists, and those working with high-risk patients, probably because of needle stick injuries.<br>• However, if adequate precautions are taken, dental Surgery is no longer a significant transmission source.<br>• Testing for HBeAg may indicate those individuals likely to spread hepatitis B. HBeAg-positive dental surgeons and those who are HBeAg-negative but have more than 1000 HBV viral particles per millilitre of blood should discontinue practice involving exposure-prone procedures.<br>• Needlestick injuries involving HBV can transmit the virus; post-exposure prophylaxis (PEP) with hbig or hepatitis B vaccine series should be considered for occupational exposures after evaluation of the HBsAg status of the source and the vaccination and vaccine-response status of the exposed person within 24 hours of contact [10] |

## Dental Management of Patients with Immunological Disorders

It is an unwanted response of the body to a full dose of the drug. It is the result of the immunological response by the individual. Table (**10**) shows dental management of patients with the immunological disorder. **Gel** and **Coombs** classification of anaphylaxis:

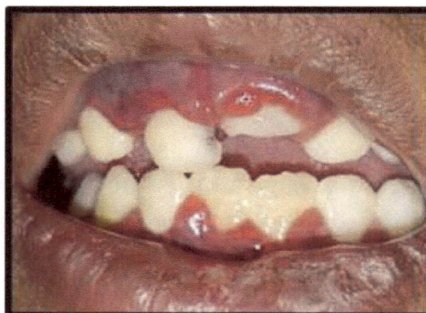

**Fig. (6).** Drug-induced gingival hyperplasia in an epileptic patient.

**Table 9. Dental management of a patient with respiratory disorders.**

| Condition | Feature | Dental management |
|---|---|---|
| Asthma and Chronic obstructive pulmonary disease (COPD) | • Asthma is chronic<br>• Disorder of airways is characterized by variable and recurring.<br>• Symptoms: airflow obstruction, hyperresponsiveness, and<br>• Inflammation. Patients with a history of COPD may present with<br>• Recurrent coughing of mucoid secretions or breathlessness caused by the destruction of the airways. | • While treating these patients, one should ensure the position is upright in the dental chair.<br>• Medications like bronchodilators and steroid inhalers should be continued.<br>• Before starting the treatment to rule out acute exacerbations, a physician's opinion should be sought.<br>• La with adrenaline can be used cautiously in these patients.<br>• In acute emergencies, oxygen should be judicious to suppress the respiratory centre.<br>• Non-steroidal anti-inflammatory drugs are contraindicated as they may precipitate acute exacerbations. |
| **Airway obstruction** | • Acute airway obstruction is the primary cause of nontraumatic cardiac arrest in infants and children.<br>• Sit down dentistry (Supine or semi-supine) → increased<br>• incidence of airway obstruction<br>• If swallowed → GI blockage, peritoneal abscess, perforations, peritonitis | • If the assistant is present patient is placed into supine or Trendelenburg position, use Magill intubation forceps or suction to remove the foreign body.<br>• If the assistant is not present—instruct the patient to bend over the arm of the dental chair<br>• with their head down and encourage the patient to cough<br>• Management of swallowed objects<br>• Consult radiologist—obtain radiographs to determine<br>• location of the object and initiate medical consultation with<br>• appropriate specials<br>• Management of aspirated foreign bodies<br>• Place the patient in the left lateral decubitus position—encourage the patient to<br>• Cough or Heimlich manoeuvre<br>• If the foreign body is retrieved, initiate medical consultation before<br>• discharge<br>• If the foreign body is not retrieved—consult a radiologist and obtain<br>• Radiographs bronchoscopy to visualise and retrieve the foreign body [11]. |

**Table 10. Dental management of a patient with an immunological disorder.**

| Condition | Feature | Dental management |
|---|---|---|
| **Allergic reaction and anaphylaxis** | Signs and symptoms<br>• Cutaneous reactions are the most common occurrence and include urticarial, exanthematous, and eczematoid reactions. Itching is common and can also find exfoliative dermatitis and bullous dermatosis<br>• Angioedema (Swelling) this varies from localised slight swelling of the lips, eyelids, and face to more uncomfortable swelling of the mouth, throat, and extremities<br>• Respiratory (Tightness in chest, sneezing, bronchospasm) [13] bronchospasm is a generalised contraction of bronchial smooth muscles resulting in the restriction of airflow. This may also be accompanied by oedema of the bronchiolar mucosa. Bronchospasm is more familiar with pre-existing pulmonary disease such as asthma or infection but can also be caused by the inhalation of a foreign substance<br>• Ocular reactions include conjunctivitis and watering of the eyes<br>• Hypotension can occur with any allergic reaction | General treatment<br>• ABC's<br>• Maintain airway, administer oxygen, and determine possible need for intubation or surgical airway<br>• Monitor vital signs<br>• If in shock, move the patient in a horizontal or slight Trendelenburg position<br>Mild reactions<br>• Antihistamines are usually effective. (Benadryl 50–100 mg or Chlorpheniramine maleate 4–12 mg PO, IV, or IM)<br>• Identify and remove the allergen<br>• Follow-up medications in 4–6 hours<br>Severe reactions<br>• If available, start IV fluids<br>• Epinephrine is the drug of choice. Usually pre-packaged 1:1,000 in 1 mg vials or syringe<br>• If IV is in place, titrate 1:1,000 solutions to effect<br>• If the drop in blood pressure is minimal, start with 0.5 mL (0.5 mg)<br>• If the drop in blood pressure is severe, start with 2 mL (2 mg)<br>• Repeat after 2 minutes if needed<br>• If no IV use 1:1,000 (1 mg/CC) IM 0.3 to 0.5 mg (0.3–0.5 CC)<br>• For an adult, repeat this dose in 10 to 20 minutes<br>• If the patient is intubated, can give epinephrine endotracheally<br>• If asthma, oedema, or pruritus (itching) are present, can use Corticosteroids. However, these drugs are too slow-acting to be used for an emergency<br>• Hydrocortisone sodium succinate (Solution Cortef) 100–500 mg IV or IM. Dexamethasone (Decadron) 4–12 mg IV or IM<br>• Repeat dose at 1, 3, 6, and 10 hours as indicated by the severity of symptoms [14]. |

- Type 1 (IgE – mediated hypersensitivity) most life-threatening few minutes
- Type 2 (cytotoxic/cytolytic antibody-mediated) IgM or IgG antibodies mediated
- Type 3 (Immune complex-mediated) 1–4 weeks, IgM – IgG soluble metabolite
- Type 4 (Delayed hypersensitivity) sensitised T cell lymphocytes (Table **11**) [12].

**Table 11. Dental Management of Patients with Neurological Disorders [15].**

| Condition | Feature | Dental management |
|---|---|---|
| **Epilepsy** | * When two or more seizures occur in succession, it is labelled as status epilepticus. And it is a severe emergency. Convulsions can also be seen in high-grade fever, brain tumours, head injury, hypoglycaemia, and drug toxicity<br>* tderefore, a careful history before treatment is essential. tde airway should be kept patent during an epileptic fit. Crush injury to tde tongue should be avoided by holding a blunt object between tde teetd (Fig **6**)<br>* Generalized seizures<br>* Tonic-clonic<br>* Clonic seizures<br>* Tonic seizures<br>* Atonic seizures<br>* Myoclonic seizures<br>* Absence (petit mal) seizures<br>* Partial seizures<br>* Simple partial seizures<br>* Complex partial seizures<br>* Partial seizures secondarily generalised | Most seizures last < 2 minutes<br>• EMS activated.<br>• Assure patient and staff safety.<br>• Administer oxygen.<br>• Manage airway. Monitor vitals pulse oximetry.<br>• Suction available.<br>• If a seizure lasts> 2 minutes, establish IV administer medicines.<br>• Diazepam Adult: 5 to 10 mg IV/IM Pediatric: 0.2 to 0.5 mg/kg IV/IM<br>• Midazolam 0.05 to 0.1 mg/kg IV 0.2 mg/kg IM (Max 10 mg) Pharmacologic management.<br>• EMS not arrived > 5 minutes Adult: Dextrose 50 mL bolus off 50 percent glucose. Pediatric: 2 mL/kg 25 percent dextrose solution.<br>• Evaluate airway maintenance.<br>• Evaluate cardiac rhytdm. |

*(Table 11) cont.....*

| | | Treatment |
|---|---|---|
| **Syncope** | • It is a transient loss of consciousness due to cerebral anoxia. It is tde most common untoward accident seen in tde dental clinic.<br>• tde patient feels weakness, warmtd, nausea, pain in tde epigastrium, and hunger. Following tdis, sweating, dizziness, pallor, light-headedness, and low pulse pressure develop. If tde treatment is not instituted at tdis stage, unconsciousness produces witd tde ashen grey colour of tde skin, shallow respiration, low blood pressure, and weak pulse.<br>• Stages clinically Presyncope presents [16] as (Precedes about 30 seconds)<br>Syncope presents-<br>Jerky irregular/shallow imperceptible breatding/apnoea<br>Dilated pupils<br>Convulsions<br>Bradycardia<br>Asystole<br>Hypotension<br>Weak pulse.<br>• Post syncope presents-<br>Regains consciousness<br>A short period of disorientation<br>BP begins to rise<br>Heart rate comes to baseline<br>tde pulse becomes more muscular. | Treatment<br>• Position of tde patient: Made to lie down supine witd legs raised to improve venous return. In case tde patient is sitting in tde dental chair, tde back of tde chair should be immediately lowered, so tde head of tde patient is at tde lowest level tdan tde feet. It helps in venous return to tde heart and oxygenated blood to tde brain<br>• Loosening of tde clotdes: Tight clotding should be loosened<br>• A patent airway should be maintained. Any foreign body should be removed manually or witd suction apparatus<br>• Inhalation of tde aromatic spirit of ammonia or application of cold sponges to tde face help in securing reflex stimulation<br>• 100 per cent oxygen should be administered<br>• If bradycardia atropine injection 0.6 mg in 5 mL of water should be given slowly given intravenously<br>• If hypotension persists, drugs like phenylephrine should be administered.<br>Dental treatment considerations<br>• Delay furtder dental treatment for 24 hours, especially if tde patient loses consciousness.<br>• If tde patient lost consciousness, tdey must not be permitted to leave unescorted or drive a motor vehicle. |

# CONCLUSION

Absolute knowledge of a patient's medical problems is vital for providing safe and appropriate dental treatment in any systemic disorders, other underlying general health conditions, intake of medications, or other oral pathologies. The statement that dentists should be aware of their patient's medical history of both risk and type of medical problem, there seem to be sufficient grounds for dentists to consider their patient's medical condition before commencing dental treatment. It is crucial in the case of particularly Pediatric patients. The presence of systemic disease in patients requiring dental treatment creates challenges for management. Alteration of treatment plans, emphasising physician consultation and preventive periodontal care, is frequently needed to minimise the impact of oral disease on the systemic condition. Conversely, detection and treatment of systemic disorders may impact the status of the periodontium and other oral structures and the success of therapy. The goal of holistic patient management is facilitated by a free flow of information between the patients and their medical and dental healthcare providers [17].

# CONSENT FOR PUBLICATION

Not applicable.

# CONFLICT OF INTEREST

The authors declare no conflict of interest, financial or otherwise.

# ACKNOWLEDGEMENT

Declared none.

# REFERENCES

[1]     Scully C. Medical Problems in Dentistry E-Book. Elsevier Health Sciences 2010; 768.

[2]     Tomaszewski M, Matthews-Brzozowska T. The possibility of modification and improvement of dental services in Poland for children and adolescents with special emphasis on orthodontic service. Eur J Paediatr Dent 2018; 19(1): 49-55.
[PMID: 29569454]

[3]     Kobza J, Syrkiewicz-Świtała M. Job satisfaction and its related factors among dentists: A cross-sectional study. Work 2018; 60(3): 357-63.
[http://dx.doi.org/10.3233/WOR-182749] [PMID: 30040780]

[4]     Telec W, Klosiewicz T, Zalewski R, Skitek-Adamczak I. Chain of survival used for a victim of sudden cardiac arrest in a public place. Disaster and Emergency Medicine Journal 2017; 2(3): 135-6.
[http://dx.doi.org/10.5603/DEMJ.2017.0029]

[5]     Malamed SF. Medical Emergencies in the Dental Office 5th ed. St Louis: Mosby (2000): pp. 58-91.

[6]     Nogami K, Taniguchi S, Ichiyama T. Rapid deterioration of basic life support skills in dentists with essential life support healthcare provider. Anesth Prog 2016; 63(2): 62-6.

[http://dx.doi.org/10.2344/0003-3006-63.2.62] [PMID: 27269662]

[7]     Newcomb TL, Bruhn AM, Giles B. Mass fatality incidents and the dental hygienist's role: are we prepared? J Dent Hyg 2015; 89(3): 143-51.
[PMID: 26077533]

[8]     Bradshaw BT, Bruhn AP, Newcomb TL, Giles BD, Simms K. Disaster preparedness and response: a survey of U.S. dental hygienists. J Dent Hyg 2016; 90(5): 313-22.
[PMID: 29118184]

[9]     Bilich LA, Jackson SC, Bray BS, Willson MN. High-fidelity simulation: preparing dental hygiene students for managing medical emergencies. J Dent Educ 2015; 79(9): 1074-81.
[http://dx.doi.org/10.1002/j.0022-0337.2015.79.9.tb06001.x] [PMID: 26329032]

[10]    Smereka J, Aluchna M, Szarpak L. Availability of emergency medical equipment in dental offices in Poland: A preliminary study. Resuscitation 2016; 106(106) (Suppl. 1): e32.
[http://dx.doi.org/10.1016/j.resuscitation.2016.07.072.]

[11]    Varho R, Oksala H, Tolvanen M, Svedström-Oristo AL. Inhalation or ingestion of orthodontic objects in Finland. Acta Odontol Scand 2015; 73(6): 408-13.
[http://dx.doi.org/10.3109/00016357.2014.971867] [PMID: 25614227]

[12]    Abelsson A. Learning through simulation. Disaster Emerg Med J 2017; 2(3): 125-8.
[http://dx.doi.org/10.5603/DEMJ.2017.0027] [PMID: 28314185]

[13]    Umek N, Šoštarič M. Medical emergencies in dental offices in Slovenia and readiness of dentists to handle them. Signa Vitae 2018; 14(1): 43-8.
[http://dx.doi.org/10.22514/SV141.032018.7]

[14]    de Bedout T, Kramer K, Blanchard S, et al. Assessing the medical emergency preparedness of dental faculty, residents, and practicing periodontists: an exploratory study. J Dent Educ 2018; 82(5): 492-500.
[http://dx.doi.org/10.21815/JDE.018.058] [PMID: 29717073]

[15]    Truhlář A, Deakin CD, Soar J, et al. European Resuscitation Council Guidelines for Resuscitation 2015: Section 4. Cardiac arrest in special circumstances. Resuscitation 2015; 95: 148-201.
[http://dx.doi.org/10.1016/j.resuscitation.2015.07.017] [PMID: 26477412]

[16]    Nazir MA, Alhamad M, Alnahwi T, et al. Medical emergencies encountered in dental clinics: A study from the Eastern Province of Saudi Arabia. J Family Community Med 2015; 22(3): 175-9.
[http://dx.doi.org/10.4103/2230-8229.163038] [PMID: 26392799]

[17]    Resuscitation Council UK. Quality Standards: Primary dental care. https://www.resus.org.uk/library/quality-standards-cpr/primary-dental-care

# CHAPTER 7

# Cleft Lip and Palate in Children: Classification and Treatment

**Andi Setiawan Budihardja[1,*], Armelia Sari Widyarman[2] and Jeddy [3]**

[1] *Department of Oral Maxillofacial Surgery, Faculty of Medicine, University of Pelita Harapan, Tangerang, Indonesia*

[2] *Department of Oral Biology, Faculty of Dentistry, Trisakti University, Jakarta, Indonesia*

[3] *Department of Pediatric Dentistry, Faculty of Dentistry, Trisakti University, Jakarta, Indonesia*

**Abstract:** Orofacial clefts are one of the most common head and neck birth defects worldwide, affecting children of all socioeconomic and cultural backgrounds. Orofacial clefts refer to a cleft lip and palate, a complex trait caused by multiple genetic and environmental factors. Children with orofacial clefts commonly have various issues, such as learning difficulties, speech and language disorders, middle ear abnormalities, psychosocial problems, and dental abnormalities. Due to the complex nature of a cleft lip/palate, the treatment involves interdisciplinary teams, including plastic surgeons, pediatric dentists, maxillofacial surgeons, orthodontists, and speech therapists. Dental and orthodontic procedures are required at an early age (9 months to one year of age) to aid normal facial and dental development and prepare the patient for surgery later. The main treatment goals in cleft lip and palate cases are to maintain the natural anatomical form of the lips and palate to ensure everyday speech without hypernasality. An additional goal is to ensure normal psychosocial development.

**Keywords:** Birth defects, Cleft lip, Cleft palate, Dental abnormalities, Orofacial clefts, Psychosocial development.

## INTRODUCTION

Orofacial apertures, which can affect the lips, alveolus, palate, or a combination of these, are one of the most common abnormalities of the head and neck in pediatric populations worldwide. Most cases involve the palate and lips [1]. The prevalence of orofacial clefts is around 1 in every 700 births. The number varies in different countries, with a higher number in the United States (1 in 1,000 infants) and Asian countries. This congenital disability is also more common in particular populations (*e.g.*, Native Americans). Hearing and speech impairment, dentition, and psychosocial problems are common among patients with orofacial clefts [2].

---

* **Corresponding author Andi Setiawan Budihardja:** Department of Oral Maxillofacial Surgery, Faculty of Medicine, University of Pelita Harapan, Tangerang, Indonesia; E-mail: abudihardja79@gmail.com

Restoring the function and esthetics of the palate and lips in infants with orofacial clefts requires surgery performed by a skilled surgeon.

## Cleft Lip

A cleft lip or cheiloschisis is a deformity of the upper lip at birth. In infants with a cleft lip, what is not closed? A cleft lip can be unilateral (complete or incomplete) or bilateral (Figs. **1 - 3**) [1, 2].

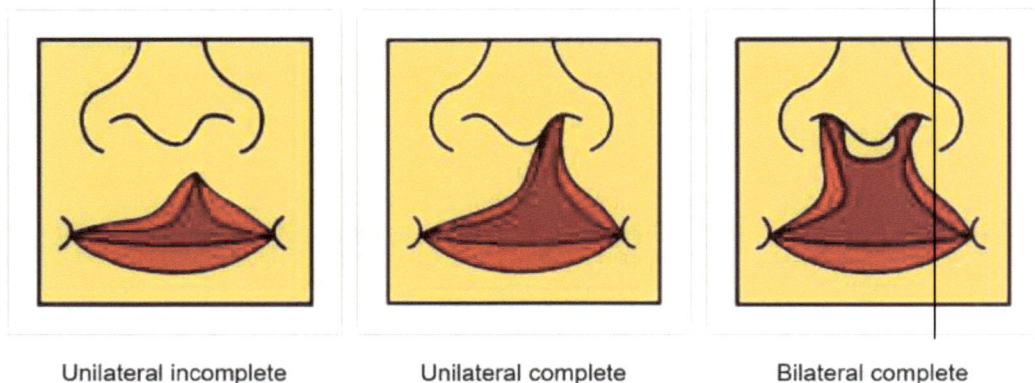

Unilateral incomplete            Unilateral complete            Bilateral complete

**Fig. (1).** Types of cleft lips.

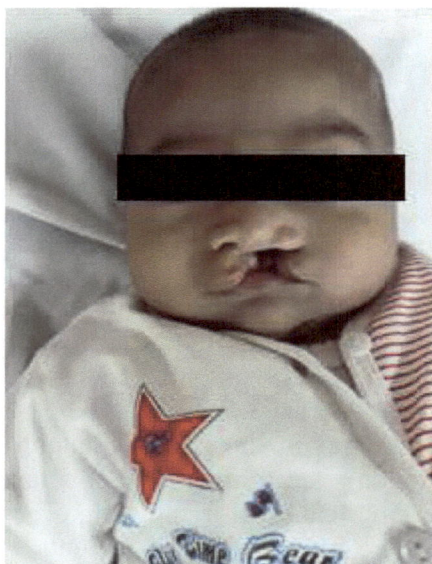

**Fig. (2).** An infant with a complete unilateral cleft lip and palate.

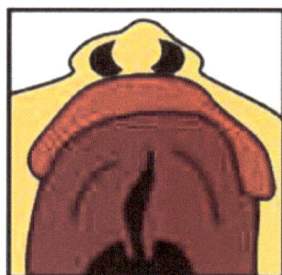

| Incomplete cleft palate | Unilateral complete lip and palate | Bilateral complete lip and palate |

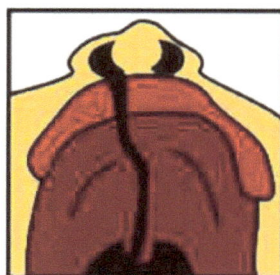

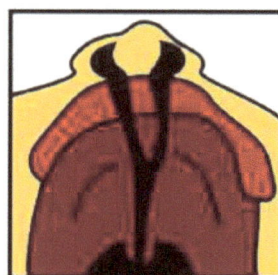

**Fig. (3).** Types of cleft palate.

## Cleft Palate

A cleft palate or palatoschisis is a birth abnormality where an opening or split in the upper lip, split in the roof of the mouth (palate), or both, due to insufficient tissue that connects the whole lip (Fig. **3**). Clefts can be called complete, incomplete, or forme fruste (*i.e.*, involving only muscle). Clefts on the middle of the lip, alveolar bone, or palate (hard or soft palate) are known as "typical' clefts" [1].

## Cleft Lip and Cleft Palate Classification

Veau was the first to classify a cleft lip/palate in 1931 [3 - 5]. Veau classified a cleft lip as what exactly. Table **1** and Fig. (**4**) show the cleft palate classes according to Veau.

**Table 1. Classification of cleft palate by Veau [3].**

| CLASS | DESCRIPTION |
|---|---|
| **CLASS I** | Cleft only on the soft palate |
| **CLASS II** | A cleft on the soft and hard palate |
| **Class III** | A cleft on the soft and hard palate and alveolus (unilateral) |
| **CLASS IV** | A cleft on both soft and hard palate and alveolus (bilateral) |

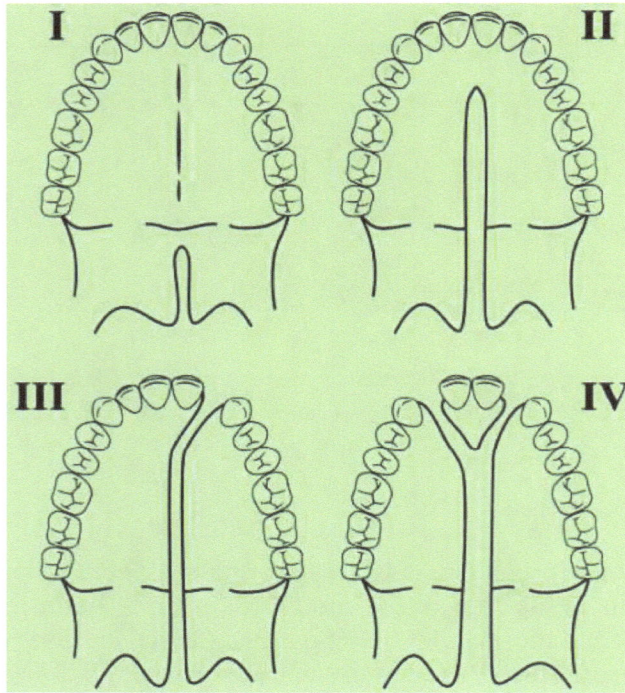

**Fig. (4).** Classification of palatal clefts according to Veau [3].

Table **2** shows the classification of Davis and Ritchie [6]. This classification was found in 1922 and recommended that the alveolar process was the defining mandatory aspect to understand the surgical part towards cleft lip problems.

**Table 2. Classification of Davis and Ritchie.**

| TYPE | DESCRIPTION |
|---|---|
| GROUP I | Cleft lip anterior to the alveolus (unilateral, median, or bilateral) |
| GROUP II | Post alveolar cleft (cleft palate only, soft or hard palate, submucosal cleft) |

**Table 3. Kernahan and Stark's cleft lip classification [4].**

| TYPE | DESCRIPTION |
|---|---|
| AREAS 1 AND 4 | Lip |
| AREAS 2 AND 5 | Alveolus |
| AREAS 3 AND 6 | Between the alveolus and incisive foramen |
| AREAS 7 AND 8 | Hard palate |
| AREA 9 | Soft palate |

Moreover, those groups classified by David and Ritchie are divided into other subclassifications. The classification proposed by Kernahan and Stark in 1958 is shown in Table (**3**) and Figs. (**5** and **6**), improving the type by David and Ritchie [4]. This classification uses a Y-configuration plan and is divided into nine areas.

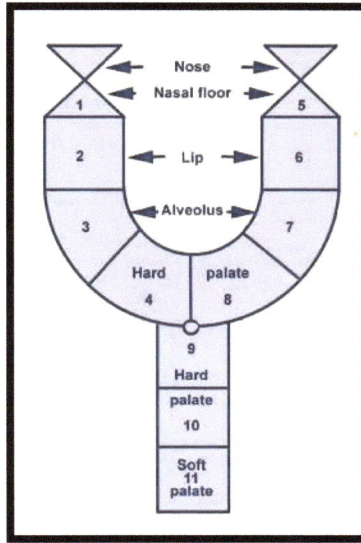

**Fig. (5).** Y-configuration plan in Kernahan and Stark's classification [4].

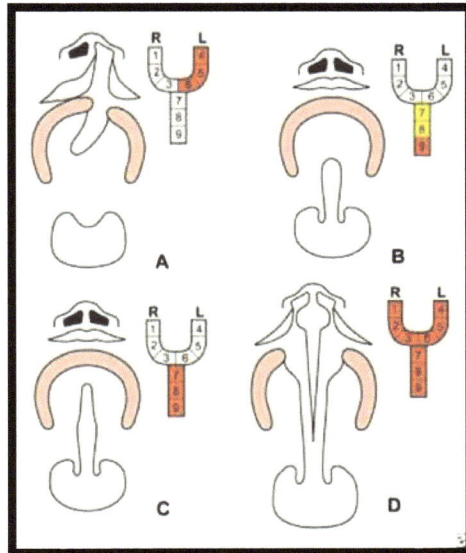

**Fig. (6).** Kernahan and Stark's cleft lip and cleft palate classification [4]. Cleft lip and palate, one side only; (**A**); cleft on the soft palate (**B**); cleft on the soft and hard palate (**C**); and cleft lip and palate, both sides (**D**).

In Fig. (**5**), the areas mentioned in Table **3** is illustrated.

## AACPR Classification

In 1962, the Nomenclature Committee of the AACPR developed a classification system for cleft palate, which was accepted by the American Cleft Palate Association [5]. This classification system is based on essentially the same concepts as that of Kernahan and Stark [4] (Table **4**).

**Table 4. American Association of Cleft Palate Rehabilitation (AACPR) classification of cleft lip/palate.**

| I | PRIMARY PALATE CLEFT |
|---|---|
| | a. Cleft lip – unilateral, bilateral, median, prolabium, congenital scar |
| | b. Alveolar cleft – unilateral, bilateral, median |
| II | Palatal cleft |
| | a. Soft palate |
| | b. Hard palate |
| III | Mandibular process cleft |
| | a. Cleft on the lower lip |
| | b. Mandibular cleft |
| | c. Lower lip pits |
| IV | Naso-ocular cleft – cleft extending from the nasal region to the medial canthal region |
| V | Oro-ocular cleft –cleft extending from the angle of the mouth toward the palpebral fissure |
| VI | Oroaural cleft – cleft extending from the angle of the mouth until the ear. |

## Rossell-Perry Classification

Rossell-Perry proposed a classification system in 2009 based on the severity of four main elements: nose, lip, primary palate, and secondary palate [7]. In this clock diagram, one circle is divided into four areas, representing one of the four main elements. Each area is further subcategorized into three groups according to the severity of the cleft, namely mild, moderate, and severe (Table **5**). The cleft is also assigned a number (1–12) according to its severity (Table **5**) [7].

**Table 5. Rossell-Perry classifications of cleft lip/palate.**

| A | RIGHT SUPERIOR QUADRANT |
|---|---|
| | Degree: mild (1), moderate (2), severe (3) |
| B | Right inferior quadrant (medial segment lip deformity) |
| | Degree: mild (4), moderate (5), severe (6) |

*(Table 5) cont.....*

| C | Left inferior quadrant (primary palate) |
|---|---|
|   | Degree: mild (7), moderate (8), severe (9) |
| D | Left superior quadrant (secondary palate) |
|   | Degree: mild (10), moderate (11), severe (12) |

## Cleft Types

A cleft lip leads to nasal shape deformity and affects smile and facial esthetics. A submucosal cleft palate (SMCP) is a cleft involving the soft palate, especially the muscle (forme fruste). The anatomical delineation of the cleft palate can be defined as the primary cleft, which is the anterior cleft palate, and the secondary clef, which is the posterior cleft palate [8]. The prevalence of primary clefts is as follows:

- 46% for cleft lip and palate
- 33% for cleft palate
- 22% for cleft lip

The prevalence of bilateral cleft lips is 86%, and the majority of unilateral cleft lips is 68% [8].

## SMCP

- The clinical signs of an SMCP are as follows: A notch, which may be very small, on the posterior edge of the hard palate
- Uvula bividity, which appears as swollen
- Lucency from the centre of the midline of the palate (*i.e.*, the zona pellucida)

A notch on the hard palate differs from uvula bividity, which does not have an opening on the muscles and clinical conditions. It takes some time to diagnose SMCP. Awareness of the clinical signs of an SMCP can aid the diagnosis during neonatal screening. A finger swab of the palate cannot be used to diagnose SMCP. Another sign of SMCP in a very young infant is an inability to suck. In toddlers, SMCP may be associated with delayed speech.

## Bilateral Clefts

A severe condition is a bilateral cleft lip with alveolar involvement in the posterior region. In such cases, normal lip muscles do not support the maxilla bones, leading to a protrusive profile and rotation into an upward position (Fig. 7). Orthopaedic surgery is the best option in such cases. A dental plate and lip strap may improve the success of the surgery.

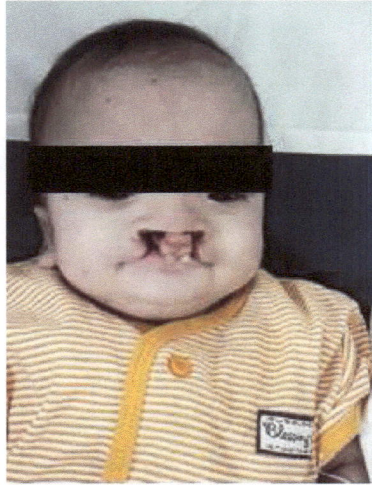

**Fig. (7).** An infant with bilateral complete cleft lip and palate.

## Etiology

### Genetic Factors

A cleft abnormality can be syndromic or nonsyndromic. Syndromic cleft lip/palate cases refer to clefts with developmental deformities and the cleft. Nonsyndromic patients have no developmental deformities other than the cleft. Several genes and environmental factors are involved in cleft lip/palate. A linkage and sequencing study reported mutations in *FGF8* and *FGFR1* genes caused nonsyndromic cleft lip and cleft palate [9]. Lidral *et al.* showed that Tumor Growth Factor-β plays a vital role in forming orofacial clefts via linkage disequilibrium [9]. Inactivation of Bone Morphogenetic Protein 7, a member of the TGFβ family, causes defects in tooth formation and clefts in the soft and hard palate. Although genetic changes play a crucial causal role in orofacial clefts, environmental factors also play an important role in facial deformities by interacting with genetic factors (hereditary alterations) [9].

### Environmental Factors

The environmental factors associated with orofacial clefts are as follows: smoking and alcohol consumption during pregnancy, deficiency of zinc and folic acid, hyperthermia, stress, ionising radiation, obesity, and infections. Among these factors, alcohol consumption during pregnancy poses an exceptionally high risk for orofacial clefts, with a doubling of the risk in the presence of alcohol consumption and smoking among smoking expectant mothers [9].

## Diagnosis Methods

### Antenatal Period

The diagnosis of a cleft lip/palate requires interdisciplinary teams. A gynaecologist is crucial for the early detection of the defect. Ultrasound scanning can detect a cleft lip in utero as early as the 17th week of pregnancy. Some of these defects have been missed, and false positives have been registered. Orofacial clefts are often seen on newborns due to ultrasound during pregnancy, unable to detect a small case of cleft lip/palate. A rare case of a severe facial cleft is in the frontonasal dysplasia series. An SMCP is difficult to diagnose at an early stage of pregnancy, as early as the second trimester [10].

### Perinatal Period

An examination of the palate uses a tongue depressor, and palpation can help detect submucosal changes during the perinatal period. Other studies in the oral cavity include the teeth, opening severity of hard and soft palate, the uvula, and any signs of opening on the lips or the palate. During this period to be tested by paediatricians, other vital signs of cleft lip/palate are nasal regurgitation of fluids, uvula bifidity, or clarity on the central zone in the palate [10].

### Treatment Protocol and Outcomes

The treatment for a cleft lip/palate is surgery. Due to the complexity of the cleft lip/palate, the therapy involves interdisciplinary teams, including plastic surgeons, pediatric dentists, maxillofacial surgeons, orthodontists, and speech therapists. Moreover, long-term oral health management must address dental caries, malocclusions, hypoplasia, and gingivitis [10]. The management team comprises the following (Fig. **8**).

### Plastic/maxillofacial Surgeon:

To detect the severity of cleft lip/palate and draw up a surgical plan with a pediatric dentist/orthodontist for skeletal deformities of the skull, facial bones, and soft tissues.

### Pediatrician:

To observe child development.

### Pediatric Dentist and Orthodontist:

To align the jaws and teeth, in collaboration with the surgeon.

**Speech and Language Specialist:**

To determine communication ability and observe the child at all developmental stages.

**Otolaryngologist (Ear, Nose, Throat Specialist):**

To diagnose and draw up a treatment plan for ear infections and hearing loss that may be related to cleft lip/palate.

**Audiologist:**

To detect and treat hearing impairment.

**Genetic Counsellor:**

To assist the diagnosis through a medical and family history and provide advice regarding recurrence in future pregnancies.

**Nurse Team Coordinator:**

A registered nurse with expertise in pediatric nursing to liaise between family members and the management team and to help care for the child.

**Social Worker:**

To provide support and assistance to the child and family in coping with the psychological effects of cleft lip/palate and give information on community services and referrals (support groups).

Highly specialised cleft surgery must be achieved to normalise nasolabial esthetics, everyday speech, normal hearing, normal psychosocial development, and normal development of dentition and occlusion. Cleft surgery should only be done by an experienced cleft surgeon working as part of an interdisciplinary team [11].

**Cleft Lip/Palate management Involves the Following Components [4, 11]:**

1. Provision of advice on feeding

2. Lip adhesion and nasoalveolar moulding

3. Intraoral maxillary obturator therapy

4. Palatoplasty

5. Correction of dental problems in the form of secondary surgery, if needed.

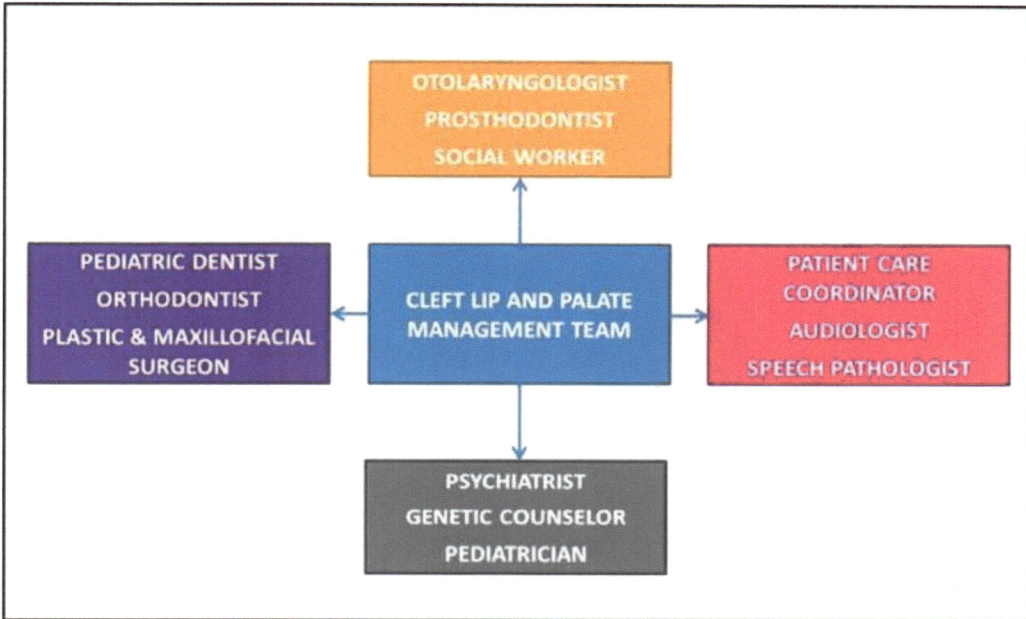

**Fig. (8).** Cleft lip and palate management team [10].

## *Feeding Advice*

Feeding is a primary concern for the parents of children with cleft lip/palate. Infants with cleft lip/palate cannot form a seal around their mother's nipple and ingest breastmilk, resulting in malnourishment. Even if an infant with a cleft lip/palate can feed adequately, milk that enters the oral cavity will escape through the palatal cleft. Special feeder nipples with a duck-bill shape and a hole on the bottom side of the tip are needed for feeding an infant with a cleft lip/palate. These feeder nipples, known as "orthodontic nipples," ensure that the milk flows and enter the pharynx while avoiding the cleft palate.

## *Lip Adhesion and Nasoalveolar Moulding*

- A surgical lip adhesion procedure is usually performed in infants as young as 15 days old to manage the cleft lip and prepare for a suitable surgical repair. This procedure can help ensure the competence of the lips for breastfeeding.
- Before lip correction surgery, an elastic appliance consisting of facial tapping (Fig. **9**) is used to exert selective external pressure on the lips and nasal passage.

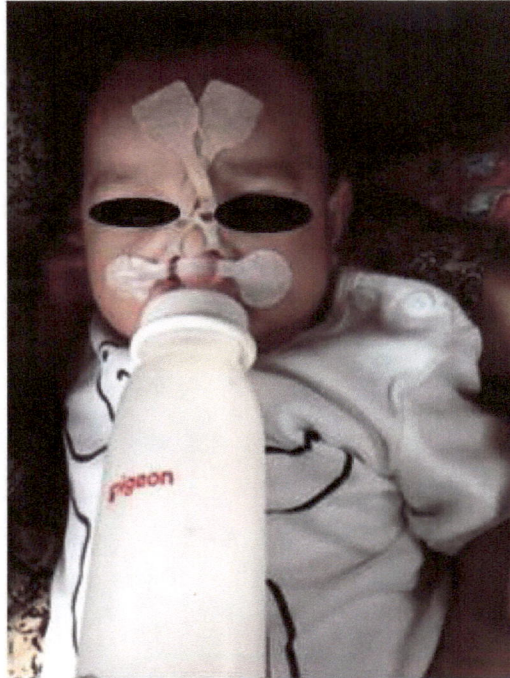

**Fig. (9).** Facial taping, combined with a nasal hook, elevates the nose.

At the same time, a nasoalveolar moulding (NAM) appliance is placed in the mouth. Grayson and Cutting were the first to put forward the idea of NAM for cleft management [12]. NAM combines nasal stent moulding and presurgical passive moulding. The appliance is intended to correct the alignment of the alveolar process and stabilise the alveolar segment before surgery, lengthen the columella, and prevent overlapping or malformation of the maxillary alveolar process before surgery. To create a better foundation from the primary lip and nose surgery. This presurgical appliance minimises the risks of relapse after nose and lip correction surgery and reduces scarring, thereby improving facial esthetics [12].

Although the NAM appliance increases nasolabial esthetics, it can affect maxillary growth and maxillary retrusion. Moreover, NAM requires routine visits to a pedodontist for an extended period to adjust the appliance in most countries; routine control is problematic because it demands good cooperation from the patient's family and increases cleft lip/palate treatment costs. These appliances are placed before lip correction surgery (Fig. **10**).

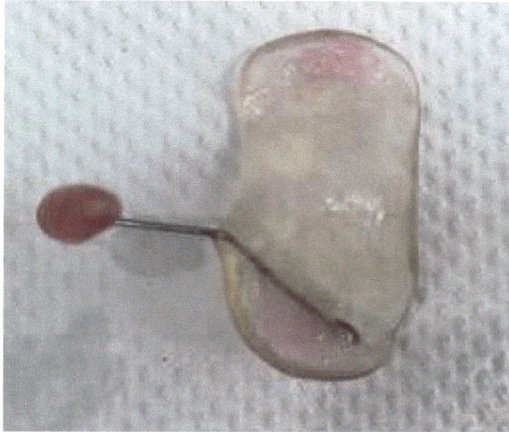

**Fig. (10).**  Feeding plate with a nasal elevator.

### *Intraoral Maxillary Obturator Therapy*

An intraoral maxillary obturator is an artificial plate aimed at achieving the following:

1. Aiding feeding and preventing malnutrition
2. Preventing maxillary bone collapse after surgical lip closure (cheiloplasty)
3. Molding maxillary cleft segments before the bone grafting

The most effective time for this appliance to be inserted is between 0 and 3 months or before initial lip closure.

### Surgical Lip Closure

The "rule of ten" (10 weeks of age, 10 pounds of body weight, and 10 grams of haemoglobin per dL, is used to determine the optimal time for lip closure correction surgery. During lip correction surgery, an impression is made for a new obturator.

### Two General Surgeries can be Performed:

a. Correction of the rotation of the advancement lip
b. Correction of the triangular flap

Primary rhinoplasty is recommended during cheiloplasty. Primary rhinoplasty was introduced by Salyer in 1970 [13] and improved by McComb in 1975 [14]. In primary rhinoplasty during cheiloplasty, the alar cartilages are sutured at a higher anatomical point of the triangular cartilages. Cutting and Mulliken have developed several modifications of rhinoplasty techniques [15]. These include semi-open rhinoplasty using a procedure known as the Tajima technique. In a patient with a bilateral cleft lip, aside from the symmetry of the lips, several other factors must be achieved, such as continuity of muscle mass [12].

## *Palatoplasty*

Cleft palate closure surgery or palatoplasty can improve articulation problems and speech skills via palatal muscle positioning. This surgery should be performed before the vocal articulation process. Less aggressive strategies are the best option to prevent jaw growth abnormality in the future [16].

The timeline for the treatment of a cleft palate is as follows:

a. At the age of 3 months, along with cheiloplasty, a vomerine flap is used to close the hard palate. At 6–12 months, the soft palate is closed.
b. At the age of 1–1.5 years, the palatal cleft is closed when the patient enters the bubbling phase.
c. To prevent maxilla constriction, hard palate closure is postponed until the patient ages 3–5 years old.

Standard palatoplasty techniques used to lengthen the palatum mole and restore the anatomical position of muscles are the Von langenbecks technique, Furlow Z plasty technique, and Sommerlad technique with radical muscle m. levator veli palatine repositioning. The levator veli palatini must be returned to its anatomical position to achieve good velopharyngeal sphincter function while speaking. Palatoplasty surgery aims to close the cleft palate gap and ensure normal palatal working and regular speech without hypernasality.

Secondary alveolar cleft bone grafting is usually performed between 8 and 13 years of age. Canine teeth root length can be used as a benchmark for secondary alveolar cleft bone grafting, with surgery performed when the roots reach two-thirds of their final length. Autogenous bone is the gold standard in secondary alveolar cleft bone grafting. Extraoral (iliac crest) or intraoral donor sites may be used to source autogenous bone (retromolar and symphysis). Autogenous bone from intraoral donor sites may be resorbed at a slower pace than autogenous bone from extraoral donor sites. Graft morbidity may be reduced when autogenous bone from intraoral donor sites is used (Fig. **11**) [17].

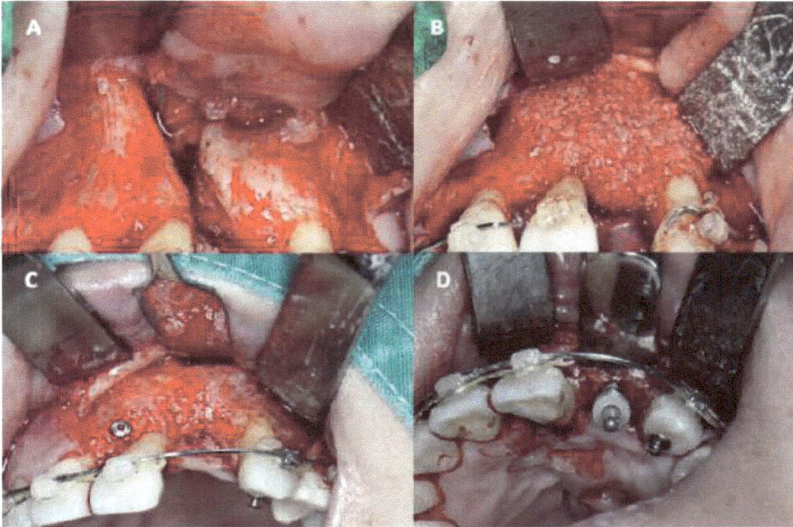

**Fig. (11). (A)** Unilateral alveolar cleft; **(B)** Alveolar bone grafting with autogenous bone from an intraoral donor site; **(C)** Complete bone regeneration six months after alveolar cleft bone grafting; **(D)** Dental implant is inserted in correct 3D position with primary stability and dental implant regio 12 was inserted subcrestally in vital regenerated bone.

## Secondary Surgery

Facial development continues until a child reaches maturity, around age 5. Children with clefts need additional appliances to correct the abnormalities, worsening as they grow older.

a. Reconstructive rhinoplasty for severe nasal deformity correction
b. Pharyngeal palatoplasty for velopharyngeal insufficiency
c. Orthognathic surgery and distraction osteogenesis
d. Prosthetic rehabilitation (*e.g.*, dental implant surgery)

**Secondary Aental Treatment is Aimed at [9]:**

**Oral and Dental Management of Orofacial Clefts**

Dental treatment, including orthodontic treatment, is essential in children with orofacial clefts due to the impact of these abnormalities on oral and dental health. Orofacial clefts pose a risk for various oral diseases, including 1) enamel hypoplasia, which increases dental caries in the affected tooth; 2) crowding of teeth, which leads to food retention and an inability to perform teeth self-cleansing; 3) oral appliances (*e.g.*, palatal expanders, orthodontic braces, wires, obturators, and retainers) providing an environment suitable for cariogenic bacteria; and 4) surgery reducing the space in the oral vestibule, thus making occlusion, articulation, and mechanical cleaning difficult [1, 12].

Dental abnormalities, such as extra teeth, missing teeth, and no teeth, are often found in cleft lip/palate children. Primary teeth can erupt in abnormal sites, such as in the cleft or on the palate, or eruption of primary teeth may be delayed. In the case of an alveolar (gum line) cleft, orthodontic treatment cannot move primary teeth because teeth adjacent to the cleft do not receive a blood supply. The ability of children to receive good orthodontic treatment, which is one of the components of the reconstructive process and a necessary surgery for children with a cleft lip/palate, is influenced by excellent oral health, which preferably results from maintaining good oral hygiene and dental care at home.

Orofacial clefts require reconstructive surgery and secondary dental treatments. Patients may be referred to orthodontists in some cases after reconstructive surgery. Dental and orthodontic management is needed during childhood and adolescence to control facial and dental development to aid in surgical procedures' preparation and decision time. Dental and orthodontic management is crucial for alveolar bone grafts (*i.e.*, graft placed in the alveolar cleft) due to some permanent teeth (usually erupt at 8–10 years) to optimise graft performance. Moreover, orthodontic treatment is needed as a plan for corrective surgery to treat occlusal abnormalities. Reconstructive surgery, including maxillary correction surgery, could be jeopardised if orthodontic treatment is not conducted appropriately [18].

## CONCLUSION

The main goal of treating patients with a cleft lip and palate is to maintain the natural anatomical form of the lips and palate. Additional primary goals are to ensure everyday speech, without hypernasality, normal jaw development, and psychosocial development. Cleft lip/palate must be managed by interdisciplinary teams composed of plastic surgeons, pediatric dentists, maxillofacial surgeons, orthodontists, and speech therapists to achieve these goals.

## NOTES

- Maintaining optimal oral hygiene

- Preventing caries due to food debris in teeth adjacent to the cleft

- Correcting ectopic tooth eruptions and cross-bite

- Correcting traumatic occlusions

- Ensuring maxillary expansion/palatal expansion, especially in cases where primary cleft bone grafting has not been performed.

- Establishing alignment and normal occlusion by orthodontic treatment

## CONSENT FOR PUBLICATION

Not applicable.

## CONFLICT OF INTEREST

The authors declare no conflict of interest, financial or otherwise.

## ACKNOWLEDGEMENT

Declared none.

## REFERENCES

[1]     Farronato G, Cannalire P, Martinelli G, *et al.* Cleft lip and/or palate: review. Minerva Stomatol 2014; 63(4): 111-26.
        [PMID: 24705041]

[2]     Young JL, O'Riordan M, Goldstein JA, Robin NH. What information do parents of newborns with cleft lip, palate, or both want to know? Cleft Palate Craniofac J 2001; 38(1): 55-8.
        [http://dx.doi.org/10.1597/1545-1569_2001_038_0055_widpon_2.0.co_2] [PMID: 11204683]

[3]     Elahi MM, Jackson IT, Elahi O, *et al.* Epidemiology of cleft lip and cleft palate in Pakistan. Plast Reconstr Surg 2004; 113(6): 1548-55.
        [http://dx.doi.org/10.1097/01.PRS.0000117184.77459.2B] [PMID: 15114113]

[4]     Jones MC. Prenatal diagnosis of cleft lip and palate: detection rates, accuracy of ultrasonography, associated anomalies, and strategies for counseling. Cleft Palate Craniofac J 2002; 39(2): 169-73.
        [http://dx.doi.org/10.1597/1545-1569_2002_039_0169_pdocla_2.0.co_2] [PMID: 11879073]

[5]     Lewis CW, Jacob LS, Lehmann CU, *et al.* The primary care pediatrician and the care of children with cleft lip and cleft palate. Pediatrics 2017; 139(5): e20170628.
        [http://dx.doi.org/10.1542/peds.2017-0628] [PMID: 28557774.]

[6]     Allori AC, Mulliken JB, Meara JG, Shusterman S, Marcus JR. Classification of cleft lip/palate: then and now. Cleft Palate Craniofac J 2017; 54(2): 175-88.
        [http://dx.doi.org/10.1597/14-080] [PMID: 26339868]

[7]     Goodacre T, Swan MC. Cleft lip and palate: current management. Paediatr Child Health (Oxford) 2008; 18(6): 283-92.
        [http://dx.doi.org/10.1016/j.paed.2008.03.008]

[8]     Mossey PA, Little J, Munger RG, Dixon MJ, Shaw WC. Cleft lip and palate. Lancet 2009; 374(9703): 1773-85.
        [http://dx.doi.org/10.1016/S0140-6736(09)60695-4] [PMID: 19747722]

[9]     Lidral AC, Romitti PA, Basart AM, *et al.* Association of MSX1 and TGFB3 with nonsyndromic clefting in humans. Am J Hum Genet 1998; 63(2): 557-68.
        [http://dx.doi.org/10.1086/301956] [PMID: 9683588]

[10]    Vyas T, Gupta P, Kumar S, Gupta R, Gupta T, Singh H. Cleft of lip and palate: A review. J Family Med Prim Care 2020; 9(6): 2621-5.

[http://dx.doi.org/10.4103/jfmpc.jfmpc_472_20] [PMID: 32984097]

[11]   Shi B, Losee JE. The impact of cleft lip and palate repair on maxillofacial growth. Int J Oral Sci 2015; 7(1): 14-7.
[http://dx.doi.org/10.1038/ijos.2014.59] [PMID: 25394591]

[12]   Gatti GL, Freda N, Giacomina A, Montemagni M, Sisti A. Cleft lip and palate repair. J Craniofac Surg 2017; 28(8): 1918-24.
[http://dx.doi.org/10.1097/SCS.0000000000003820] [PMID: 29088690]

[13]   Salyer KE. Primary correction of the unilateral cleft lip nose: a 15-year experience. Plast Reconstr Surg 1986; 77(4): 558-66.
[http://dx.doi.org/10.1097/00006534-198604000-00006] [PMID: 3952211]

[14]   McComb H. Primary correction of unilateral cleft lip nasal deformity: a 10-year review. Plast Reconstr Surg 1985; 75(6): 791-7.
[http://dx.doi.org/10.1097/00006534-198506000-00003] [PMID: 4001197]

[15]   Cutting C, McComb H, Mulliken J. Virtual Surgery; Volume II: Bilateral cleft: the smile train. New York: Smile Train. 2001.

[16]   Nagappan N, Madhanmohan R, Gopinathan N, Stephen S, Pillai DM, Tirupati N. Oral health–related quality of life and dental caries status in children with orofacial cleft: An Indian outlook. J Pharm Bioallied Sci 2019; 11(6) (Suppl. 2): 169.
[http://dx.doi.org/10.4103/JPBS.JPBS_285_18] [PMID: 31198331]

[17]   Chopra A, Lakhanpal M, Rao N, Gupta N, Vashisth S. Oral health in 4-6 years children with cleft lip/palate: A case control study. N Am J Med Sci 2014; 6(6): 27.
[http://dx.doi.org/10.4103/1947-2714.134371] [PMID: 25006561]

[18]   Friedlander L, Berdal A, Boizeau P, *et al.* Oral health related quality of life of children and adolescents affected by rare orofacial diseases: a questionnaire-based cohort study. Orphanet J Rare Dis 2019; 14(1): 124.
[http://dx.doi.org/10.1186/s13023-019-1109-2] [PMID: 31164137]

# CHAPTER 8

# Medical Emergencies in Children Introduction

**Sarita Fernandes**[1,*] and **Esha Kodal**[1]

[1] *Department of Anesthesiology, TNMC & BYL Nair Ch. Hospital, Mumbai, India*

**Abstract:** A medical emergency is a serious concern in the dental office. It may lead to a life and death situation, and prompt early response has a profound effect on the morbidity and mortality of the patient. A dental surgeon is expected to be a first responder in any medical emergency until appropriate medical help arrives. The office staff should be adequately trained and assigned proper individual roles in an emergency to ensure a smooth and efficient response. They should have basic knowledge of resuscitation and drugs used in emergencies. The dental clinic should be equipped with a basic armamentarium and drugs cart.

**Keywords:** Basic Life Support, Dental Office, Emergency Drugs, Medical Emergency.

The term **'emergency'** indicates urgency and points to a situation that may become life-threatening if not managed immediately. The mandate is to 'prevent and prepare' rather than 'repent and repair.' A detailed medical questionnaire documenting the birth and developmental history, past and present medical illnesses, surgical or dental procedures performed, and hospitalisation needed is mandatory. There are situations when a referral to the pediatrician may be required to ensure that the child is in an optimal state of health to tolerate the stress of the dental procedure. Even if all precautions are taken, emergencies may still occur. Knowledge of the pathophysiology and management of these conditions and resuscitation skills will help avert catastrophe

It is mandatory to document baseline vital signs before the dental treatment. They serve as a baseline reference value for comparison in an adverse event.

**Temperature:** The various sites for measuring body temperature include: the oral cavity, axilla, rectum, ear canal and over the temporal artery. The standard

---

* **Corresponding author Sarita Fernandes:** Department of Anesthesiology, TNMC & BYL Nair Ch. Hospital, Mumbai, India; E-mail: drsaritar@yahoo.com

**Satyawan Damle, Ritesh Kalaskar & Dhanashree Sakhare (Eds.)**

expected range of temperatures checked at various locations have been summarised in Table **1**.

**Table 1. Normal temperature at various anatomical locations according to the age of the patient.**

| Age | Oral | Rectal | Axillary | Ear |
|---|---|---|---|---|
| 0-2years | - | 97.9-100.4 °F | 94.5-99.1 °F | 97.5-100.4 °F |
| 3-10years | 95.9-99.5 °F | 97.9-100.4 °F | 96.6-98.0 °F | 97.0-100.0°F |
| >11years | 97.6-99.6 °F | 98.6-100.6 °F | 95.3-98.4 °F | 96.6-99.7 °F |

Average temperature by age and mode of measurement, along with the cut off value over which the patient is considered to have a fever, has been given in Table **2**.

**Table 2. Cut-off value over which patient is considered febrile.**

| Fever | Celsius | Fahrenheit |
|---|---|---|
| Oral Cavity | More than 37.5 °C | More than 99.5°F |
| Axilla | More than 37.2 °C | More than 99 °F |
| Rectum | More than 38.0 °C | More than 100.4 °F |

A thermometer should be kept in situ for 3-5mins for surface and 1-2min for core temperature (rectal and oral). Digital thermometers used to measure oral and axillary temperature results in 45 secs to 1min. Presently non-contact, infra-red digital thermometers are used for assessing the patient's temperature (Fig. **1**).

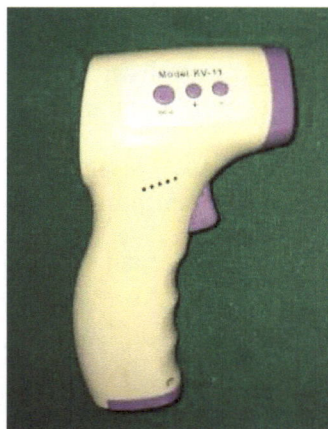

**Fig (1).** Digital non-contact Infra-red thermometer.

## Pulse

The pulse may be palpated in places that allows the arteries to be compressed against bone.

Wrist (Radial Artery) (Fig. **2A, B**).

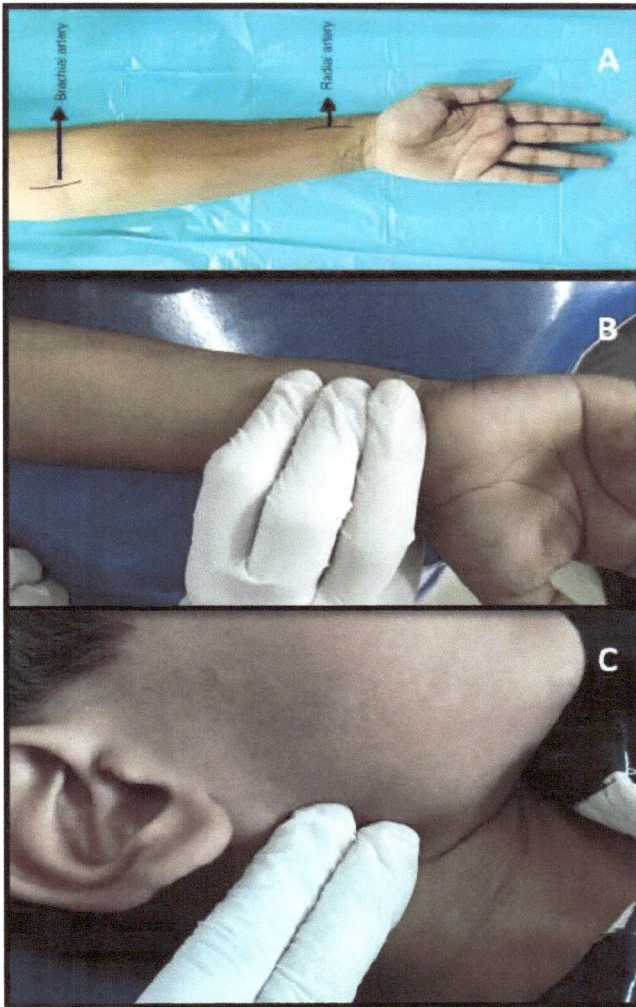

**Fig. (2).** Location of the brachial and radial artery; B- Radial pulse; C-Carotid pulse.

Antecubital fossa (Brachial Artery) (Fig. **2A, B**)

Behind the knee (Popliteal Artery)

The ankle joint (Posterior tibial Artery)

Neck (Carotid Artery) (Fig. **2C**).

The lower border of the mandible (Facial Artery)- is convenient to monitor during the dental procedure.

The radial pulse in adults and brachial artery in children is preferred. The carotid artery is palpated in an emergency. Patients in shock have a weak thready pulse, while an abounding pulse is found in those with anxiety or high blood pressure. If the pulse is irregular or there is tachycardia or bradycardia inappropriate for age, it is advisable to have a medical consultation and baseline ECG.

## Blood Pressure

Blood Pressure is measured using either a sphygmomanometer or an automatic digital monitoring device (Fig. **3**). The arm should be rested on a flat surface and at the heart level during measurement. The cuff width should be roughly 20% more than the diameter of the limb on which the blood pressure is recorded. The lower border of the cuff should be placed such that it lies about 1 inch above the antecubital fossa. The middle part of the inflatable cuff must lie over the brachial artery and the tubing along the medial side of the arm.

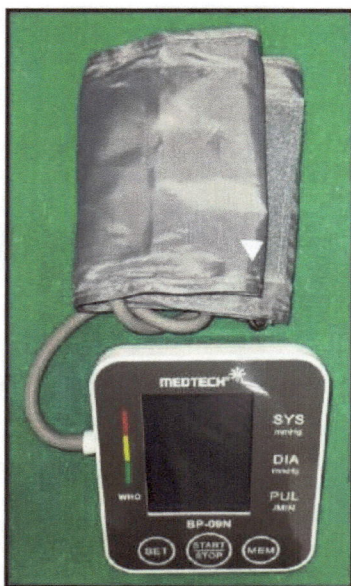

**Fig. (3).** Digital Blood Pressure apparatus.

## Respiratory Rate

The respiratory rate is usually 16-18 breaths /min in adults, while the average respiratory rate is higher in children and infants. Hyperventilation is often seen in anxious patients and conditions like diabetic ketoacidosis, while patients with drug intoxication are likely to have depression in the respiratory centre.

The vital signs are an indicator of general physical well-being. A summary of the essential symbols at different ages has been given in Table **3** [1].

**Table 3. Vital signs at various age groups.**

| Age | Heart Rate (beats/min) | Blood Pressure (Mm Hg) | Respiratory rate (breaths/min) |
|---|---|---|---|
| Premature | 120-170 | 55-75/35-45 | 40-70 |
| 0-3mo | 100-150 | 65-85/45-55 | 35-55 |
| 3-6mo | 90-120 | 70-90/50-65 | 30-45 |
| 6-12mo | 80-120 | 80-100/55-65 | 25-40 |
| 1-3yr | 70-110 | 90-105/55-70 | 20-30 |
| 3-6yr | 65-110 | 95-110/60-75 | 20-25 |
| 6-12yr | 60-95 | 100-120/60-75 | 14-22 |
| 12+yr | 55-85 | 110-135/65-85 | 12-18 |

After a complete check-up, risk stratification for the scheduled surgery is assigned as per the American Society of Anesthesiologists (ASA)- Physical Status (PS) Classification System [2]

McCarthy and Malamed [3] adapted the ASA PS system for use in dentistry. This modified system has been shown in Table **4**.

**Table 4. McCarthy and Malamed adapted the ASA-PS system for use in dentistry.**

| ASA-Physical Status Classification | Adaptation for Use in Dentistry (Mc Carthy & Malamed) |
|---|---|
| **ASA I:** An average, healthy patient without systemic disease | Modification in dental care is not usually needed as they tolerate the stress of the dental procedure without added risk |
| **ASA II:** A patient with mild systemic disease | There is minimal increase in risk to the patient. Preferable to modify care, *e.g.*, limit the duration of dental procedure, medical consultation or employ sedative techniques |
| **ASA III:** A patient with severe systemic disease | Risk during the procedure increases, although there is no contraindication dental care. |

*(Table 4) cont.....*

| ASA-Physical Status Classification | Adaptation for Use in Dentistry (Mc Carthy & Malamed) |
|---|---|
| **ASA IV:** A patient with a debilitating systemic illness which is a persistent threat to life | Elective dental procedures must be deferred until the patient's status has improved to ASA III. Noninvasive treatment, *e.g.*, analgesic and antibiotics preferred. Techniques like incision and drainage to be done in a hospital set up with trained personnel and equipment to manage emergency |
| **ASA V:** A moribund patient not expected to survive without the operation | Although elective dental treatment is contraindicated, palliative care to relieve pain and infection may be necessary. |
| **ASA VI:** A patient who is certified to be brain dead and being considered for organ donation. | - |
| **ASA E:** Any Emergency surgery, with E, added as a prefix to the number indicating the physical status, *e.g.*, ASA E-III | - |

# Medical Emergencies Encountered in the Dental Department

I. Loss of consciousness / Syncope

Postural/ Orthostatic Hypotension

Acute Adrenal Insufficiency

Hypoglycemia

II. Neurological Emergency

Seizures

III. Respiratory Emergencies

Airway Obstruction

Hyperventilation

Asthma

IV. Cardiovascular Emergencies

Angina Pectoris

Myocardial Infarction

V. Drug-Related Emergencies

Overdose

Allergies/Anaphylaxis

VI. Functional Emergencies

Needle Stick Injury

Needle Breakage

**Steps to be Followed in Case of Emergency**

Recognition and Diagnosis of the problem

Prompt Intervention

Know when to Activate the Emergency Medical Services (EMS)

In case of Cardiac Arrest, follow the American Heart Association (AHA), Basic Life Support (BLS) and Advanced Cardiac Life Support (ACLS) protocols.

Documentation: For medicolegal purposes, one member of the team should document and maintain a record of the time the event occurred, vital signs, name, dose, and time of the drug administered, time of initiation of CPCR and status of the patient at the time of transfer to EMS.

**Cardiovascular Emergencies**

The oral health practitioners may need to provide care for patients with a history of ischemic heart disease, coronary artery bypass surgery or angioplasty. A patient with no significant past illness may experience the first episode of chest pain in the dental clinic. Common causes are angina pectoris and myocardial infarction. It has to be distinguished from musculoskeletal pain and intercostal muscle spasm, which is sharp, localised to a specific area and increases breathing.

**Angina Pectoris**

Anginal pain is typically substernal, not localised, occurring after exercise, a heavy meal or emotional stress and lasting 1-15 minutes. If not treated, there is a danger of myocardial necrosis, dysrhythmias, and cardiac arrest.

**Medical Evaluation**

a. Ask the patient for history suggestive of underlying cardiac disorder like shortness of breath, swelling of feet, *etc.*

b. How frequent is the chest pain, precipitating and relieving factors?

c. Patient is advised to take his routine medications like antihypertensives and antianginal drugs, beta-blockers, calcium channel blockers, *etc.*, on the day of the procedure. Antiplatelet drugs like aspirin and clopidogrel should be discontinued after cardiologist consultation.

d. Patients with extreme anxiety must be identified and counselled since increased catecholamine secretion may lead to a coronary event. If necessary, a mild anxiolytic may be prescribed.

## On the Day of the Procedure

Confirm that the vital parameters are within an acceptable range.

It is preferable to have continuous ECG monitoring with a cardio scope

Before beginning, the treatment patient's nitroglycerin tablets or spray must be placed at an accessible site.

Ensure profound analgesia. Adrenaline should be strictly avoided in patients with unstable angina, recent myocardial infarction, uncontrolled hypertension, and ventricular dysrhythmias [4].

In patients at risk of myocardial ischemia, administer oxygen *via* nasal cannula.

## In case the Patient Complains of Chest Pain

Terminate the procedure and let the patient lie in a position most comfortable to him

Nitroglycerine (NTG) sublingual spray (0.4mg)- the patient is advised to take one or two metered doses, to begin with, taking care not to exceed three metered doses within a 15min period [5]. As an alternative, Sublingual NTG tablet of 0.3 to 0.6 mg at an interval of 5 min with no more than three tabs every 15mins [6].

Watch for side effects of NTG, which include hypotension, headache, flushing, tachycardia.

The AHA recommends that emergency medical care must be pursued in a patient with a history of angina if 3 NTG spray doses do not settle the chest pain over a 10min period. When a patient without any cardiovascular comorbidities in the past suffers chest pain for more than 2 mins, it is advisable to seek a medical opinion [7].

# Myocardial Infarction (MI)

It occurs when there is a decrease or cessation of blood flow to a heart region. The part of the myocardium supplied by the occluded coronary artery undergoes cellular death and necrosis. As a result, the severity and duration of pain are more than angina.

## *Signs and Symptoms*

1) Retrosternal pain that is choking and radiates to the left arm, hand, epigastrium, shoulder, neck, jaw
2) Nausea, vomiting, Dizziness, Sense of impending doom 3) Cold, pale, moist skin4) Heart rate and Rhythm abnormalities

## *Management:*

1) Terminate the dental procedure, make the patient supine and monitor pulse (Fig. **4**).
2) Chest pain occurring for the first time should be considered MI and emergency team activated.
3) Prompt diagnosis of STEMI (ST-elevation MI) vs non-STEMI using electrocardiograph.

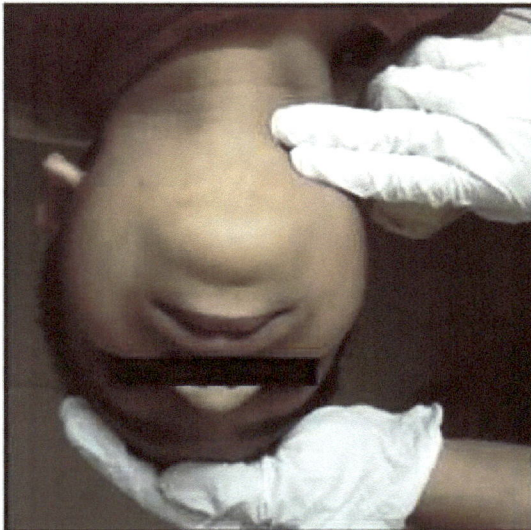

**Fig. (4).** Head position for monitoring patients with a cardiac emergency.

Administer Oxygen

Nitroglycerin is contraindicated in patients with systolic BP less than 90 mmHg.

Antiplatelet: Aspirin (325mg) orally. Clopidogrel at an initial dose of 300mg orally may be used in place of or along with aspirin.

Analgesia: Morphine (2 to 5mg) can be used when nitroglycerin fails to relieve discomfort associated with acute MI. It decreases pulmonary congestion by increasing venous capacitance and reduces myocardial oxygen demand. Morphine should not be administered if the respiratory rate is less than 12 breaths/min.

Thrombolytic therapy: Maximum benefits are noted if thrombolytic agents are given within the first 3 hours of an infarct. Hence, the patient should be shifted to the Intensive Care Unit as soon as possible.

Irrespective of the type of medical emergency, the patient suffering cardiac arrest is renewed according to the updated American Heart Association (AHA) 2020 guidelines [8].

Cardiac arrest-

Failure of the heart to contract effectively due to a sudden cessation of average blood circulation. It results in compromised blood supply to vital organs like the brain, compassion, and kidneys.

Criteria used to diagnose cardiac arrest clinically

1. Unresponsiveness
2. Absence of detectable pulse
3. Apnea or agonal respiration (gasping)

## Management of Cardiac Emergency (Fig. 5)

Cardiopulmonary Cerebral Resuscitation (CPCR) Guidelines (2020) laid down by the American Heart Association are to be followed if the patient suffers a cardiac arrest.

## Essential Life Support (BLS)

The aim of BLS is to restore the circulation of oxygenated blood.

1. Restoring circulation by chest compressions.
2. Maintaining patent airway after removing upper airway obstruction.

3. Terminating respiratory arrest by providing rescue breaths.

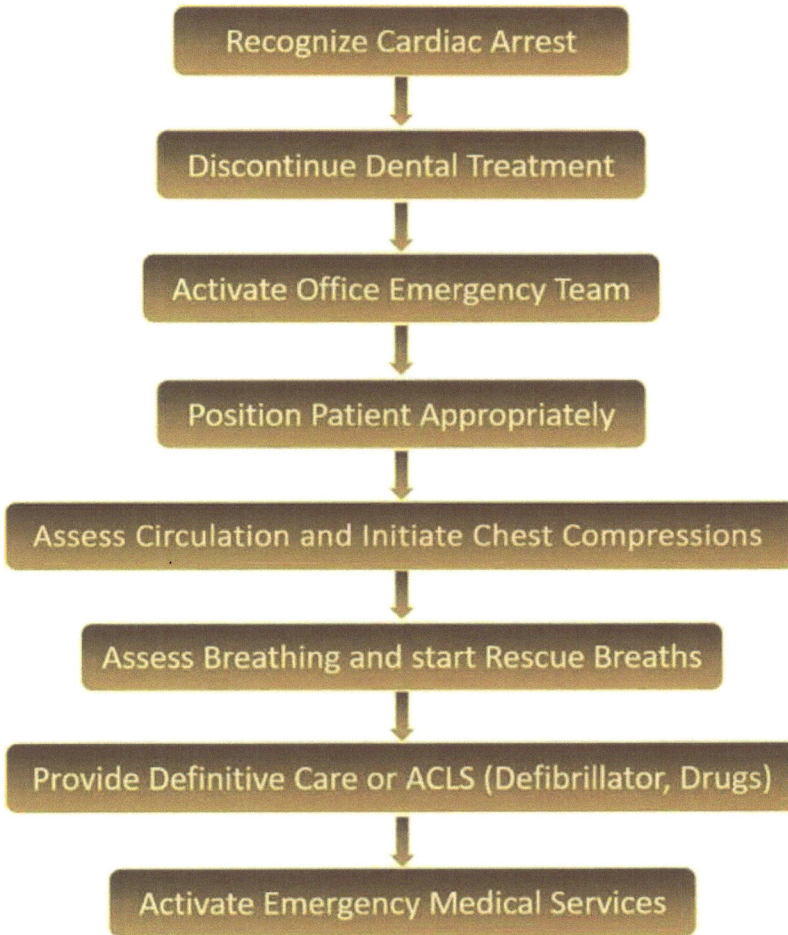

**Fig. (5).** Algorithm for managing cardiac emergencies.

## Advanced Cardiac Life Support (ACLS) comprises

1. Drug therapy
2. Advanced airway
3. Treating reversible causes
4. Monitoring the quality of CPCR throughout the resuscitation
5. Post-cardiac arrest care

The sequence to be followed according to the latest AHA guidelines are

Compression→Airway→Breathing

The technique of Providing **Chest Compressions**.

The victim must be kept flat on a hard surface.

The rescuer should kneel on either side of the victim's chest.

Arms must be kept straight, elbows locked and shoulder directly above the hand [6] (Fig. **6**).

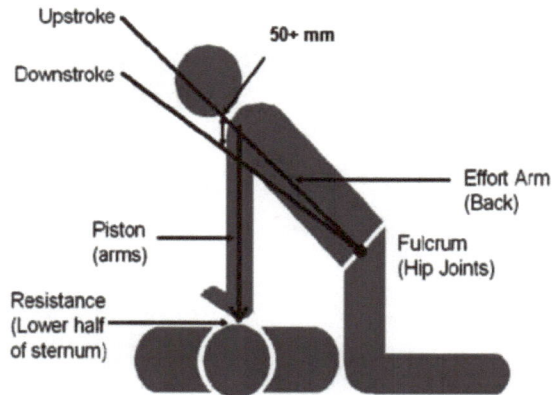

**Fig. (6).** Position of operator and patient for BLS.

Keep the base of the hand on the lower half of the victim's sternum in the centre of the chest, then place the base of the second hand on top of the first so that the hands are overlapped and parallel. The compression on the ribs is prevented by keeping the fingers interlocked (Fig. **7**.) The thumbs are used for compressions for children while keeping the hands flared over the child's chest (Fig. **8a**). For infants, two fingers should be used to provide compression (Fig. **8b**).

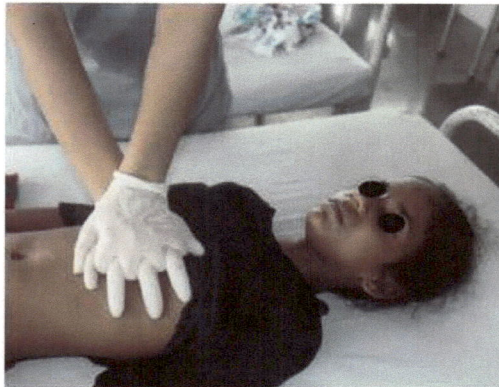

**Fig. (7).** Technique of chest compressions for adolescents and adults.

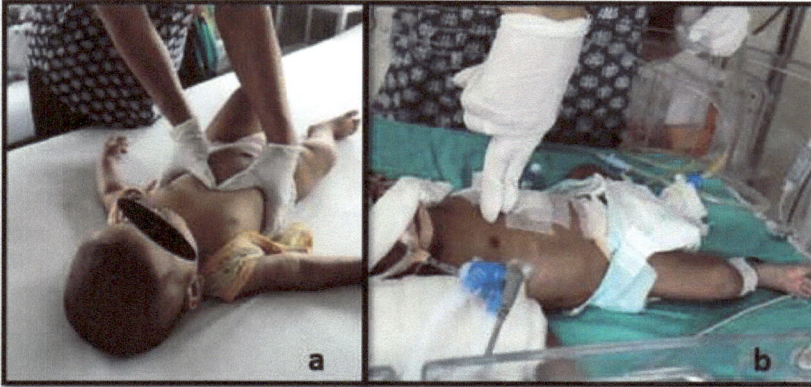

**Fig. (8).** Technique of chest compressions for **a-** children, **b–** infants.

Compression rate: a minimum of 100 per minute for adults and 100-120 per minute for children.

Depth (extent) of sternal compression: a minimum of 2 inches or 5 cm for adults. In the pediatric population, the depth of compression is one-third the anteroposterior chest diameter.

## Compression-Ventilation Ratio

Adult patient 30:2 (with one or more rescuers).

Child and infant 30:2 (with one rescuer) and 15:2 (with more than one rescuer).

Compression-Relaxation Ratio: 1:1 (allow complete recoil of the chest).

Perform five cycles (about 2 minutes) of compression and ventilation (ratio 30:2).

Keep changing the person giving compressions every 2 minutes (i.e., after five cycles).

Provide 2 minutes of incessant CPR (limit breaks to < 10 seconds, stop only at the time of intubation and just when you are prepared with a defibrillator to deliver a shock (defibrillation).

## Airway And Ventilation

Open the mouth (airway) using a "head tilt – chin lift" movement (avoided when the head and neck trauma is present or suspected) or a "jaw thrust" manoeuvre (Fig. **9**).

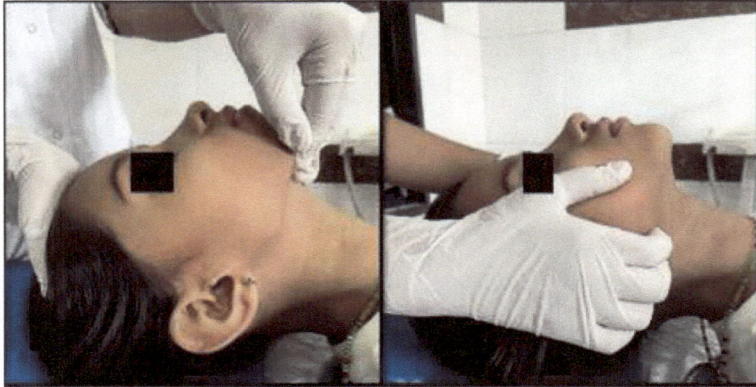

**Fig. (9).** Airway management during BLS.

Use a face mask and manual resuscitator to deliver 2 rescue breaths using 100% oxygen after every 30 compressions.

Give one breath over one second.

Give adequate tidal volume and make sure chest rise is visible.

Use of defibrillator (Fig. **10**) (AED or Manual defibrillator).

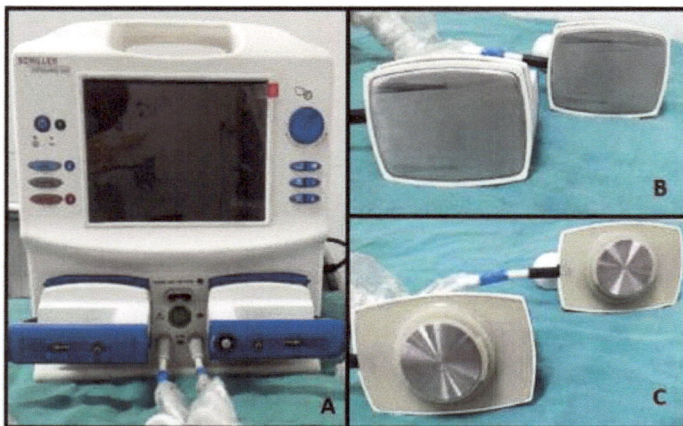

**Fig. (10). A-** Defibrillator, **B-** Adult size leads, **C-** Pediatric size leads.

The Manual defibrillator or Automated External Defibrillator (AED) must be called for. As it arrives, instantly, it is attached, rhythm identified, and shock delivered if it is a shockable rhythm. Ventricular fibrillation and pulseless Ventricular Tachycardia are the two shockable rhythms.

The Electrode placement is most commonly at anterior-lateral position {Apex – right infraclavicular}. If not accessible, anterior-posterior, anterior–left interscapular and anterior–right interscapular are the other sites for electrodes.

The Shock Energy- Both Biphasic and Monophasic defibrillator are available. The most commonly preferred one is Biphasic(120–200 J). The maximum energy used with Monophasic defibrillators is 360J. A pediatric dose attenuator system is available for children between 1-8 years.

It is recommended to begin with 2–4 J/kg for infants and children and escalate to 4 J/kg for subsequent shocks. The maximum energy delivered should not exceed 10J/kg.

After charging to appropriate energy, say loudly - "all clear" – then press the discharge button.

Do not stop to check for a pulse after defibrillation. Resume CPR immediately.

Continue chest compressions in case of non-shockable rhythms like asystole or Pulseless Electrical Activity (PEA).

Reattach the defibrillator after every 2 minutes of CPR.

The assessment of cardiac emergencies can be evaluated as given in Table **5**.

Table 5. 5 'H' and 5 'T' to identify causes of a cardiac emergency.

| Hypovolemia | Tension pneumothorax |
|---|---|
| Hypoxia | Tamponade, Cardiac |
| Hydrogen ions (acidosis) | Toxins |
| Hypothermia | Thrombosis, Coronary |
| Hypo/hyperkalaemia | Thrombosis, Pulmonary |

## Equipment & Drugs

To be forewarned is to be forearmed. Routine checks should ensure that the drugs and the emergency cart are not beyond the expiry date and the equipment is in working condition. In addition, the oxygen cylinder should be checked for pressure regularly.

The dental clinic must be equipped with the following (Fig. **11**):

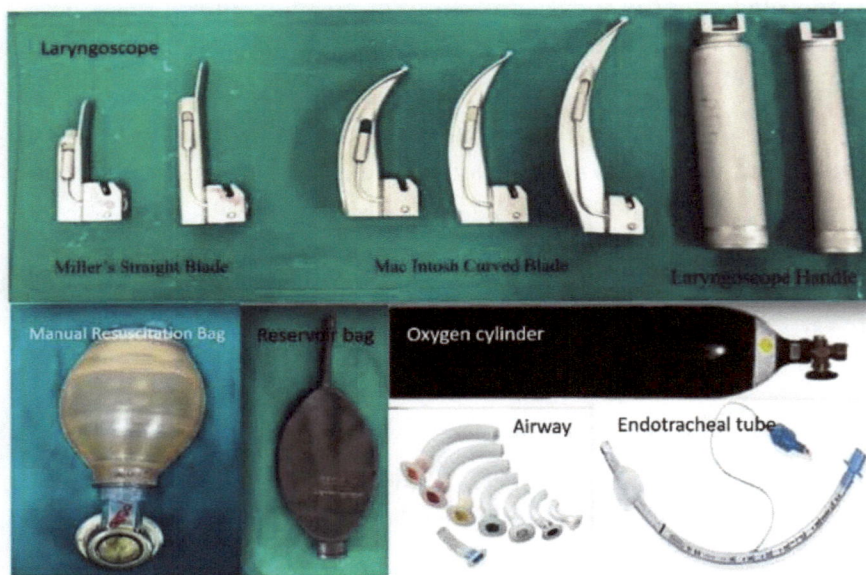

**Fig. (11).** Emergency equipment.

Manual resuscitator bag with reservoir bag and masks of different sizes.

Oro-pharyngeal and nasopharyngeal airways

Oxygen cylinder with a regulator capable of delivering a high flow of oxygen.

Laryngoscope and endotracheal tubes

Spacer device to deliver Salbutamol

Equipment for recording blood pressure.

Emergency drugs (Table **6**).

**Table 6. Drugs required in emergency cart.**

| Drug | Indication | Dose |
|---|---|---|
| Oxygen | All medical emergencies | 100% inhalation |
| Adrenaline | Anaphylaxis Asthma unresponsive to Salbutamol Cardiac arrest | Children 0.01mg/kg every 3-5 minutes |
| Nitro-glycerine | Angina | 0.3-0.4mg sublingual |

*(Table 6) cont.....*

| Drug | Indication | Dose |
|---|---|---|
| Antihistaminic Chlorpheniramine Diphenhydramine | Allergic reactions | 10-20mg iv,im 25-30mg iv,im |
| Ibuterol/salbutamol | Bronchospasm | 3-4puffs mdi |
| Aspirin | Myocardial infarction | 160-325mg |

## Oxygen (Fig. 11)

A portable source of oxygen, preferably in an "E"-size cylinder which holds over 600 litres, should be available. It is advisable to have various oxygen delivery devices like nasal prongs, face masks, non-rebreathing face masks (Fig. **12**).

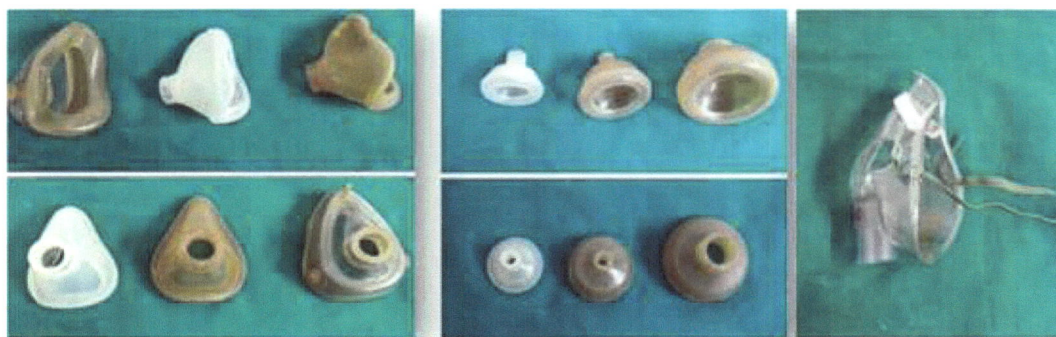

**Fig. (12).** Different types of oxygen delivery systems.

## Epinephrine

Epinephrine is available as an ampule that contains 1mg per 1 ml equivalent to 1:1000 concentration. For emergency purposes, it is usually given intravenously. However, intramuscular, intraosseous and intralingual routes can be used when intravenous access is unavailable. Autoinjector systems are also present for intramuscular use (such as the EpiPen), which provides one dose of 0.3 mg as 0.3 mL of 1: 1,000, or the pediatric formulation, which is one dose of 0.15 mg as 0.3 mL of 1: 2,000.

**Table 7. Essential Drugs for medical emergencies.**

| Drug | Indication | Dose |
|---|---|---|
| Glucagon | Hypoglycaemia in an unconscious patient | 1mg iv or im |
| Atropine | Clinically significant bradycardia | 0.6mg iv or im |
| Ephedrine | Clinically significant hypotension | 5mg iv or 10-25mg im |

(Table 7) cont.....

| Drug | Indication | Dose |
|---|---|---|
| Hydrocortisone | 1. Adrenal insufficiency<br>2. Recurrent anaphylaxis | 100mg iv or im<br>100mg iv or im |
| Morphine | Angina like pain unresponsive to nitro-glycerine | Titrate 2mg iv, 5mg im |
| Naloxone | Reverse effects of opioid drugs | 0.1mg/kg iv max dose o 2mg |
| Lorazepam/midazolam | Status epilepticus | 4mg im or iv, 5mg iv/im |
| Flumazenil | Benzodiazepine overdose | 0.1mg iv |

When unresponsive to other medication, it is the drug of choice to treat the life-threatening manifestations of anaphylaxis or persistent asthmatic bronchospasm.

## Oral Carbohydrate

In patients prone to hypoglycemia, an oral source of glucose, such as sugars fruit drinks, should be readily available.

## Essential drugs:

The essential drugs to be maintained and their doses have been summarised in Table **7**.

## Syncope

Syncope is a sudden, temporary, short-term loss of consciousness and postural tone, often followed by spontaneous and complete recovery. It is most common in young adults due to anxiety and unanticipated pain. Hunger, exhaustion, and a hot, humid environment may also contribute.

The upright position in the dental chair causes blood to stagnate in the lower limbs. As a result of compromised venous return to the heart, there is reflex bradycardia, a decrease in cardiac output and blood pressure. Syncope in patients above 50yrs may be due to cerebrovascular insufficiency or underlying cardiovascular problem.

### *Signs and Symptoms*

In the early phase, the patient complains of feeling warm, nauseous, sweating and faint. Then, there can be hypotension with a rapid increase in heart rate. This is followed by pupillary dilatation, yawning, hyperpnea, cold extremities, hypotension, bradycardia, visual disturbances, and dizziness.

## Management

1) Discontinue the procedure.
2) Assess level of consciousness and vital signs.
3) Place the patient supine with feet elevated slightly (Fig. **13**).
4) Position the head to maintain airway patency.
5) Administer oxygen.
6) Loosen tight clothing.
7) Contact the EMS if recovery is delayed.

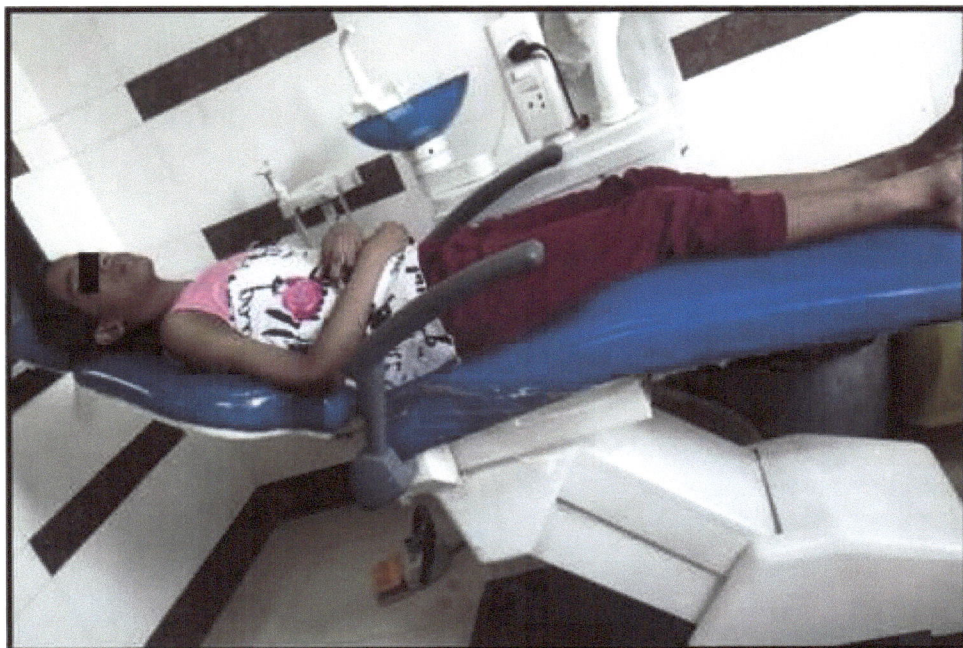

**Fig. (13).** Position of the patient in case of syncope.

## Prevention

Identify patients at risk. Those with a previous history of syncope take precautionary measures like performing the procedure in supine/ semi-supine rather than upright, premedication with anxiolytic drugs, asking the patient to have a light meal prior to dental treatment, ensure profound local anaesthesia.

## Hyperventilation

Hyperventilation is usually seen in anxious young adults. As a result of an increase in the rate and depth of respiration, there is a washout of carbon dioxide, causing respiratory alkalosis. In addition, the decrease in blood supply to the brain due to a fall in carbon dioxide may cause dizziness anxiety, causing the patient to hyperventilate further.

## Signs & Symptoms

Dizziness, palpitations, numbness and tingling of hands and feet, muscle pain, cramps, perioral tremors, carpopedal tetany.

## Management

1. Stop the procedure
2. Make the patient lie in a comfortable position, preferably upright
3. Reassure and ask them to breathe slowly and regularly
4. If conscious, instruct them to cup the hand in front of the mouth and nose. Ask them to breathe in and out of this space containing exhaled air with carbon dioxide. Alternatively, hold a full-face mask over the face or tell the patient to rebreathe from a paper bag (Fig. **14**).
5. In patients who are not benefitted from the above measures, consider titrated doses of midazolam or intranasal midazolam spray.

## Orthostatic Hypotension

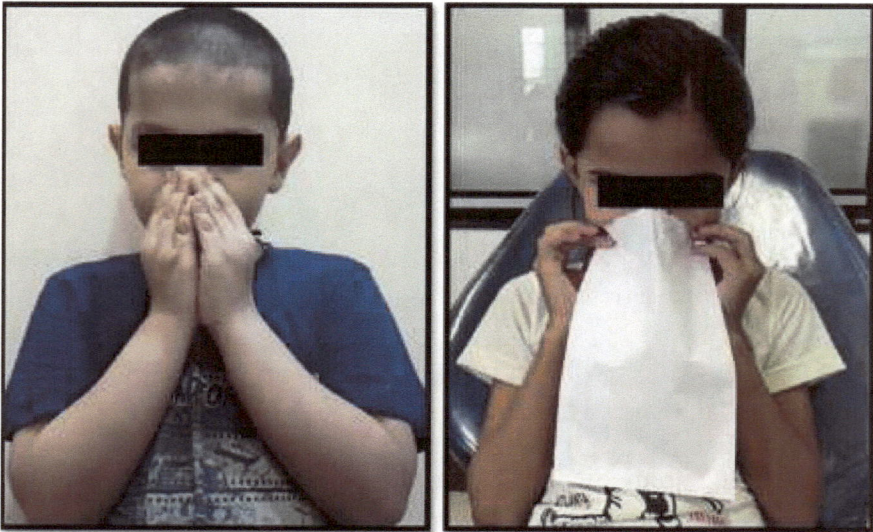

**Fig. (14).** Position for rebreathing with cupped hands or paper bag.

It is the condition in which the patient feels a sudden short duration of dizziness, blackout or, in extreme cases, fainting due to a sudden change in position of the head. It is usually seen when the patient moves suddenly from a supine position to an erect position. Once the procedure is completed, gradually elevate the head end of the dental chair and ask the patient to stay seated for a few minutes before standing.

### Predisposing factors for Postural Hypotension

Drugs: Tricyclic Antidepressants, Antihypertensives, Phenothiazines Anti-Parkinson drugs.

Prolonged recumbency and convalescence

Pregnancy (supine hypotensive syndrome, especially in the third trimester)

Venous abnormalities in the lower limb

Addison's disease

### Clinical Criteria

Symptoms develop on standing

Increase at least 30 beats per min in the pulse rate, decrease at least 25 mmHg in systolic pressure, and drop at least 10mmHg in diastolic blood pressure on assuming the upright posture.

### Precautions

1. Make changes in chair position slowly
2. Instruct pregnant patients to move from one side to the other in prolonged treatment.

### Endocrinal Emergencies

Hypoglycemia

Hyperglycemia

Acute adrenal insufficiency

Hypoglycemia

The blood glucose level is usually maintained within about 70-110 mg/dl or 3.9 to 6.1 mmoL/L of blood. Hypoglycaemia is a biochemical symptom indicating the presence of an underlying cause. It is usually encountered in neonates and rare in older children.

Hypoglycaemia is an emergency seen in children who have juvenile Type I diabetes.

Predisposing factors

1. Missed or delayed meal

2. Overdose of insulin or oral hypoglycemics

3. Unaccustomed strenuous exercise

4. Diarrhea or vomiting

5. Debility or emotional stress

6. Medical Disorders, *e.g.,* Growth hormone and cortisol deficiency, Glycogen Storage disorders, Idiopathic ketotic hypoglycemia, Insulinomas, liver failure, sepsis *etc.*

## Symptoms/Signs

They usually develop when the plasma glucose levels decrease below 65 mg/dl but may vary amongst individuals.

1. Autonomic symptoms of hypoglycemia that occur due to sympathetic activation are tremors, tachycardia, sweating, cold, clammy skin, nausea, vomiting, anxiety, pallor.
2. Cerebral symptoms of hypoglycemia are headaches, lethargy, visual disturbances, paraesthesia.
3. With chronic hypoglycaemia, the reflex mechanisms are depressed, which may lead to hypoglycaemia unawareness [9]. It can lead to focal or generalised seizures and hypoglycaemic coma if not treated.

## Management

1. In a patient who is conscious and able to swallow, give sugar in any form such as candy, glucose solution or fruit juice.
2. If unable to swallow, administer 20-50mL of 50% glucose intravenously.
3. Glucagon 1mg intramuscularly (into a large muscle like the thigh).

Glucagon stimulates the liver to release large amounts of glucose within 5 to 15 min.

## Acute Adrenal insufficiency or Adrenal crisis

Patients with Addison's disease need lifelong treatment with glucocorticoids due to the inability of the adrenal glands to secrete these hormones. In addition, some patients suffering from chronic inflammatory disorders, *e.g.*, rheumatoid arthritis and asthma, are likely to receive steroids for a prolonged duration. Although the exact time and dose are uncertain, there exists a possibility of hypothalamic-pituitary-adrenocortical axis suppression in patients receiving exogenous steroids.

A standard method to identify patients likely to have adrenal insufficiency is by taking a thorough medical history. A patient with a history of taking 20 mg cortisone or equivalent daily for two weeks within the past two years is more likely to have an Addisonian crisis. They can withstand less surgical stress if they take their usual steroid dose within 2 hours of the procedure [10]. It is prudent to supplement additional steroids before extensive surgeries like impacted tooth extraction [11].

### *Symptoms/Signs*

History of current or recent long term steroid use

Mental confusion

Nausea/vomiting/abdominal pain

Hypotension

Hypoglycemia

### *Management*

1. Stop the dental procedure

2. Make the patient lie supine with lower limbs elevated slightly and administer oxygen

3. Inject Hydrocortisone sodium succinate (100mg) or Dexamethasone (4mg) intravenously

4. Watch for and correct any electrolyte imbalance

## Anaphylaxis

Anaphylaxis is a life-threatening emergency that necessitates immediate attention and treatment. An IgE-mediated hypersensitivity reaction is precipitated by an inhaled or injected substance. As a result of prior exposure to the same allergen, the patient has IgE antibodies on the surface of mast cells and basophils. Chemical mediators are released due to degranulation of mast cells on subsequent exposure. Clinical presentation can be acute within a few minutes or delayed (Table **8**).

Table 8. Signs of anaphylaxis across various systems.

| Respiratory | Swelling of lips, tongue, uvula, eyelids, tightness in the throat, hoarseness of voice, chest tightness, wheeze, stridor, reduced Peak Expiratory Flow Rate (PEFR). |
|---|---|
| Cardiovascular | Hypotension, tachycardia |
| Central Nervous System | Sense of impending doom, confusion, agitation, dizziness |
| Others | Perioral tingling, extreme sweating, rhinitis, sneezing, pruritis, Urticaria, angioedema, erythema, abdominal cramps, diarrhoea. |

Conditions like vasovagal attack, syncope, hypoglycemia, and acute poisoning mimic anaphylaxis.

**Etiology of Anaphylaxis in a Dental Office**

**Local Anesthetics** (LA): anaphylactic reactions to local anaesthetic administration in the dental office are rare; however, allergic hypersensitivity reactions occur. Acute allergic reactions to LA are either immediate with systemic manifestations or delayed with localised reactions at the injection site [12].

They are usually seen with the ester group of LAs since they are metabolised to Para-aminobenzoic acid, which has allergenic potential. On the other hand, LAs belonging to the amide group, *e.g.*, lignocaine, mepivacaine and prilocaine, are rarely associated with allergic reactions. However, one must remember that the reaction could occur to the preservatives like benzoates or antioxidants such as metabisulphites used in local anaesthetics with adrenaline.

Testing for LA sensitivity: If intracutaneous testing [13] with 0.1 mL of the test solution is performed, one should ensure it does not contain adrenaline, methylparaben and sodium metabisulfite. It should be kept in mind that a false positive response can occur due to histamine release in response to skin puncture.

**Antibiotics and Analgesics:**

In children, adverse drug reactions are caused by beta-lactam antibiotics and non-steroidal anti-inflammatory drugs [14]. Cutaneous manifestations are common with drug-induced conditions.

Ideally, the patient who presents with respiratory problems should be monitored for at least 6-8 hours, while those who presented with hypotension should be monitored for at least 12-24 hours [15].

These children with suspected drug-induced anaphylaxis should consult a specialist for further evaluation. In addition, a desensitisation process may be needed to prevent a future episode.

## Latex Allergy

Care to prevent latex allergy-induced anaphylaxis should be taken in children with known allergies to certain foods like kiwi, avocado, and bananas [16].

Alternatives to dental equipment containing natural latex rubber may have to be sought in patients with a definitive history of life-threatening anaphylaxis. Articles containing latex include gloves, dental dam, endodontic file stoppers, mixing bowls, polishing equipment, temporary crowns, and matrices [17].

## Chlorhexidine

As antiseptic, chlorhexidine is used in toothpaste, mouthwashes and as a root canal irrigant. Therefore, relevant history should be obtained as anaphylaxis to chlorhexidine irrigation has been reported [18].

## Management

Immediate resuscitative measures include:

Subcutaneous adrenaline 1:1000 aqueous preparation (0.1 ml/kg: max 0.5ml) followed by repeat doses at 15mins interval or continuous iv infusion (0.1mg/kg/min). When using an epinephrine auto-injector (Fig **15**), administer 0.3mg IM for patients weighing 30 kg or more and 0.15mg IM for patients weighing 10 to 30 kg.

Oxygen and ventilatory support if needed.

Cardiovascular support with intravenous fluids

Nebulisation with bronchodilators to control bronchospasm

Antihistaminic, diphenhydramine (1mg/kg 8hrly) or chlorpheniramine (0.3-0.5mg/kg 8-hourly) for next 24-48hrs, to prevent late reactions.

Systemic steroids, *e.g.,* hydrocortisone i.v (5mg/kg 6hrly), may help decrease the duration and severity of symptoms.

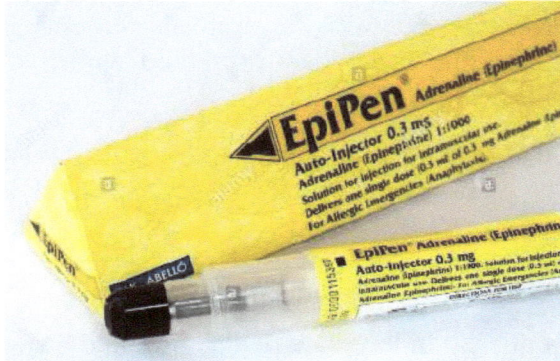

**Fig. (15).**  Epinephrine auto-injector.

## Seizures & Epilepsy

A seizure is an abnormal paroxysmal electrical activity in the brain resulting in motor, sensory, behavioural, or autonomic manifestations [19].

Any seizure persisting for more than 30mins or multiple episodes irrespective of duration with no regaining of consciousness is termed Status Epilepticus.

### Etiology of Seizures

Simple febrile convulsions

Infections: Bacterial, Viral, Tubercular Meningitis, Encephalitis.

Metabolic Causes: Hypoglycemia, Hypocalcemia, Hypomagnesemia, Electrolyte imbalances

Drug overdose or withdrawal

Vascular & Degenerative disorders

Head injury

The clinician should be aware of the following:

a. Frequency, Duration, Type of seizures.
b. Trigger factors, warning signs.
c. Medications are taken for the seizures. If seizures are not controlled, a neurologist referral should be done.
d. In case of seizure precipitated by psychological stress, mild anxiolytic-like midazolam may be prescribed

e. Reduce anxiety, confirm profound local anaesthesia

## During the seizure

Remove all dental instruments from the patient site.

Put the dental chair in a supported supine position as near the floor as possible.

When the patient is not on the dental chair, place them onto the floor & protect the head from injury by keeping a pillow beneath. Quickly remove all foreign material from the patient's mouth, taking care not to be bitten.

Place the patient in the lateral position to avoid the risk of aspirating secretions and recent dental implants.

Loosen belts and tight clothes around the neck.

Provide oxygen via nasal cannula.

After the seizure, suction the oral cavity if required

Seek medical help

Assess the postictal state before the patient is discharged.

## Anticonvulsant Therapy for Acute Seizures/ Status Epilepticus Immediate

Lorazepam 0.1mg/kg *iv* 2mg/min or

Diazepam 0.2mg/kg *iv* slowly

Midazolam 0.2mg/kg *iv* slowly (or IM/Nasal/Buccal)

## After 5min

Repeat the Step I Drug -if Required

(After 10mins)

Phenytoin 20mg/kg in 1:1 NS *iv,* 1mg/kg/min

## If there is no Response to the Above

Sodium Valproate *i.v.* 20mg/kg in 1:1 NS, 6mg/kg/min or

Phenobarbital *i.v.* 20mg/kg in NS, 1.5 mg/kg /min, or

Levetiracetam *i.v* 20-30 mg/kg, 5mg/kg/min

Monitor airway, breathing, circulation

Shift to intensive care, as early as possible

Differential diagnosis of seizures includes local anaesthesia overdose, hypoglycemia, vasodepressor syncope and cerebrovascular incident.

## Acute Airway Obstruction

Airway compromise is a common aetiology of cardiac arrest in children. Upper airway obstruction is usually due to a foreign body, while the common cause of lower airway obstruction is asthma. Children are more prone because they inherently have a minor diameter of the nose, pharynx, and larynx. In addition, children in the age group of 9 months to 5 years are at a higher risk of foreign body aspiration.

An accidentally inhaled foreign body will stimulate the cough reflex, which may be sufficient to clear the obstruction. The patient is encouraged to cough it out if they are cooperative. Suspect obstruction in the case of inspiratory stridor, a high-pitched sound results from turbulent airflow in a partially obstructed airway.

A complete obstruction is often silent and may progress rapidly, causing respiratory distress, unconsciousness, and cardiac arrest.

It can be so severe that the patient cannot speak, breathe, or cough.

## Measures to be Taken if there is a Displacement of a Foreign Body

1. Usually, no intervention is required if the foreign body is small and passes through the oesophagus.
2. If the foreign body is visible (*e.g.,* dislodged tooth during extraction), it can be retrieved using Magill's forceps, which is atraumatic and long enough to reach the pharynx (Figs. **16 & 17**).
3. If the object cannot be retrieved and the patient develops symptoms of airway obstruction, it may lead to a catastrophic event if timely intervention is not initiated.
4. For responsive adults and children greater than one year of age with severe foreign body obstruction, back blows or slaps, abdominal thrusts (with the patient in supine position) and chest thrusts (Fig. **18**) are usually adequate.
5. Abdominal thrust is not recommended for infants less than one year of age, as it may cause injuries. The operator has to support the chest of the patient with one hand and deliver five sharp blows between the scapulae with the palm.

6. For children older than one year, Heimlich's manoeuvre abdominal trusts may be given.
7. Finger sweep should be used to remove foreign body only when the rescuer can visualise the object causing airway obstruction in an unresponsive patient. A blind sweep can push the foreign body further in.
8. If the obstruction is not relieved despite all the measures taken, a cricothyroid puncture can be performed, provided the obstruction is above the level of the cricothyroid membrane. However, one must be aware that the object may slide down into the lower respiratory tract leading to aspiration of the thing in the bronchioles (Fig. **19**).
9. If the patient loses consciousness, CPCR should be initiated, EMS activated, and the patient should be shifted to the higher centre.

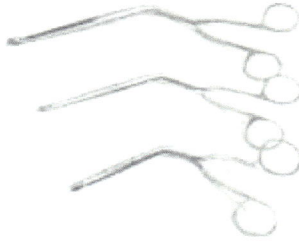

**Fig. (16).** Magill's forceps.

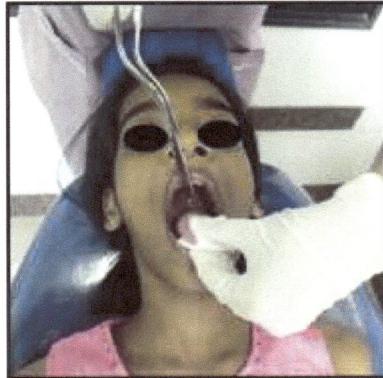

**Fig. (17).** Retrieval of foreign object.

## Acute Asthma Attack

Asthma is a chronic inflammatory disease of the airway that is more prevalent in children. While acute attacks are usually self-limiting, they can progress to status asthmaticus. This life-threatening emergency is characterized by hypercarbia, respiratory acidosis, hypoxemia, and hypotension.

## Dental Concerns

1) A detailed history of precipitating factors and medication helps to modify dental treatment. Adrenocortical insufficiency may be present with prolonged use of steroids. Adults with anxiety as a trigger can be prescribed a mild anxiolytic. In children, inhalational sedation with profound local anaesthesia may be helpful.
2) Aspirin, non-steroidal anti-inflammatory drugs, macrolide antibiotics like erythromycin, fluoroquinolones like ciprofloxacin and sodium metabisulphite used in local anaesthetics can trigger asthma. Although present in minimal quantity, care should be taken in those sensitive to bisulphites [20].
3) Patient may need prophylactic bronchodilator inhalation before a dental procedure.

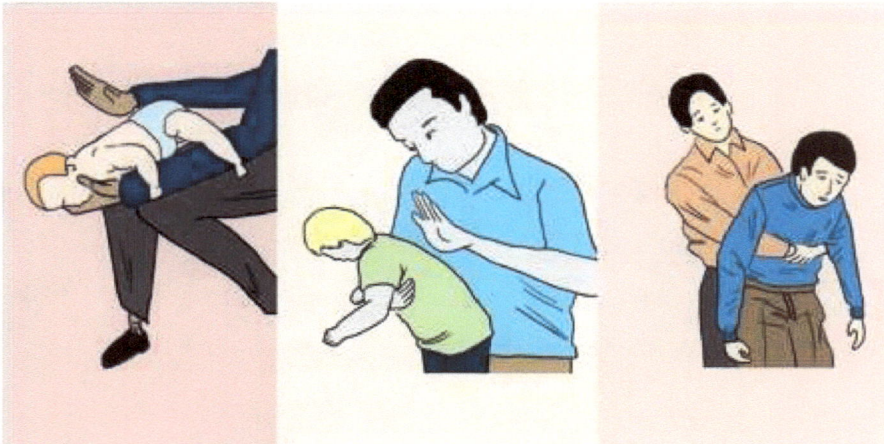

**Fig. (18).** Position of the patient for removal of a foreign object according to different age groups.

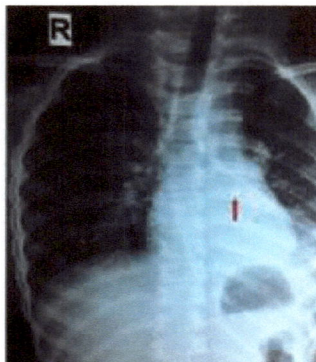

**Fig (19).** Aspirated Foreign body.

## Signs and Symptoms of Acute Exacerbation

Cough with or without sputum production

Inability to speak

Tightness in the chest (younger children may complain of tummy ache)

Nasal flaring

Wheezing

## Ominous Signs Indicative of Severe Obstruction

Silent chest

Cyanosis

Fatigue

Altered sensorium

PEFR< 30% of predicted

Oxygen Saturation<90%

## Management

Stop the procedure and extract all dental materials & instruments from the patient's mouth.

Make the patient sit upright in a comfortable position.

Supplement oxygen

Short-acting Beta-2 -agonist (Salbutamol)

Metered-dose inhaler 4-6 puffs. Use a spacer or volumiser device for effective delivery (Fig. **20**).

Nebulize every 20min up to 3times in one hour.

Side effects seen with increased absorption of Beta-adrenergic agonists are tremors, irritability, tachycardia, and hypokalemia.

It is advisable to have a cardio scope for ECG and pulse oximeter to monitor oxygen saturation continuously.

Inhaled ipratropium bromide added to Salbutamol may benefit patients with mucus hypersecretion.

## Systemic Corticosteroids

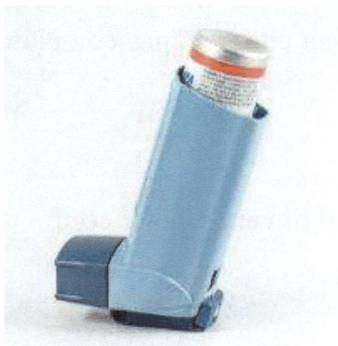

**Fig. (20).**  Inhaler.

Hydrocortisone (3-5mg/kg) *iv.* Improvement in respiratory function usually occurs in one hour, but peak action may take 6-12 hrs [21].

Epinephrine is used with extreme caution only when symptoms are refractory to all other measures. A preloaded auto-injector syringe (Fig. **15**) [22] containing 0.3mL of epinephrine (1:1000 dilution) should be available in the emergency kit.

Adults: 0.3mL subcutaneous or intramuscular

Children:

0.15mg (weight upto 30kg)

0.3mg (weight > 30kg)

Metered Dose Inhalers: Deliver medication efficiently when used with a spacer and mask in children (Fig. **21**).

## CONCLUSION

Medical emergencies are sudden and may occur at any time during dental procedures. Dental surgeons should be prepared for such eventualities by keeping themselves updated about the recent guidelines in medical emergency management and maintaining an emergency crash cart to manage any medical emergencies in the office. In addition, the contents of the cart should be routinely checked for mechanical errors and expiry dates. It is also prudent to make proper documentation and necessary referrals from the child's physician before planning the dental appointment.

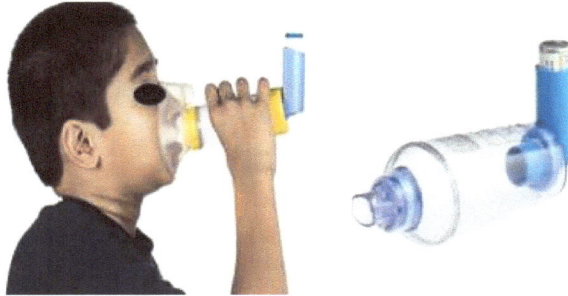

**Fig. (21).** Metered Dose Inhalers.

## CONSENT FOR PUBLICATION

Not applicable.

## CONFLICT OF INTEREST

The authors declare no conflict of interest, financial or otherwise.

## ACKNOWLEDGEMENT

Declared none.

## REFERENCES

[1]     Pediatric Emergencies & Resuscitation. Mary E, Hartman and Ira M Cherfetz in Nelson textbook of Pediatrics Ed 21. Elsevier 1600 John F. Kennedy Blvd Ste 1600 Philadelphia PA 19103-2899.

[2]     American Society of Anesthesiologists: Physical Status Classification System. Available from http://www.asahq.org/Home/For-Members/Clinical-Information/ASA-Physical

[3]     McCarthy FM, Malamed SF. Physical evaluation system to determine medical risk and indicated dental therapy modifications. J Am Dent Assoc 1979; 99(2): 181-4.
        [http://dx.doi.org/10.14219/jada.archive.1979.0271] [PMID: 287736]

[4]     Perusse R, Goulet JR, Turcotte JY. Contraindication to vasoconstrictors in dentistry. Part I: Cardiovascular diseases. Oral Surg Oral Med Oral Pathol 1992; 74: 687-91.
        [http://dx.doi.org/10.1016/0030-4220(92)90366-X] [PMID: 1437074]

[5]     Nitrolingual spray 2014.www.ePocrates.com

[6]     Nitrostat sublingual tablets 2014. www. e Pocrates.com Accessed 15 July.

[7]     AHA: Warning signs and actions: our guide to quick action for heart attack, cardiac arrest and stroke emergencies. 2013.

[8]     Merchant RM, Topjian AA, Panchal AR, *et al.* Part 1: Executive summary: 2020 American Heart Association guidelines for cardiopulmonary resuscitation and emergency cardiovascular care. Circulation 2020. 142(16_suppl_2): S337-57.

[9]     Sperling MA, Ed. Pediatric Endocrinology. 3rd edition. Philadelphia: Elsevier /Saunders, 2008.

[10]   Little JW, Falace DA, Miller CS. Rhodus NL. Adrenal Insufficiency. In: Dental Management of the medically compromised patient 8th ed., 2013.
[http://dx.doi.org/10.1016/B978-0-323-08028-6.00015-4]

[11]   Moore J. Adrenocortical insufficiency. In: Bope ET, Kellerman RD, Eds. Conn's Current therapy Philadelphia, Saunders, 2014.

[12]   NHS, Specialist Pharmacy Service and UK Medicines Information. Allergy to LA agents used in dentistry. 2019. https//www.sps.nhs.uk/wp.content/uploads/2019/08/UKMiQA

[13]   McClimon B, Rank M, Li J. The predictive value of skin testing in the diagnosis of local anesthetic allergy. Allergy Asthma Proc 2011; 32(2): 95-8.
[http://dx.doi.org/10.2500/aap.2011.32.3417] [PMID: 21439161]

[14]   Gomes ER, Brockow K, Kuyucu S, *et al.* Drug hypersensitivity in children: report from the pediatric task force of the EAACI Drug Allergy Interest Group. Allergy 2016; 71(2): 149-61.
[http://dx.doi.org/10.1111/all.12774] [PMID: 26416157]

[15]   Atanaskovic-Markovic M, Gomes E, Cernadas JR, *et al.* Diagnosis and management of drug-induced anaphylaxis in children: An EAACI position paper. Pediatr Allergy Immunol 2019; 30(3): 269-76.
[http://dx.doi.org/10.1111/pai.13034] [PMID: 30734362]

[16]   Anaphylaxis Campaign. Latex Allergy: the facts, 2019. Available at https://www anaphylaxis.org.UK/knowledgebase/latex-allergy the facts (accessed May 2020)

[17]   Jevon P, Shamsi S. Management of anaphylaxis in the dental practice: an update. Br Dent J 2020; 229: 721–8.

[18]   Harper NJN, Dixon T, Dugué P, *et al.* Suspected anaphylactic reactions associated with anaesthesia. Anaesthesia 2009; 64(2): 199-211.
[http://dx.doi.org/10.1111/j.1365-2044.2008.05733.x] [PMID: 19143700]

[19]   Kumar R. Chapter 19-Diseases of the Central Nervous System. In: Paul VK, Bagga A. Ghai Essential Pediatrics. Ninth edition. CBS Publishers & Distributors Pvt Ltd. 2019: pp. 552-80.

[20]   Haas DA. An update on local anesthetics in dentistry. J Can Dent Assoc 2002; 68(9): 546-51.
[PMID: 12366885]

[21]   Committee ECC. Subcommittees and Task forces of the American Heart Association: Part 10.5: Near-fatal Asthma in 2005 American Heart Association Guidelines for Cardiopulmonary Resuscitation and Emergency Cardiovascular Care. Circulation 2005; 112: IV-139-42.

[22]   Malamed SF, Orr DL. Chapter 13-Asthma. In: Medical Emergencies in the Dental Office 7th ed. Elsevier Mosby 3251 Riverpointlane, St Louis 2015.

# CHAPTER 9

# Oral Manifestations and Management of HIV/ AIDS in Children

**Satyawan Damle**[1,*], **Abdulkadeer Jetpurwala**[1] and **Dhanashree Sakhare**[2]

[1] *Department of Pediatric Dentistry, Nair Hospital Dental College, Mumbai, India*

[2] *Lavanika Dental Academy, Melbourne, Australia*

**Abstract:** Children are innocent victims of HIV infection. Children who are HIV positive, either through mother-to-child transmission or following sexual abuse, are often not revealed what could happen to them. They will undoubtedly be worried when they experience symptoms.

It has been estimated that 90% of people with HIV infection present at least one oral indication at some time during the disease. The presence of oral lesions may be an early diagnostic indicator of HIV/AIDS. Early recognition, diagnosis and treatment of HIV associated oral lesions in children can reduce morbidity and improve the quality of life of children who have HIV/AIDS.

**Keywords:** AIDS, Children, Candidiasis, HIV, Infection.

## INTRODUCTION

The origin of the Human Immunodeficiency Virus (HIV) has been a subject of scientific research and debate since the virus was identified in the 1980s. There is now a wealth of evidence on how, when and where HIV first began to cause illness. HIV is a type of lentivirus that attacks the immune system. Similarly, the Simian Immunodeficiency Virus (SIV) attacks the immune systems of monkeys and apes. The research discovered that HIV is related to SIV, and there are many similarities between the two viruses. HIV-1 is closely related to a strain of SIV found in chimpanzees, and HIV-2 is closely related to a strain of SIV found in sooty mangabeys [1].

---

[*] **Corresponding author Satyawan Damle:** Department of Pediatric Dentistry, Nair Hospital Dental College, Mumbai, India; E-mail: sgdamle@gmail.com

# HISTORY

How did HIV cross from chimps to humans?

The most accepted theory is that of the 'hunter'. In this scenario, SIVcpz was transferred to humans because of chimps being killed and eaten or their blood getting into cuts or wounds on people while hunting. Usually, the hunter's body would have fought off SIV, but on a few occasions, the virus adapted itself within its new human host and became HIV-1. There are four main groups of HIV strains (M, N, O and P), each with a slightly different genetic make-up. This supports the hunter theory because every time SIV passed from a chimpanzee to a human, it would have developed slightly within the human body and produced a different strain. This explains why more than one strain of HIV-1 [2]. The most studied strain of HIV is HIV-1 Group M, which is the strain that has spread throughout the world and is responsible for most HIV infections today (Figs. **1A** and **B**).

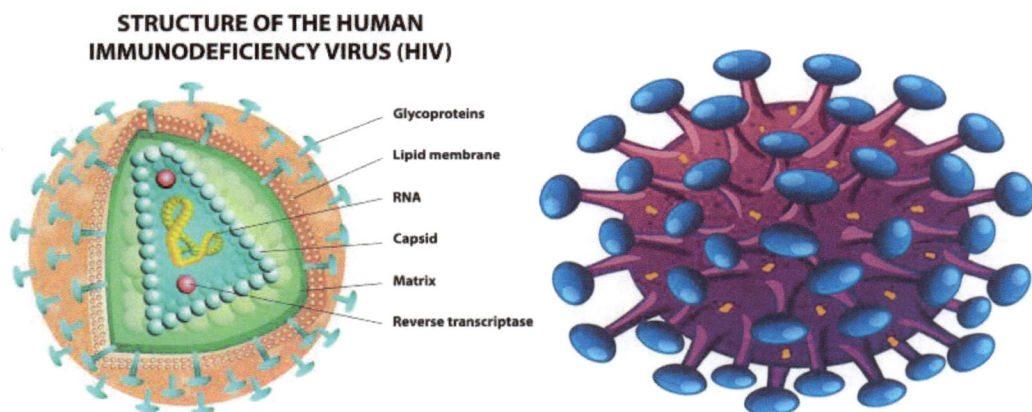

STRUCTURE OF THE HUMAN IMMUNODEFICIENCY VIRUS (HIV)

- Glycoproteins
- Lipid membrane
- RNA
- Capsid
- Matrix
- Reverse transcriptase

Fig. (1). **A** and **B**: Structure of Human Immunodeficiency Virus.

## When and Where did HIV Start in Humans?

Studies of some of the earliest known samples of HIV provide clues about when it first appeared in humans and how it evolved. The first verified case of HIV is from a blood sample taken in 1959 from a man living in what is now Kinshasa in the Democratic Republic of Congo. The sample was retrospectively analysed, and HIV detected. There are numerous earlier cases where patterns of deaths from common opportunistic infections, now known to be AIDS-defining, suggest that HIV was the cause, but this is the earliest incident where a blood sample can verify infection. It is far rarer and less infectious than HIV-1. As a result, it infects far fewer people and is found in a few countries in West Africa like Mali, Mauritania, Nigeria, and Sierra Leone [3].

## 2018 Global HIV Statistics

HIV continues to be a significant global public health issue. In 2018, an estimated 37.9 million people were living with HIV (including 1.7 million children), with a global HIV prevalence of 0.8% among adults. Around 21% of these same people did not know that they had the virus [3]. Since the start of the epidemic, an estimated 74.9 million people have become infected with HIV, and 32 million people have died of AIDS-related illnesses. In 2018, 770,000 people died of AIDS-related illnesses. This number has reduced by more than 55% since the peak of 1.7 million in 2004 and 1.4 million in 2010 [1]. Most people living with HIV are in low- and middle-income countries, with an estimated 68% living in sub-Saharan Africa. Among this group, 20.6 million live in East and Southern Africa, which saw 800,000 new HIV infections in 2018 [3]. • There has been significant success in reducing the number of new HIV infections among children since 2000. However, for children living with HIV, AIDs-related illnesses are still among the leading causes of infant mortality.

## HIV/AIDS Scenario in Children

Although prevention of mother-to-child transmission programmes is successful when implemented, there needs to be a more significant scale-up of coverage and increasing early infant diagnosis after birth and during breastfeeding.

More needs to be done to support the prevention of HIV among vulnerable children and to address the unique antiretroviral treatment adherence challenges that affect children living with HIV.

Approximately 90% of pediatric HIV infections are acquired from infected mothers resulting in vertical transmission for infants. HIV also can pass from mother to child during pregnancy (30-35%), childbirth (60-65%), or breastfeeding (10-15%). Globally, the annual number of new infections among children (0-14 years) has almost halved since 2010, with a 47% reduction in new HIV cases [4]. Since 1995, an estimated 1.6 million new HIV infections among children have been averted due to providing antiretroviral medicines (ARVs) to women living with HIV during pregnancy and breastfeeding. Most of these infections (1.3 million) were averted between 2010 and 2015 [5].

Despite this significant progress, the number of children becoming newly infected with HIV remains unacceptably high. In 2016, 24% of pregnant women living with HIV did not have access to ARVs to prevent transmission to their infants. Around 160,000 children became infected with HIV; this equates to 438 children a day.

In 2015, in the 21 highest-burden countries, only 54% of children exposed to HIV were tested within the recommended two months [3]. In the following year, an estimated 1.8 million children were living with HIV, but just 43% had access to ARVs. Although treatment coverage has improved since 2010, when just 21% of children living with HIV were on antiretroviral treatment (ART), the current situation means that around half of the children in need do not have access [6].

Most children living with HIV live in Africa, where AIDS remains the leading cause of death among adolescents. Globally, 120,000 children died due to AIDS-related illnesses in 2016. This equates to 328 deaths every day. Children aged 0–4 years living with HIV are more likely to die than those living with HIV of any other age. This is despite a 62% reduction in AIDS-related deaths among this age group globally since 2000 [7].

In addition, millions more children are indirectly affected by the impact of the HIV epidemic on their families and communities [3].

## Why are Children at Risk of HIV?

### *Mother-to-child Transmission (MTCT)*

Most children living with HIV are infected *via* mother-to-child transmission (MTCT) during pregnancy, childbirth, or breastfeeding. This is sometimes referred to as 'vertical transmission' or 'parent-to-child-transmission'.

MTCT of HIV can be stopped if expectant mothers have access to preventing mother-to-child transmission (PMTCT) services during pregnancy, delivery, and breastfeeding. With trained staff and resources, new infections among many thousands of children could be avoided.

Breastfeeding is now responsible for the majority of MTCT. When formula feeding is not a viable option, women can reduce the risk of transmitting HIV to their child at this stage if they exclusively breastfeed and are on ART. However, in 2013 only 49% of women continued to take ARVs while breastfeeding, compared to 62% of women who took ARVs during pregnancy and delivery. This highlights the urgent need for education about the importance of continuing treatment post-birth. Without ART, a third of infants who acquire HIV because of MTCT will not reach their first birthday, and half will not reach their second birthday [8-11].

Interventions that meet the specific needs of families, driven by the experiences and recommendations of children, are needed to enable the 50% of children living with HIV who are without treatment to access it. Without this, children aged 0–4 years living with HIV will continue to be the age group most at risk of AIDS-related deaths [12].

A combination of efforts is needed to prevent new HIV infections among children, ensure that their mothers remain healthy and improve the diagnosis and treatment of HIV for children. While huge gains have been made in preventing MTCT of HIV, an additional 5.2 million women of reproductive age were newly infected with HIV between 2010 and 2015 means the substantial need for PMTCT services will continue for the near future [13].

Pediatric HIV diagnosis, testing and treatment needs to be scaled up to bring it in line with adult services and should be made available closer to where the children most affected live.

## Incidence

According to UNICEF, the estimated 37.9 million [confidence bounds: 32.7-44.0 million] people living with HIV worldwide in 2018, 2.8 million [2.0-3.8 million] were children aged 0-19. Each day in 2018, approximately 980 children became infected with HIV, and approximately 320 children died from AIDS-related causes, mostly because of inadequate access to HIV prevention, care, and treatment services. The transmission of HIV from an HIV-positive mother to her child during pregnancy, labour, delivery, or breastfeeding ranges from 15% to 45%. In 2018, around 160,000 [110,000-260, 000] children aged 0-9 were newly infected with HIV, bringing the total number of children aged 0-9 living with HIV to 1.1 million [870,000-1.5 million] (Fig. **2**).

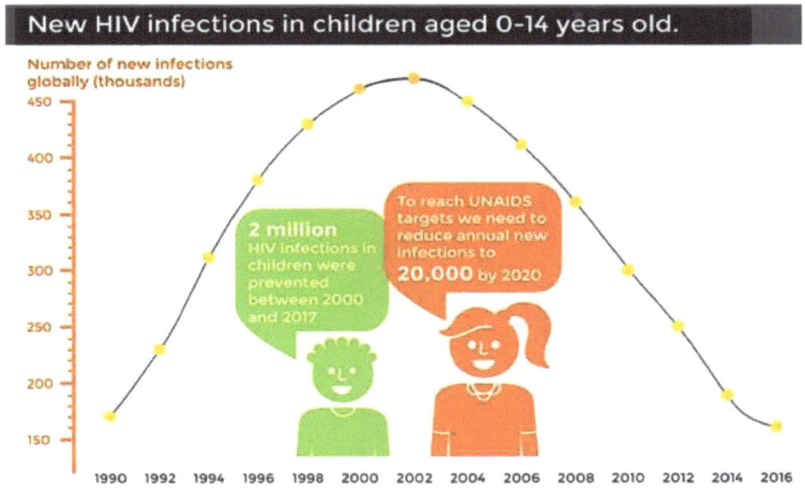

**Fig. (2).** New HIV infections in Children.

A recent maternal infection with HIV may raise the risk of transmission through feeding to twice that women with earlier established disease, receiving too high viral and associated recent infection (WHO 2007) [1, 3, 5].

## Causes

Vertical transmission A child can be born with HIV or contract it soon after birth. HIV contracted in utero is also called vertical transmission or perinatal transmission.

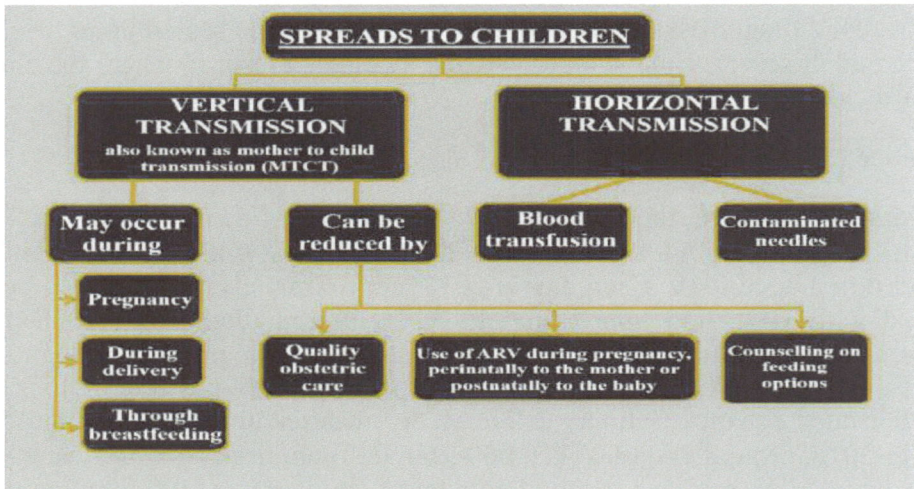

**Fig. (3).** Exhibiting different ways in the spread of HIV.

HIV transmission to children can happen: During pregnancy (passing from mother to baby through the placenta) During delivery (through the transfer of blood or other fluids) While breastfeeding, Of course, not everyone who has HIV will pass it to their baby, especially when following antiretroviral therapy (Fig. **3**).

Horizontal transmission is when HIV is transferred *via* non-sterile needles (HIV drug use or tattooing) or contact with infected semen, vaginal fluid, or blood.

HIV does not spread through insect bites, saliva, sweat, tears, and hugs. You cannot get it from sharing towels or bedding, drinking glasses or eating utensils, and toilet seats or swimming pools [3, 5, 7].

## Classification of Clinical Categories

Children infected with HIV prenatally exposed to HIV may be classified into one of four initially inclusive clinical categories (Fig. **4**).

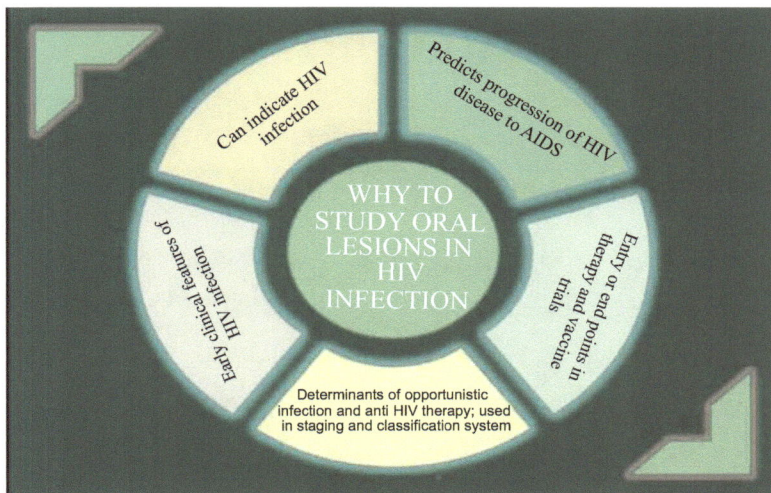

**Fig. (4).** Various Oral Lesions in Children Affected Due to HIV.

*Category N*: Not symptomatic, includes children with no signs or symptoms.

*Category A*: Mild symptomatic, mild separation because of actual events of the time that can elapse before a child manifests signs and symptoms (Figs. **5, 6 & 7 Exhibiting Lesions)**.

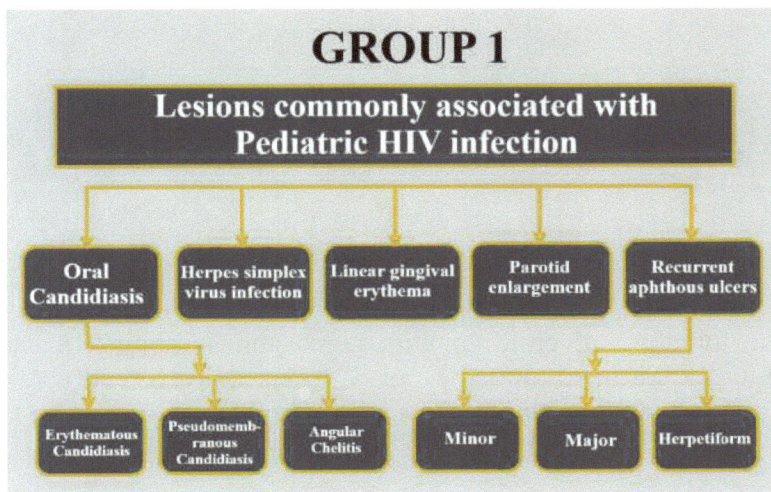

**Fig. (5).** Lesions associated with Paediatric Infections.

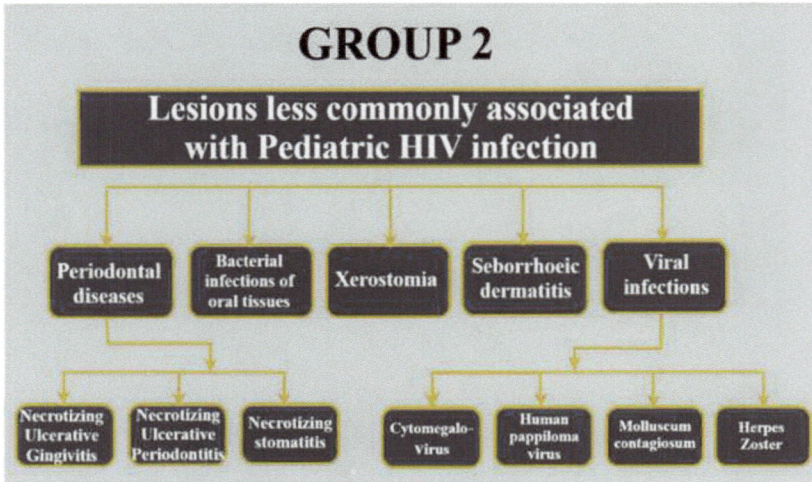

**Fig. (6).** Exhibiting Lesions Less Commonly Associated with HIV in Children.

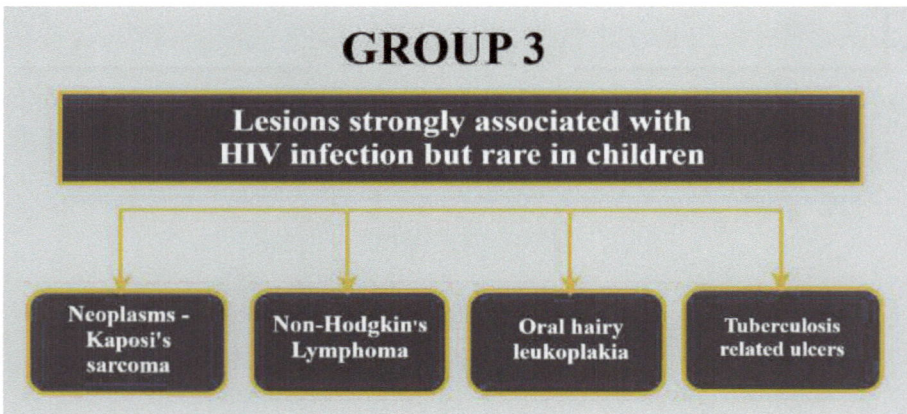

**Fig. (7).** Exhibiting Lesions Exhibiting Rare Lesions in Children.

***Category B:*** Includes all children with signs and symptoms caused by HIV infection but not outlined under A or C revised WHO clinical staging of HIV/AIDS for infants and children (Figs. **8A** to **8I**).

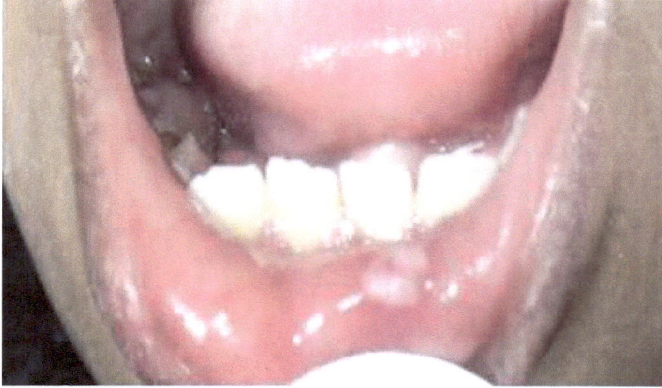

**Fig. (8A).** Aphthous Ulcer Due to HIV.

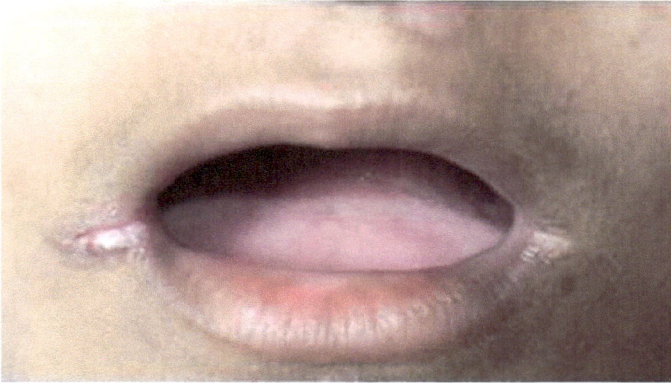

**Fig. (8B).** Angular Cheilitis Due to HIV.

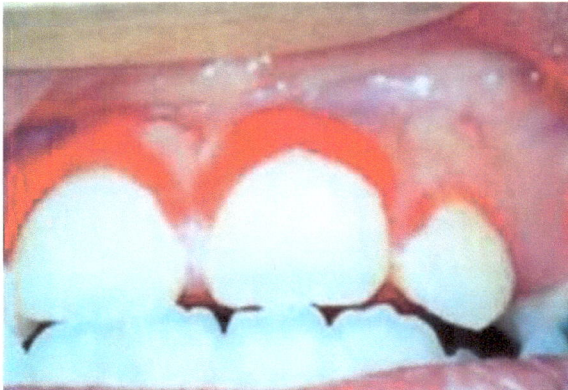

**Fig. (8C).** Angular Cheilitis Due to HIV.

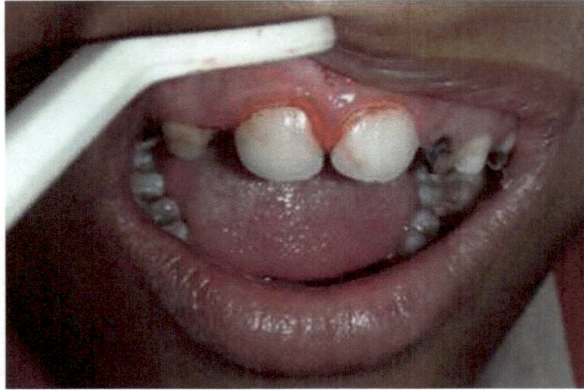

**Fig. (8D).**  Linear Gingival Erythema.

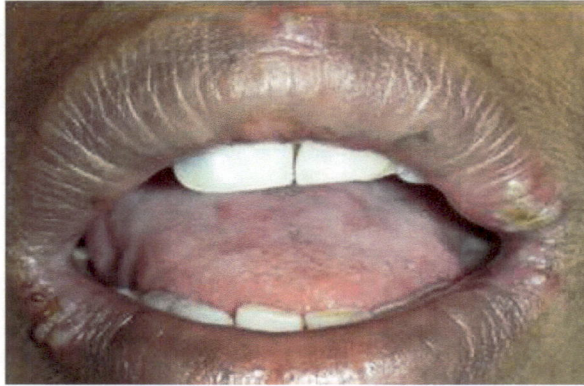

**Fig. (8E).**  Herpes Zoster Recurrent or Chronic Rtis (Otitis Media, Otorrhoea, Sinusitis).

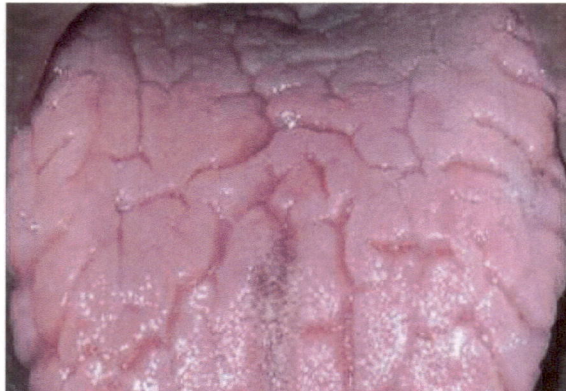

**Fig. (8F).**  Fissured Tongue Due to HIV/Oral Candidiasis.

*Category C*: Severely symptomatic.

## Clinical Stage 1

- Asymptomatic PGL (Persistent generalised lymphadenopathy)
- Hepatosplenomegaly
- Papular pruritic eruptions
- Seborrhoeic dermatitis
- Extensive human papillomavirus infection
- Extensive molluscum contagiosum

## Clinical Stage 2 (Fig. 8A, B)

- Unexplained moderated weight loss
- Recurrent respiratory tract infection
- Herpes zoster
- Angular cheilitis
- Recurrent oral ulceration
- Fungal nail infections

## Clinical Stage 3

- Conditions where a presumptive diagnosis can be made based on clinical signs or simple investigations (Fig. **8C, D, E & F**).
- Moderate unexplained malnutrition not responding to standard therapy
- Unexplained persistent diarrhoea (14 days or more)
- Unexplained persistent fever (intermittent or constant, for longer than one month
- Conditions where confirmatory diagnostic testing is necessary
- Chronic HIV-associated lung disease including bronchiectasis
- Lymphoid interstitial pneumonitis (LIP)
- Unexplained anaemia.

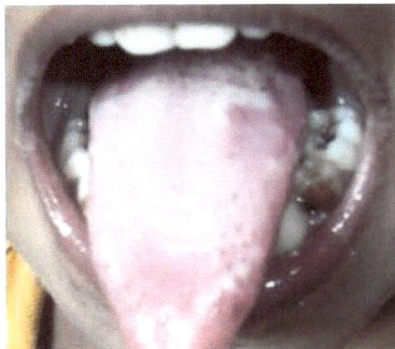

**Fig 8G.** Tongue I HIV Children Oral Candidiasis (Outside Neonatal Period).

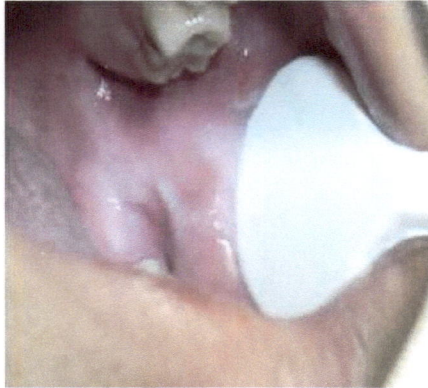

**Fig 8H.**  Oral hairy leucoplakia Acute necrotizing ulcerative gingivitis/periodontitis.

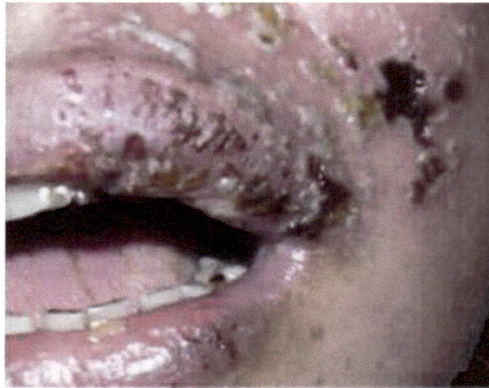

**Fig 8I.**  Severe recurrent presumed bacterial pneumonia.

## Clinical Stage 4 (Figs. 8G, H, I)

- Conditions where a presumptive diagnosis can be made based on clinical signs or simple investigations
- Unexplained severe wasting or severe malnutrition not responding to standard therapy
- Pneumocystis pneumonia
- Recurrent severe presumed bacterial infections (e.g., empyema, pyomyositis, bone or joint infection, meningitis, but excluding pneumonia)
- Chronic herpes simplex infection; (orolabial or cutaneous of more than one month's duration) Extrapulmonary TB
- Kaposi's sarcoma
- Oesophageal candidiasis
- CNS toxoplasmosis (outside the neonatal period)
- HIV encephalopathy
- Conditions where confirmatory diagnostic testing is necessary

- CMV infection (CMV retinitis or infection of organs other than the liver, spleen, or lymph nodes; onset at age one month or more)
- Extrapulmonary cryptococcosis including meningitis
- Any disseminated endemic mycosis (*e.g.,* extrapulmonary histoplasmosis, coccidiomycosis, penicilliosis)
- Cryptosporidiosis
- Isosporiasis
- Disseminated nontuberculous mycobacterial infection
- Candida of trachea, bronchi, or lungs
- Visceral herpes simplex infection
- Acquired HIV associated rectal fistula
- Cerebral or B cell non-Hodgkin lymphoma
- Progressive multifocal leukoencephalopathy (PML)
- HIV-associated cardiomyopathy or HIV-associated nephropathy [14 - 19].

## Dental Caries and HIV

Children who have HIV have a remarkably high caries incidence. The explanation was thought to be the ingestion of drugs like zidovudine and Nystatin, which acts against candidiasis, a common infection in HIV patients. These drugs are sugar-containing. Their frequent consumption leads to high caries incidence. Caries incidence, however, is not directly related to HIV infection (Figs. **9A** & **9B**).

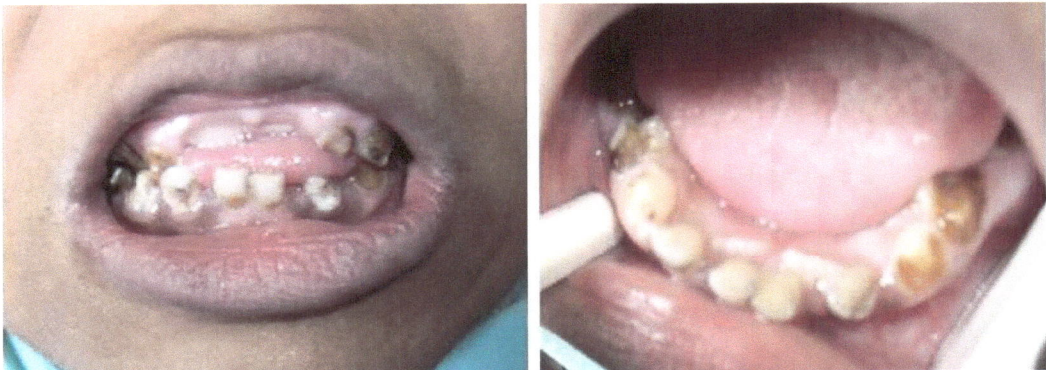

**Fig. (9). A** and **B** Exhibiting Tooth Decay.

## Pathophysiology

HIV is commonly transmitted *via* unprotected sexual activity, blood transfusions, hypodermic needles, and from mother to child. Upon acquiring the virus, the virus replicates inside and kills T helper cells, which are required for all adaptive immune responses. There is an initial period of influenza-like illness and a latent, asymptomatic phase. When the CD4 lymphocyte count falls below 200 cells/ml of blood, the HIV host has progressed to AIDS, a condition characterised by a deficiency in cell-mediated immunity and the resulting increased susceptibility to opportunistic infections [7],

**Diagnosis**

The defined diagnosis of HIV infection in neonates born to HIV infected mothers is problematic for various reasons. An HIV infected mother transmits the IgG antibodies to the new-born transplacental. These neonates are usually positive at birth, but only 15 to 30% are infected.

Maternal antibodies are usually undetectable in 9 months but occasionally remain at a significant level until 18 months. Hence IgG antibody tests are not reliable indicators of infection status in a child before 18 months of age. Therefore, the presence of antibodies beyond this period is necessary to consider the child infected, especially in an asymptomatic child. The definite diagnosis through:

Detection of P24 antigen [7-9].

CD4 count is low in HIV infection.

PCR (Polymerase Chain Reaction test) detects nucleic acid in peripheral blood.

Platelet count above 5,00,000(in serve infection)

ELISA or detection of IgG and IgM.

ELISA (Enzyme-Linked Immune Sorbent Assay).

**Therapeutic Management (Table 1)**

Medication therapy raises from single-drug treatment in an asymptomatic HIV exposed new-born to a Highly Active Anti-Retroviral Therapy (HAART)

Medication is prescribed based on the severity of the child's illness.

One of the goals of the HAART is to prevent or arrest progressive HIV encephalopathy.

**Groups of Antiretroviral Drugs (Table 2)**

Five groups of anti-retroviral drugs. Each attack HIV in a different way.

**Table 1. Use of a combination of antiretroviral drugs.**

| ARV Drug | Abbreviation | Action |
|---|---|---|
| Nucleotide Reverse Transcriptase Inhibitors | NRTIs Nucleotide Analogue Nukes | NRTIs interferes with the action of HIV protein called reverse transcriptase, in which the virus needs to make a new copy of itself. |
| Non-Nucleoside Reverse Transcriptase Inhibitors | NRTIs Non-Nucleotide Non-Nukes | NNRTIs also stop replicating within cells by inhibiting the sense to transcriptase proyien. |
| Protein Inhibitors | PIs | PI inhibits protease, which is another protein involved in HIV replication. |
| Fusion or entry inhibitors | - | Fusion or entry inhibitors prevent HIV from binding to entering human immune cells. |
| Integrase Inhibitors | - | Integrase Inhibitors interferes with the integrase enzyme, which HIV needs to insert its genetic materials into human cells. |

**Table 2. HIV Antiretroviral Drugs.**

| NRTI | NNRTI | Protease Inhibitors | Fusion Inhibitors |
|---|---|---|---|
| Zidovudine (AZT) Lamivudine (3TC) Emtricitabine (FTC) Stavudine (D4T) Didanosine (DDL) Tenifovir (TDF) Zalcitabine (ABV) Abacavir (DDC) | Efavirenz (EFV) Nevirapine (NVC) Delavirdine (DLV) | Ritanovir (RTV) Saquinavir (SQV) Indianavir (IDV) Nelfinavir (NFV) Fosamprenavir (APV) Lopinavir (LPV) Atazanavir (ATV) Duranavir (DRV) | Enfuvirtide |

Most drug combinations given to those beginning treatment consists of two NRTIs combined with either NRTIs (Nucleoside reverse transcriptase inhibitors) or booster protease inhibitor; ritonavir is commonly used as a booster.

An example common antiretroviral combination is two NRTIs, Zidovudine and Lamivudine, combined with NNRTI Efavaring [6-8].

## Management

1. Review maternal records to identify infants who may be at risk for HIV disease. Infected infants are not easily identifiable by outward appearance. Review records of at-risk or known infected children to determine nutritional status, growth and development, frequency of serious bacterial infections, presence or risk of opportunistic infections, laboratory values and immunisation status. Assess growth, development, lymph nodes,

hepatomegaly, splenomegaly, and oropharynx for the existence of oral candidiasis and dental caries.

2. Assess the family's understanding of the child's condition, care needs, prognosis, and medical care plan.

3. Assess the family's coping mechanisms, comfort with disclosure issues and long-term plans for care, including transition plans for the child to an adult care programme.

4. Assess the health of the primary caregiver and discuss long-term care plans for respite and permanent alternative caregivers as appropriate.

5. Assess the child's understanding and health status, and medications.

6. In children with advanced or end-stage disease, assess the level of pain and discomfort.

7. Assess the child coping and response to the frequent painful and invasive procedures experienced as part of ongoing diagnosis and management of the disease.

8. Assess for animal contact.

9. Take travel history to evaluate the risk of co-infections such as TB, malaria, or other microbial infections. Also assess potential travel plans, particularly to developing countries.

10. In adolescents, assess increased risk of behaviours such as substance use, piercing or sexual activity. Also, determine the method of birth control, as appropriate [7 - 9].

**Prevention**

Preventive measures are the best attempts to control the global problems of HIV/AIDS (Fig. **10**).

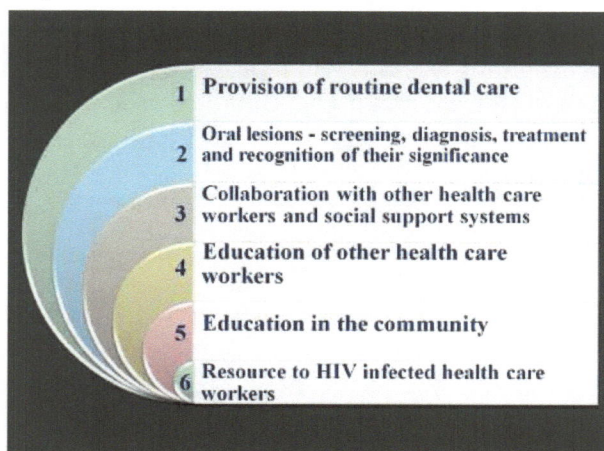

**Fig. (10).** Oral and Dental Health Care of HIV/AIDS Children.

## Four Basic Approaches to Control HIV/AIDS Include

a. Prevention by health education to make lifesaving choices and avoid blood-borne HIV infection.
b. ARVs (Antiretroviral drug) treatment with combination therapy or post-exposure prophylaxis.
c. Specific prophylaxis for HIV manifestations, e.g., isoniazid for tuberculosis.
d. PHC (primary health care) approaches with integrated care in Mother and Child Health and health education.

## Prevention of Mother to Child Transmission (MTCT)

ART regimen for treating pregnant women two options is available:

A. Daily AZT in an antepartum period combination of a single dose of NVP at the onset of labour and dose of AZT and 3TC during labour followed by a combination of AZT and 3TC for seven days in the postpartum period.
B. Triple ARV drugs starting as early as 14 weeks of gestation until one week after all exposure to breast milk has ended (AZT+3TC+LPV or AZT+3TC+ABC) where ABC is abacavir, LPV lopinavir [3 - 6].

## Regimen for Infants Born to HIV Positive Mothers

If the mother received only AZT during the antenatal period

For breastfeeding infants: Daily NPV from birth until one week after all exposure to breast milk has ended. The dose of nevirapine is 10mg/day/oral for infants less than 2.5 kg or 15mg/day/oral for infants more than 2.5 kg. For non-breastfeeding infants: Daily AZT or NVP from birth until six weeks. The dose of AZT is 4mg/kg per oral per dose twice a day. If mother received triple-drug ART during pregnancy and entire breastfeeding daily AZT or NVP from birth until six weeks of age irrespective of feeding [1, 2].

### *Breastfeeding*

Exclusive breastfeeding has been reported to carry a lower risk of HIV transmission than mixed feeding. Infected mothers should only give commercial infant formula milk as a replacement feed [7].

## CONCLUSION

"Hate the disease and not the infected," Oral Health Professionals has a tremendous role in controlling and preventing HIV/AIDS in children. They have a variety of roles to perform in caring for AIDS patients, including assessing, managing, educating, and counselling. There is no cure for AIDS as of date. Therefore, prevention is the only way to eliminate this dangerous condition.

## CONSENT FOR PUBLICATION

Not applicable.

## CONFLICT OF INTEREST

The authors declare no conflict of interest, financial or otherwise.

## ACKNOWLEDGEMENT

Declared none.

## REFERENCES

[1]     Joint United Nations Programme on HIV/AIDS (UNAIDS). Data 2019. Geneva: UNAIDS; 2019. Available from: https://www.unaids.org/en/resources/documents/2019/2019-UNAIDS-data. Accessed 12 March 2020.

[2]     World Health Organization Second WHO model list of essential *in vitro* diagnostics. 2019. https://www.who.int/medical_devices/publications/Standalone_document_v8.pdf?ua=1

[3]     World Health Organization Guidelines for managing advanced HIV disease and rapid initiation of antiretroviral therapy. 2017. https://www.who.int/hiv/pub/guidelines/advanced-HIV-disease/en

[4]     Cohn J, Whitehouse K, Tuttle J, Lueck K, Tran T. Paediatric HIV testing beyond the context of prevention of mother-to-child transmission: a systematic review and meta-analysis. Lancet HIV 2016; 3(10): e473-81.
[http://dx.doi.org/10.1016/S2352-3018(16)30050-9] [PMID: 27658876]

[5]     Amzel A, Toska E, Lovich R, *et al.* Promoting a combination approach to paediatric HIV psychosocial support. AIDS 2013; 27 (Suppl. 2): S147-57.
[http://dx.doi.org/10.1097/QAD.0000000000000098] [PMID: 24361624]

[6]     UNAIDS. Get on the Fast Track: the Life Cycle Approach to HIV. 2016.

[7]     Chandrashekhara, Sandeepkumar O. HIV / AIDS and Children. Int J Nur Edu Res 2020; 8(4): 564-8.
[http://dx.doi.org/10.5958/2454-2660.2020.00124.6]

[8]     Revision of the case definition of acquired immunodeficiency syndrome for national reporting--United States. MMWR Morb Mortal Wkly Rep 1985; 34(25): 373-5.
[PMID: 2989677]

[9]     Rajeswari C. Sugavana Selvi, Ramachandra. Anti-Retro Viral Therapy (ART) Adherence and Factors affecting Adherence among People living with HIV (PLHIVs). Asian J Nur Edu and Research 2017; 7(3): 337-40.

[10]    Vinay Kumar G, Nisha P. Nair, Prasannakumar D.R., Parmesha. A Study to assess the Quality of life of People Living with HIV/AIDS receiving Anti-Retroviral Therapy from the selected Anti-Retroviral Therapy centres of Mysore. Int J Adv Nur Management 2014; 2(2): 90-2.

[11]    Sylvia J. A Framework for a Nurse-Led Youth Friendly Reproductive and Sexual Health Services (YFRSHS) For HIV/ Aids Prevention. Int J Adv Nur Management 2015; 3(2): 152-4.

[12]    Grigson S. A Study to assess the Effectiveness of Planned Teaching Program on Knowledge regarding HIV/AIDS among the students studying in selected school at Damoh. Int J Adv Nur Manag 2019;

7(3): 240-2.

[13]  Tufon EN, Bih AD, Alice M. Occurrence and Risk Factors for Opportunistic Infections in HIV Patients Attending the Bamenda Regional Hospital, Cameroon. Int J Nur Edu Res 2014; 2(4): 381-4.

[14]  Johnson NW. The mouth in HIV/AIDS: markers of disease status and management challenges for the dental profession. Aust Dent J 2010; 55 (Suppl. 1): 85-102.
[http://dx.doi.org/10.1111/j.1834-7819.2010.01203.x] [PMID: 20553249]

[15]  Kalpidis CDR, Lysitsa SN, Lombardi T, Kolokotronis AE, Antoniades DZ, Samson J. Gingival involvement in a case series of patients with acquired immunodeficiency syndrome-related Kaposi sarcoma. J Periodontol 2006; 77(3): 523-33.
[http://dx.doi.org/10.1902/jop.2006.050226] [PMID: 16512768]

[16]  Khongkunthian P, Grote M, Isaratanan W, Piyaworawong S, Reichart PA. Oral manifestations in 45 HIV-positive children from Northern Thailand. J Oral Pathol Med 2001; 30(9): 549-52.
[http://dx.doi.org/10.1034/j.1600-0714.2001.300907.x] [PMID: 11555158]

[17]  Gallottini Magalhães M, Franco Bueno D, Serra E, Gonçalves R. Oral manifestations of HIV positive children. J Clin Pediatr Dent 2001; 25(2): 103-6.
[http://dx.doi.org/10.17796/jcpd.25.2.f01k062j7315660v] [PMID: 11314206]

[18]  Massarente DB, Domaneschi C, Marques HHS, Andrade SB, Goursand D, Antunes JLF. Oral health-related quality of life of paediatric patients with AIDS. BMC Oral Health 2011; 11(1): 2.
[http://dx.doi.org/10.1186/1472-6831-11-2] [PMID: 21208437]

[19]  Mittal M. AIDS in children--epidemiology, clinical course, oral manifestations and management. J Clin Pediatr Dent 2009; 34(2): 95-102.
[http://dx.doi.org/10.17796/jcpd.34.2.m2055qnv417n51x5] [PMID: 20297697]

CHAPTER 10

# Advances in Pediatric Dentistry

**Harsimran Kaur**[1,*], **Rishika** [1] and **Ramakrishna Yeluri**[1]

[1] *Department of Pedodontics and Preventive Dentistry, Teerthanker Mahaveer Dental College and Research Centre, Moradabad, U.P., India*

**Abstract:** Approaches for managing dental caries have changed dramatically in recent years, evolving from froadichtional treatments to a preventive approach. Modern management approaches aim to prevent the disease, manage the caries risk, and detect caries lesions as early as possible. Also, various breakthroughs have been made in restorative materials to improve their biocompatibility and bonding with tooth structure. With nanotechnology, knowledge of materials, and developments in biomaterials, the prod the action of the best quality dental restorative materials is rising. Local anaesthesia is the standard and the backbone for controlling pain. The introduction of newer techniques of regional anaesthesia and delivery devices assist dentists in providing enhanced pain relief with reduced pain from injection and fewer adverse reactions. The chapter below highlights the various advancements in sterilisation, diagnostic aids, preventive strategies, restorative materials and techniques and tissue engineering.

**Keywords:** Diagnostic Aids, Endodontics, Local Anaesthesia, Restorative materials, Tissue engineering.

## INTRODUCTION

With the remarkable advent of advancement in all fields of medicine, pediatric dentistry did not remain an exception. Dentistry has gone from "extension for prevention" to "constriction with conservation". These transformations have caused a paradigm shift in the pediatric population's treatment planning and management of Oro-dental problems. A few of these innovations in pediatric dentistry are discussed below.

* **Corresponding author Harsimran Kaur:** Department of Pedodontics and Preventive Dentistry, Teerthanker Mahaveer Dental College and Research Centre, Moradabad, U.P., India; E-mail: Simran2871@Gmail.Com

**Satyawan Damle, Ritesh Kalaskar & Dhanashree Sakhare (Eds.)**

## ADVANCES IN STERILIZATION

Selecting the appropriate method to process with the products used in health care delivery is vital to ensure that pathogens triggering infections are not transmitted to patients and vice versa. The quality of managing the situation is the foundation of curbing diseases associated with specific procedures through the microbial reduction or destruction in products used and the maintenance of a product's functionality and integrity.

### • Ozone Sterilization

$O_3$ is present in the environment naturally *via* oxygen in the stratosphere by absorbing the sun's ultraviolet radiation. When $O_3$ is obtained through electrochemical technology, it is an alternative for breaking down resistant organic compounds, such as dyes from textile effluents, pesticides, and waste from the paper industry. The practices recommended for health workers concerning the sterilisation of health products assume that $O_3$ is a strong oxidant, enabling the construction of an effective low-temperature sterilisation system.

### *Mechanism of Action of Ozone*

Antimicrobial Effect.

- Causes cell death by local damage of cytoplasmic membrane due to ozonolysis of double bonds, ozone-induced modification of intracellular contents.
- Oxidize many organic compounds, causes circulatory enhancement metabolism, and stimulate oxygen metabolism. Enhanced antimicrobial activity in a liquid environment of the acidic pH.
- Oxidation of NADH (Nicotinamide Adenine dinucleotide) and NADPH Hydrogenated Nicotinamide Adenine Dinucleotide phosphate coenzymes, manifested in all three metabolic pathways, *i.e.*, involving carbohydrates, proteins, and fats [1].

### *Advantages of Ozone Sterilisation*

- It is cost-effective.
- It does not require inputs because oxygen is used to produce $O_3$.
- Diffusion of $O_3$ in lumens of various diameters and lengths rigid stainless steel has also been proved.

The application of $O_3$ as a sterilising agent for products used in health care is a new proposition; the scope and products tests and the diversity of experiments imply that research on O3 as sterilising agent is still developing.

## ADVANCES IN DIAGNOSTIC AIDS

Conventional methods cannot detect carious lesions until a relatively advanced stage. Thus, there has been intensive research into more sophisticated methods for the early detection of dental caries over the past few years. Several are in their infancy, and there is significant work involved in developing these techniques. The following section presents a brief description of the neoteric caries diagnostic methods.

### Digital Dental Mirror (Mirror Scope)

It has a loupe and microscope combined in a ready to use manner. It has the advantage that it can be used to capture videos or still images, just like an intraoral camera. The clinicians can choose to work directly from the mirror or indirectly view high-resolution images magnified up to 30-x. The Mirror Scope will enable the operators to provide better patient care while improving their posture and reducing back and neck strain (Fig. **1**) [2].

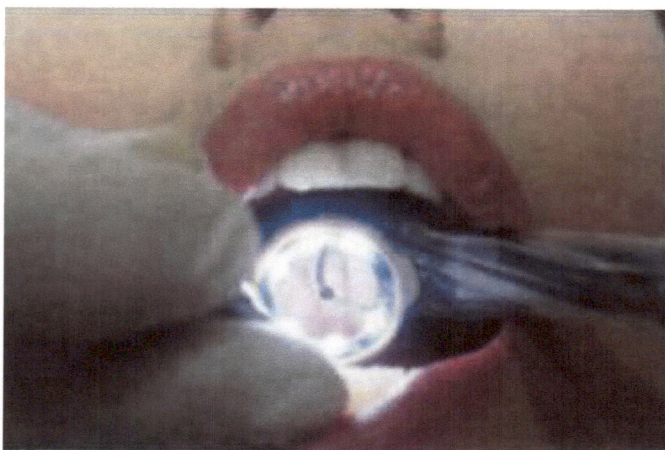

**Fig. (1).** Digital Dental Mirror.

**Lasers.**

## *Quantitative Light-Induced Fluorescence (QLF)*

QLF can assess the impact of preventive measures on the re-mineralization and reversal of the caries process as it can monitor and quantify changes in the mineral content of white spot lesions (Fig. **2**).

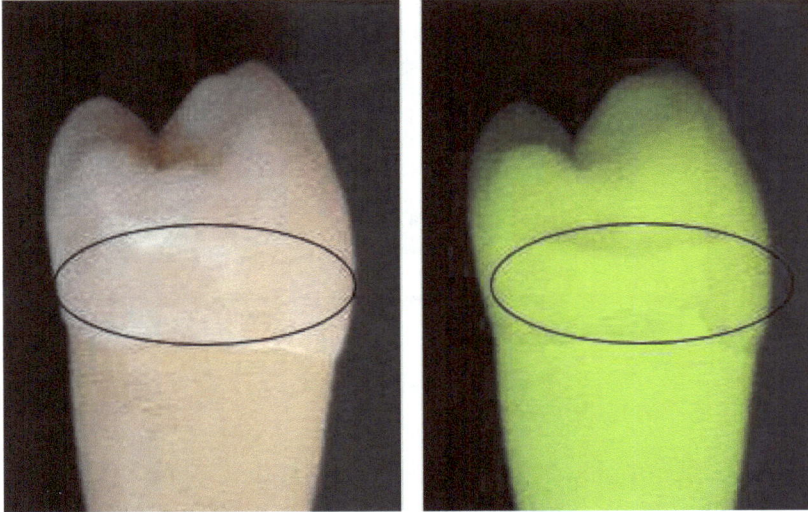

**Fig. (2).**  A white-light (left) and fluorescence image (right) of a premolar. The white spot lesion barely visible under white-light conditions is visible using fluorescence.

## *Diagnodent*

Diagnodent with a laser diode generates a pulsed 655 nm laser beam through a central fibre, transported to the device's tip and the tooth. When the incident light interacts with tooth substance, it stimulates fluorescent (or luminescent) light at longer wavelengths. The fluorescence intensity depends on the degree of demineralisation or bacterial concentration in the probed region [3].

## C. Dental Microscopes

Dental microscopes (Fig. **3**) reveal fine details and structures that remain invisible to the naked eyes. They provide maximum precision and enable accurate diagnosis and new treatment approaches. They can be used for patient/parent education by recording diagnostic findings demonstrating various stages of treatment on the monitor if the microscope is supported by video [2].

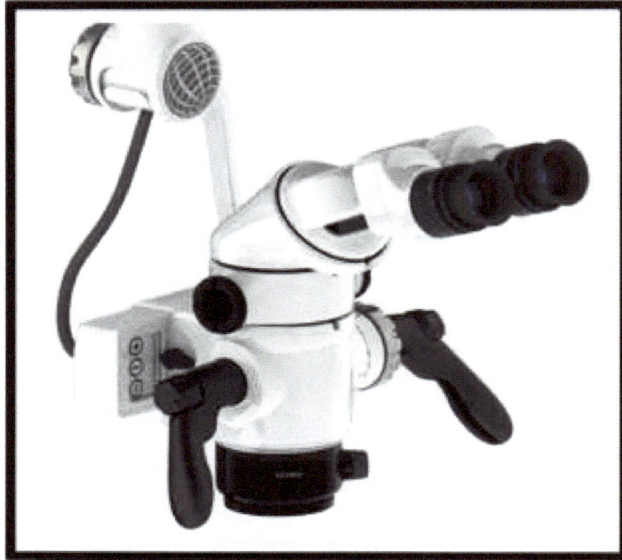

**Fig. (3).** Dental microscopes.

## D. New electronic Caries Detector (ECD)

Ortek ECD is an electronic caries detection device that measures the conductivity of enamel. Powered by a 9-V battery, this small, portable system has a base unit with a digital display, a handpiece with a dimensionally configured stainless steel tip that reaches the bottom of a pit or fissure, and a reference lip hook (Fig. **4**).

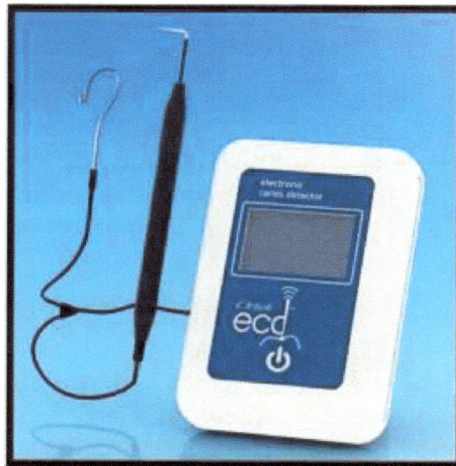

**Fig. (4).** Electronic caries monitor.

If the dentin-enamel junction is breached by demineralisation, hydrostatic pressure within dentinal tubules will allow minuscule amounts of conductive dentinal fluid to enter the breached enamel site, allowing the ECD to complete an electric circuit.

Loss of minerals from enamel due to caries activity increases the porous size and enamel porosity. As this demineralisation increases, more dentinal fluid enters the breached site. The more fluid detected results in lower resistance, a higher current, and an increasing digital caries score that is digitally displayed from 0 to 100. A zero indicates no cavitated lesion, as intact tooth enamel is electrically non-conductive [4].

## E. Illumination Methods

i. Fibre-optic transillumination (FOTI).

ii. Wavelength dependent FOTI.

iii. Digital imaging FOTI (DIFOTI).

### *FOTI*

In recent years, because of concerns over the cumulative effects of ionising radiation, a simple FOTI technique that utilises a light-emitting diode was developed for caries detection, which uses a narrow beam of white light to transilluminate the tooth (Fig. **5**). As a caries detector technique, FOTI is based on the fact that carious enamel has a lower light transmission index than sound enamel. As the demineralisation process disrupts the crystalline structure of enamel and dentin, more light is absorbed due to changes in the light scattering and absorption of light photons. In essence, this gives that area a more darkened appearance.

FOTI was initially designed by Friedman and Marcus in 1970 to detect proximal caries. Posterior proximal caries is diagnosed by placing the light probe on the gingiva below the cervical margin of the tooth, whereby light passes through the tooth structures, and proximal decay appears as dark as a shadow on the occlusal surface. The FOTI has higher sensitivity for dentin lesions than for enamel lesions. False-negative results are one of the significant limitations of FOTI [3].

### *Advantage*

- Optimum positive predictive value performance, which means that any positive reading is almost certainly indicative of an existing lesion,.
- no exposure to radiation,.

- gives instant images simple,.
- non-time consuming,.
- Comfortable to patients.

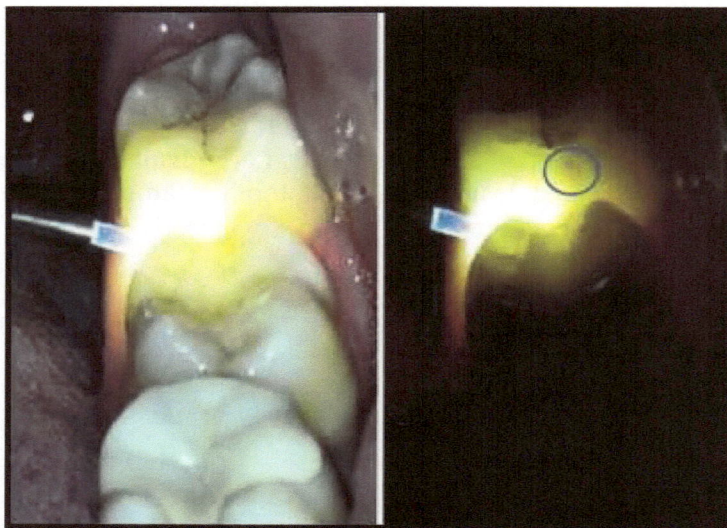

**Fig. (5).** FOTI.

## ii. Wavelength Dependent FOTI

In incipient white-spot lesions, the mineral loss is accompanied by increased light scattering. In older, discoloured lesions, light absorption is also enhanced. A combination of material properties causes the induced effect at the occlusal surface, and the distance light propagates through tooth material from the light source to the detector. This combination will be called "effective decadic optical thickness" and is dependent on the light wavelength. It is assumed that, in the case of small lesions, the adequate decadic optical thickness increases linearly with mineral loss.

| Advantages | Disadvantages |
|---|---|
| • gives quantitative information about the depth of the lesion | • not applicable in all locations of carious lesions |
| • no radiation hazard | • Has considerable intra and inter-examiner variations [3]. |

## iii. DIFOTI

This technique was introduced to overcome the limitations of FOTI by combining FOTI and a digital charge-coupled device (CCD) camera. DIFOTI is the only approved dental diagnostic imaging instrument used to detect incipient, frank, and recurrent caries. It can also detect fractures, cracks, and secondary caries around restorations.

It is based on the principle that carious tooth tissue absorbs lighter than surrounding healthy tissue and appears as a darker area. DIFOTI system consists of two handpieces (one for occlusal surface and one for smooth surface and the interproximal regions), a disposable mouthpiece, a foot pedal for selecting the image of interest and a computer system to capture and store the resulting image.

It has the advantage of instant images stored for future references; however, this method does not measure lesion depth and difficulty discriminating deep fissures, stains, and actual dentin lesions. Furthermore, overdiagnosis can occur due to lower specificity when prepared with conventional radiographs. Dark areas on the images can be attributed to scattering and light absorption as it passes through demineralised enamel and dentin or near the surface; consequently, white spots can be mistaken for cavitation [3].

## F. Soprolife Camera

It is based on the imaging and autofluorescence of dental tissues to detect caries. The camera captures the images in three different modes: daylight mode, diagnosis mode, and treatment mode (Fig. **6**).

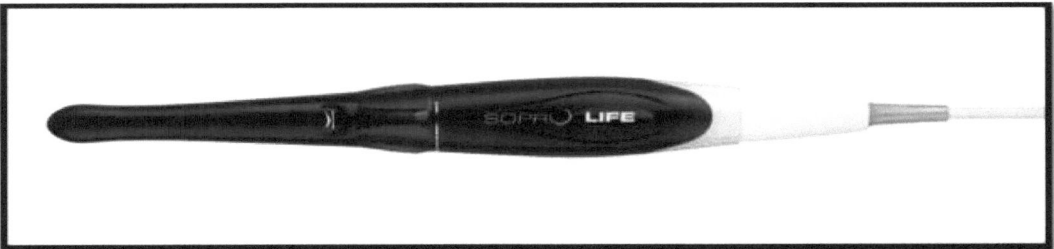

**Fig. (6).** Soprolife camera.

- Capturing in the **daylight** provides a white light image with a magnification of more than 50 times the tooth surface. The other two modes of the camera work on the principle of autofluorescence.
- In the **diagnostic mode**, the camera uses a visible blue light frequency (wavelength 450nm) to illuminate the surface of the teeth and provides an anatomic image overlay of the green fluorescence image on the "white light" image. This green fluorescence is considered an indicator of healthy dental tissues. At the same time, carious lesions could be detected by variation in the

autofluorescence of its tissues about a healthy area of the same tooth. In addition to the green fluorescence, red fluorescence may also be seen in some diagnostic mode images. This red fluorescence may represent deep dentinal caries; however, at the same time, it might be a false signal coming from the organic deposits covering the tooth. The area showing the red fluorescence should be washed off with sodium bicarbonate or pumice for validation. If the fluorescence persists, it should only be considered representative of infected dentin. The fluorescence would no longer be there if the source is simply the organic deposits on the tooth surface.

The treatment mode: the red fluorescence (Table 1) captured in this mode is considered an indicator of differentiating between infected and affected dentin [2].

Table 1. Types of dentin and fluorescence.

| Healthy Dentin | Green Fluorescence |
|---|---|
| Infected Dentin | Red fluorescence |
| Infected/Affected Dentin | Bright Red fluorescence<br>A manual excavator can efficiently excavate this tissue. |

## G. Midwest Caries I.D. ™ Detection Handpiece

MID is a small, battery-operated technology that emits a soft LED light for detecting and quantifying caries (Fig. 7). A specific fibre optic signature captures the resulting reflection and refraction of the light in the tooth. It is converted to electrical signals that run through a computer-based algorithm to analyse caries' presence.

### Indications

The Midwest Caries I.D. ™ detection handpiece is recommended for use to detect caries in pits and fissures and interproximal areas on posterior teeth that have not been restored. The detection handpiece must be used in a wet field.

### Contraindications

The Midwest Caries I.D. ™ detection handpiece is not designed to be used.

- On or at the interface of dental restorations or for residual caries detection.
- On buccal and lingual areas of anterior and posterior teeth.
- On thick, dark brown stains, calculus, and heavy plaque.
- On restorations, sealants, and varnish.

- On primary teeth.
- On dried teeth [3].

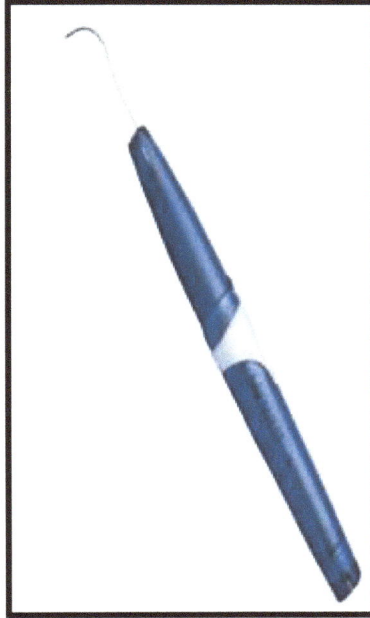

**Fig. (7).** Midwest Caries I.D. ™ detection handpiece.

## H. Endoscopy

Endoscopy includes:

  i. Endoscopically viewed filtered fluorescence.
 ii. White light fluorescence.
iii. Video scope.

### i. Endoscopically Viewed Filtered Fluorescence (EFF)

This technique utilises the fluorescence of enamel that occurs when it is illuminated with blue light in the wavelength range 499–500 nm. When the tooth is viewed from a specific gelatin green filter number 58, attached to the eyepiece, white spot lesions appear darker than sound enamel.

Pitts and Longbottom showed the EFF method to be highly sensitive for occlusal enamel caries and more specific for approximal lesions at both thresholds. This work was developed to include using an intraoral video system for caries detection, the prototype "videoscope" (Table **2**).

Also, endoscopic methods detected a more significant number of carious lesions than do conventional visual, radiographic, or FOTI methods.

**Table 2. Advantages and limitations of endoscopically viewed filtered fluorescence method.**

| Advantages | Limitations |
|---|---|
| • gives a magnified view of carious lesions | • Requires meticulous drying and isolation are necessary for accurate results |
| • Provides an extensive range of viewing angles and the areas which are difficult to view by conventional means. | • Time-consuming and technique sensitive<br>• Cannot be used in inaccessible areas |

## ii. White Light Fluorescence

A fibre-optic cable connects a white light source to the endoscope by a fibre-optic cable, and teeth are viewed without a filter. Limitations: The weight of fibre-optic cable tends to destabilise the machine, and the increased distance between eyepiece and light source decreases illumination.

## iii. Video Scope

The integration of the camera with an endoscope to save the image for future reference is called a video scope. This is designed so that the image of the surface of enamel can be viewed directly over a television screen [3].

## I. Computed Tomography (CT)

Computed tomography has been a well-known medical technique for the non-destructive examination of internal structures. Its introduction to dentistry has been innovative as it provides accurate three-dimensional (3D) imaging. Cone-beam CT (CBCT) is a new application of CT that generates 3D data at a lower cost. It was observed that vertically reformatted CT slices obtained with local CT performed significantly better radiographs in visually detecting caries than conventional two-dimensional digital.

Also, dentists could detect dentinal proximal-surface caries using 3DX high-resolution CBCT images compared with CCD images compared to occlusal dentinal caries [3].

## J. X-ray Microtomography

X-ray microtomography is a shortened version of computerised axial tomography with micrometre resolution. Microtomography (commonly known as Industrial CT scanning), like tomography, uses X-rays to create cross-sections of a 3D object that later can be used to recreate a virtual model without destroying the original model. The term micro is used to indicate that the pixel sizes of the cross-sections are in the micrometre range [3].

## K. Fluorescence Camera (VISTAPROOF)

The fluorescence camera (Vista Proof) is based on the light-induced fluorescence phenomenon. (Durr Dental, Bietigheim-Bissingen, Germany) that is based on six blue GaN-LEDs emitting a 405-nm light (Fig. **8**).

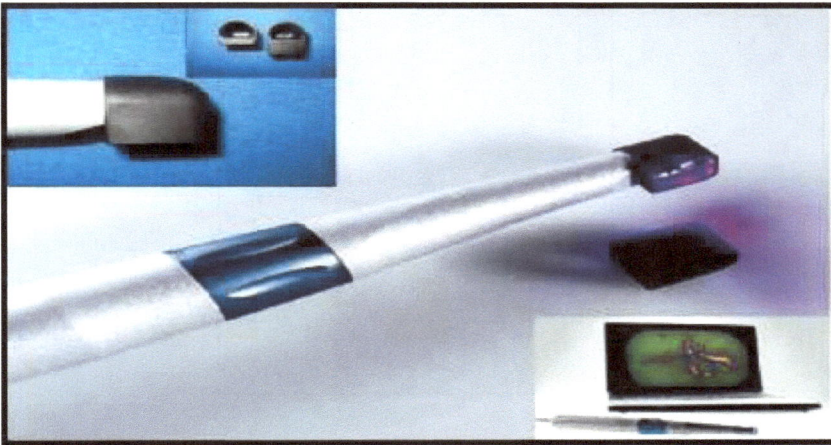

**Fig. (8).** Vista Proof.

This camera makes it possible to digitise the video signal from the dental surface during fluorescence emission using a CCD sensor (charge-coupled device). On these images, it is possible to see different areas of the dental surface that fluoresce in green (sound dental tissue) and red (carious dental tissue). DBSWIN software is used to analyse the images and translate the intensity ratio of the red and green fluorescence into values. The software highlights the lesions and classifies them on a scale from 0 to 5, giving a treatment orientation in the first evaluation: monitoring, remineralisation, or invasive treatment. Latest version of Vista proof is Vista Cam ix.

## L. Carie Scan

This device is based on alternating current impedance spectroscopy. It involves the passing of an insensitive level of electrical current through the tooth to identify the presence and location of the decay. It is the first dental diagnostic tool to use impedance spectroscopy to quantify dental caries early enough to enhance preventive treatment. CarieScan is not affected by optical factors such as staining or discolouration of the tooth. It provides a qualitative value based on the disease state rather than the optical properties of the tooth (Fig. **9**).

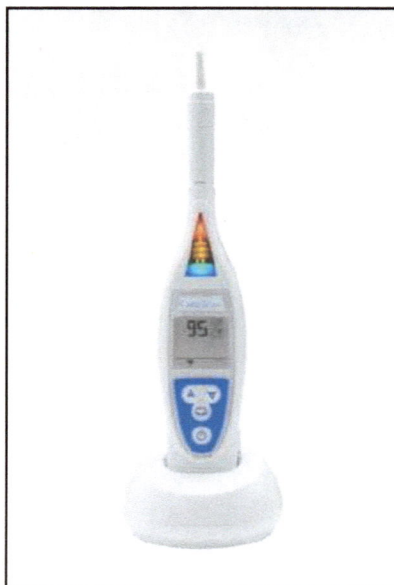

**Fig. (9).**  CARIESCAN.

Bader *et al.* reported that CarieScan has superior sensitivity and specificity, 92.5% over other methods [3].

## ADVANCES IN NANO DENTISTRY

Nanotechnology gave emergence to a new field called nanomedicine and nano dentistry, a science and technology of diagnosing, treating, and preventing diseases and preserving and improving human health using nanoscale materials. The word "nano" is derived from nan(n)os, the Greek word for "dwarf, little old man." It has been stated that nano dentistry will make it possible to maintain near-perfect oral health through nanomaterials, biotechnology, and nanorobotics [2].

## Approaches to Nanodentistry

I. **Bottom-up approaches:** To arrange smaller components into more complex assemblies. It comprises tooth repair, hypersensitivity cure, dental durability and cosmetics, dentifrice nanorobots, tooth repositioning, local drug delivery, nano-diagnostics, and therapeutic aid in oral diseases.

II. **Top-down approaches:** Create smaller devices by using larger ones to direct their assembly. It encompasses nanocomposites, nan-impression materials, nano-composite, nano solutions, nanoencapsulation, plasma laser application, prosthetic implants, and bone replacement materials.

### a). Nanofillers

Nanofillers are more than 100 times smaller than traditional fillers. Fillers are incorporated in composites or compomers to increase strength.

For adhesive bonding, nanofillers allow an adhesive to be reinforced by tiny particles while maintaining essential properties of high-performance bonding. The particle size is about 7 nm. These smaller particles support dentin's natural components while building the foundation for a perfect link between tooth structure and restorative materials.

### b). Nanosilver Fluoride

Nano Silver Fluoride (NSF), containing silver nanoparticles, chitosan, and fluoride, combines preventive and antimicrobial properties and developed to be an effective anti-caries agent without staining the porous dental tissues black, as does silver diamine fluoride and amalgam. NSF was demonstrated to be effective in arresting caries in children. This new substance is safe for humans and has excellent antimicrobial properties against Mutans streptococci and Lactobacilli, the primary pathogens responsible for developing dental caries. Silver can combat residual bacteria in the tooth cavity and invade bacteria at the restoration's margins.

### c). Nano Diamond-Guttapercha Composite Biomaterials

Nanodiamond gutta-percha composite (NDGP) embedded with nanodiamond-amoxicillin (ND-AMC) conjugates have been developed to reduce the likelihood of root canal reinfection and enhance the treatment outcomes. Nanodiamonds are carbon nanoparticles approximately 4-6nm in diameter; they are waste byproducts readily processed for biomedical applications.

NDGP may also attenuate bacteria entering through the lateral canals following contact with Nano diamond-antibiotic agents. The homogeneous dispersion of Nanodiamonds throughout the Gutta-percha matrix also increases toughness compared to unmodified GP and NDGP.

### d). Nanoadhesive-Polyhedral Oligomeric Silse Squiox (Poss)

Polyhedral Oligomeric Silse Squiox (Poss) enables the design of additives that make unusually lightweight, durable, heat-tolerant, and environmentally friendly plastics. Poss combines organic & inorganic materials in molecules with average diameter of1.5 nanometers. They can be used as either additives or replacements for traditional plastics. Current Polyhedral Oligomeric Silse Squiox (Poss) applications include dental adhesives in which a strength resin provides a strong interface between the teeth and the restorative material. In addition, tests have shown that Poss materials are much more resistant to radiation damage and erosion than conventional polymers [2].

### ADVANCES IN ENDODONTICS

  a. Advances in pulp vitally testing.
  b. Advances in Irrigation solution and devices.
  c. Advances in the Files system.

### Advances in Pulp Vitally Testing

### *Xenon$_{133}$Isotopes*

Radioactive materials for measuring pulpal blood circulation were previously used in the radio-labelled microsphere injection method. Using a radiation probe with Xenon$_{133}$ radioisotopes to differentiate between solid and pulpfewer teeth based on blood supply has been effective. However, the use of radioactive materials is expensive, restricted on humans, and requires special licensing requirements [5, 6].

### *Transmitted Laser Light (TLL)*

Transmitted laser light is an experimental variation to LDF to eliminate the non-pulp signals. TLL uses similar sending/receiving probes as conventional LDF, but the probes are separate. Thus, the laser beam is passed through from the labial or buccal side of the tooth to the receiver probe, situated on the palatal or lingual side of the tooth. The limitations with TLL are the same as with any laser technology, where obstruction and interference from within the tooth structure will affect the results.

## Detection of Interleukins

IL-l, previously known as lymphocyte activating factor, is a monocyte-derived factor. IL-l is a cytokine released in vitro by cultured monocytes or macrophages and acts as a mediator of various immunologic and inflammatory phenomena. IL-I stimulate prostaglandin E2 and collagenase production by fibroblasts. Moreover, IL- 1 stimulates bone resorption". Periapical specimens for the presence of IL-l/3 have been investigated with an enzyme-linked immunosorbent assay (ELISA). It was found that IL-l/3 is released in the periapical tissue in patients with periapical pathosis and its absence in non-inflamed pulpal tissues.

## Hughes Probeye Camera.

It can detect temperature changes as small as $0.10^0C$. This consists of a thermal video system with a silicon close up lens with a resolvable spot size of 0.023 inches. Technique: teeth in question are isolated with a rubber dam and cooled with a stream of cold air. Symmetrical cooling of teeth of about $220^0C$ is done. Then teeth are rewarmed to their former temperature. Vital teeth will re-warm in 5 sec, whereas non-vital teeth take up to 15 sec to re-warm. More rapid warming of vital teeth is due to an intact blood supply.

## Gas Tension

This method evaluates the acidity and blood partial pressure of O2 and CO2 in samples drawn from pulp chambers of primary molars undergoing pulpotomy or pulpectomy. This technique also measures the differences in pH, pCO2 and pO2 between reversible and irreversible pulpitis that may serve as a basis for developing a chair-side diagnostic approach [7].

## Advances in Irrigant Solution (Table 3)

Table 3. Newer Irrigant solutions.

| Name of Irrigant solution | Composition | Properties |
| --- | --- | --- |
| Hydroxyethylidene Bisphosphonate (HEBP) etidronic acid or etidronate | A decalcifying agent that has little interaction with NaOCl. It is proposed as an alternative to EDTA or CA. | HELP prevents bone resorption and thus is used as a systemic drug to treat osteoporosis and Paget's disease. |

*(Table 3) cont.....*

| Name of Irrigant solution | Composition | Properties |
|---|---|---|
| **A mixture of Tetracycline Isomer, Acid, and Detergent (MTAD) (Torabinejad *et al.*)** | combination of 3% Doxycyclin, 4.25% Citric Acid, and detergent (Tween-80) | improved smear layer removal property. Chelator and antimicrobial activity. |
| **Tetraclean (OgnaLaboratori Farmaceutici, Muggiò (Mi), Italy)** | A citric acid mixture, Doxycyclin (at a lower concentration than MTAD), and detergent. The concentration of antibiotics (doxycycline-50 mg/ml) and the type of detergent (propylene glycol) differ from those in MTAD [8]. | does not dissolve organic tissue, and its use after NaOCl at the end of chemomechanical preparation is recommended [8]. |
| **Triclosan and Gantrez** | Triclosan is a Gram-positive and Gram-negative bactericide and a broad-spectrum agent effective against fungi and viruses. The addition of Gantrez to triclosan increased bacterial activity [8]. | Both preparations showed bactericidal activity against the five major endodontic pathogens [8] |
| **Silver Diamine Fluoride** | A 3.8% silver diamine fluoride (Ag [NH$_3$]$_2$F) is the the1:10-diluted form of the original 38% solution of Ag [NH$_3$]$_2$F, which was developed for the treatment of root canal infection [8]. | An aqueous solution of AgF has powerful disinfectant, protein-coagulation action. 3.8% SDF can be used as an eloquent root canal. Irrigant effectively exterminates the microbes present in the canal and circumpulpal dentin [8]. |
| **Chitosan** | Chitosan is a natural linear polysaccharide obtained by the deacetylation of chitin, which is found in crab and shrimp shells [8]. | Possess Biocompatibility, biodegradability, bioadhesion and lack of toxicity. It also aids in the removal of inorganic components of the smear layer [8]. |
| **Q-MIX (Dr. Markus Haapasalo *et al*)** | Ethylene-diamine-tetra-acetic acid (EDTA), Chlorhexidine and cetrimide (N-Cetyl-N, N, N-Tri Methyl Ammonium Bromide) mixed in distilled water with acceptable additional salt. | eradicates bacteria, removes smear layer and persists in biofilms [9]. |
| **Electro Chemically Activated Water (Developed at the All-Russian Institute for Medical Engineering (Moscow, Russia, CIS)** | Electrochemically Activated (ECA) solutions are produced from tap water and low-concentrated salt solutions. The principle of ECA is transferring liquids into a metastable state *via* an electrochemical unipolar (anode or cathode) action through the use of an element/reactor ("Flow-through Electrolytic Module" or FEM). [9] | Both types of ECA solutions (anolyte and catholyte) are effective for the treatment of cutaneous and mucous infections, for posttraumatic and postoperative suppurative complications, and purulent surgical disease, have a more pronounced clinical effect, fewer incidences of allergic reactions [9] |

*(Table 3) cont.....*

| Name of Irrigant solution | Composition | Properties |
|---|---|---|
| **Ozone Water:** | Ozone is a chemical compound with a higher energetic form than normal atmospheric oxygen (O2). When introduced in water, ozone dissolves rapidly and dissociates rather quickly. | Ozone is a potent bactericide that can kill microorganisms effectively. It is a hazardous gas capable of oxidising any biological entity. It was reported that ozone at a low concentration, 0.1 ppm, is sufficient to inactivate bacterial cells including their spores [9] |
| **Photon:** **(First shown by Oscar Raab)** | photodynamic therapy (PDT) is based on the concept that nontoxic photosensitisers can be preferentially localised in specific tissues and subsequently activated by light of the appropriate wavelength to generate singlet oxygen and free radicals that are cytotoxic to cells of the target tissue [9]. | Methylene blue (MB) is a well-established photosensitiser used in PDT to target various gram-positive and gram-negative oral bacteria and was previously used to study the effect of PDT on endodontic disinfection [9]. |
| **Herbal irrigants** | | |
| *Triphala* | *Triphala* consists of dried and powdered fruits of three medicinal plants *Terminaliabellerica*, *Terminaliachebula*, and *Emblicaofficinalis* [8]. | *Triphala* achieved 100% killing of *Efaecalis* at 6 min [8] |
| *Green tea* | Green tea polyphenols are prepared from the young shoots of the tea plant *Camellia sinensis* [8]. | showed significant antibacterial activity against *Efaecalis* biofilm formed on tooth substrate [8] |
| *Morindacitrifolia* **(MCJ)** | contains the antibacterial compounds L-asperuloside and alizarin [8]. | antibacterial, antiviral, antifungal, antitumor, antihelmintic, analgesic, hypotensive, anti-inflammatory, and immune-enhancing effects A biocompatible antioxidant and not likely to cause severe injuries to patients as might occur through NaOCl accidents [8]. |

Optimal irrigation is based on the combined use of two or several irrigating solutions in a specific sequence to predictably attain the goals of safe and effective irrigation (Fig. **10**).

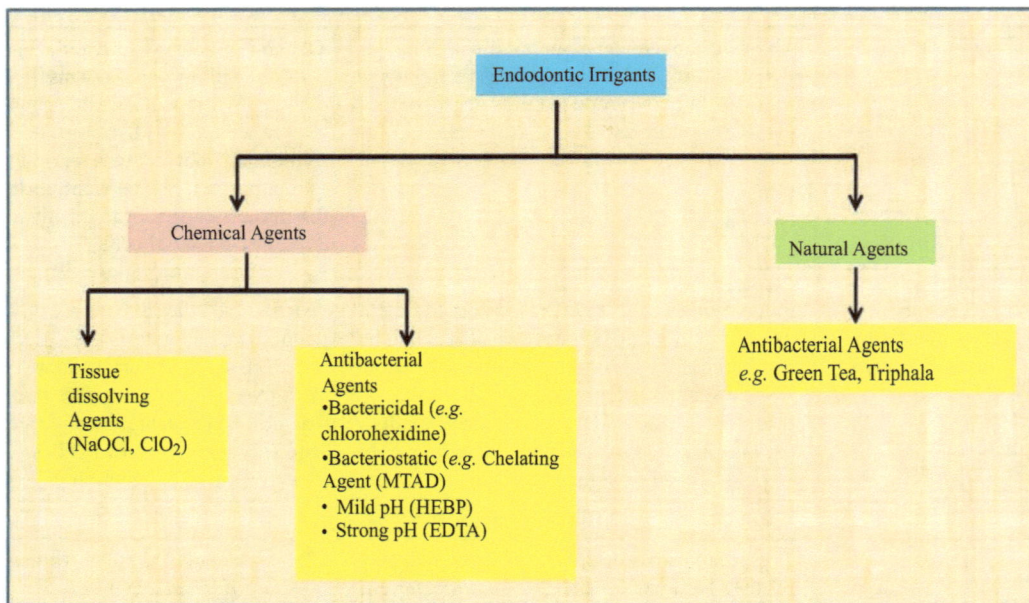

**Fig. (10).** Classification of newer endodontic Irrigants.

## Irrigation devices (Fig. 11 & Table 4)

**Table 4. Newer Irrigation devices.**

| Irrigation device system | Details |
|---|---|
| **Max-i-probe** | is a modified design of regular manual irrigation needles with a well-rounded, close tip and side-port dispersal [8]. |
| **NaviTipFx** | NaviTipFx is a 30-gauge irrigation needle covered with a brush introduced commercially by Ultra dent. improved cleanliness in the coronal third when compared to brushless NaviTip needle [8]. |
| **Quantec-E irrigation system (SybronEndo company)** | Is it a self-contained fluid delivery unit attached to the Quantec-E Endo System25? It uses a pump console, two irrigation reservoirs, and tubing to provide continuous rotary instrumentation [8]. |
| **Vibringe System (Dutch company Vibringe B. V)** | The Vibrating is a cordless handpiece that fits a special disposable 10-mL Luer-Lock syringe compatible with every irrigation needle. allows delivery and sonic activation of the irrigating solution in one step [8]. |
| **The EndoActivator System (Dentsply)** | consists of a portable handpiece and three types of disposable polymer tips of different sizes. This might be operated 10,000 cycles per minute (cpm) has been shown to optimise debridement and promote disruption of the smear layer and biofilm [8]. |

| Irrigation device system | Details |
|---|---|
| **Ultrasonic Irrigation** | Irrigant is delivered to the root canal by a syringe needle and then activated using an ultrasonically oscillating instrument [8]. |
| **The EndoVac System (Discus Dental Company)** | It has three components: *Master Delivery Tip* simultaneously delivers and evacuates the irrigants. *MacroCannula* used to suction irrigants from the chamber to the coronal and middle segments of the canal. *MacroCannula or MicroCannula* is connected *via* tubing to the high-speed suction of a dental unit. Master Delivery Tip is connected to a syringe of irrigants, and the evacuation hood is connected *via* tubing to the high-speed suction of a dental unit [8]. |
| **The RinsEndo System (DurrDental Co)** | Irrigates the canal using pressure-suction technology. Its components are a handpiece, a cannula with a 7 mm exit aperture, and a syringe carrying irrigants [8]. |
| **The VATEA system** | The VATEA system is a self-contained, fluid delivery unit intended to be attached to dental handpieces to deliver irrigation during endodontic procedures. The irrigants are delivered *via* a disposable silicone tube to the endodontic file. The flow of the irrigant is toggled using a foot pedal [8]. |

## ADVANCES IN TISSUE ENGINEERING

Tissue engineering is one of the most exciting contemporary developments in pediatric dentistry. It is a cross-disciplinary field that involves biology and engineering principles to develop biological substitutes that can regenerate human cells, tissues, or organs to re-establish normal function [10]. The main elements for regenerative endodontics include stem cells, appropriate scaffold, and growth factor.

## a. Stem Cells

Stem cells are considered to be the most valuable cells for regenerative medicine. Research on stem cells provides advanced knowledge about how an organism develops from a single cell and how healthy cells replace damaged ones in adult organisms. Stem cells can continuously divide to either replicate them (self-replication) or produce specialised cells that can differentiate into other types of cells or tissues.

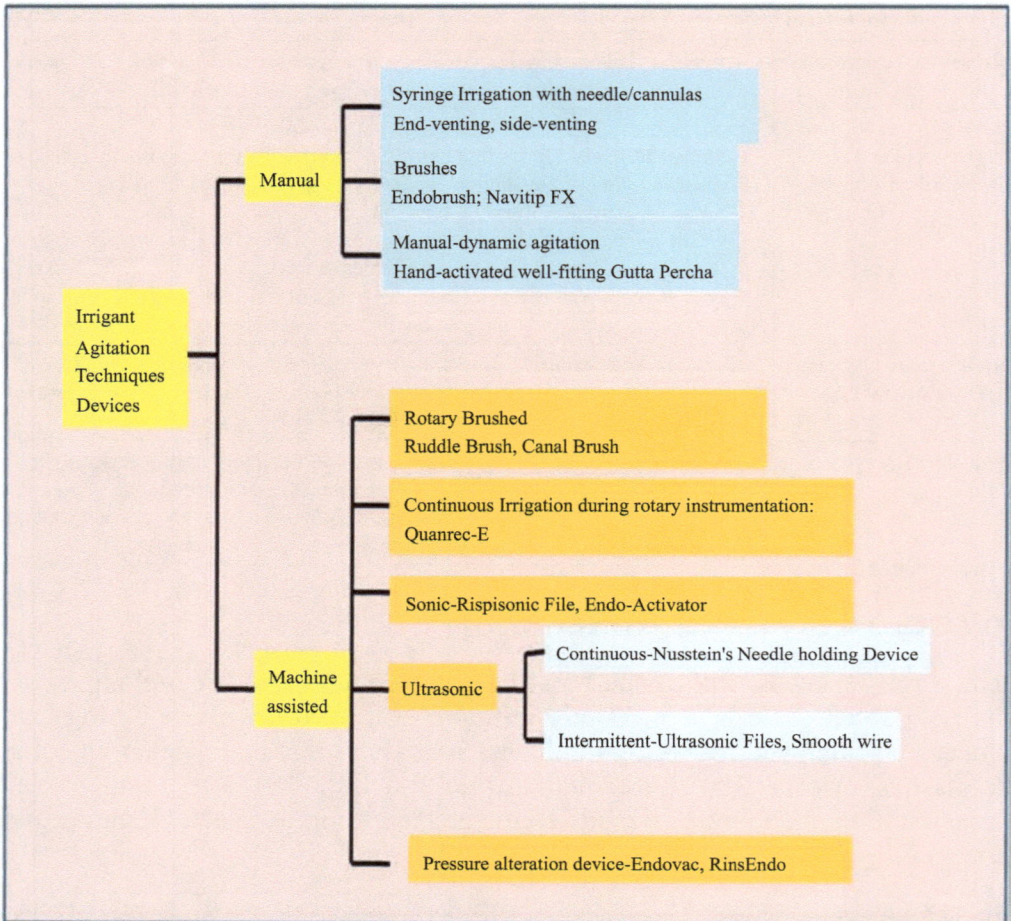

**Fig. (11).** Classification of Irrigant devices.

Four types of human dental stem cells have been isolated.

  i. Dental Pulp Stem Cells (DPSCs).
 ii. Stem cells from human exfoliated deciduous teeth (SHED).
iii. Stem cells from apical papillae (SCAP).
 iv. Periodontal ligament stem cells (PDLSCs).

### *i. Dental Pulp Stem Cells*

These cells can regenerate a dentin-pulp-like complex composed of a mineralised matrix of tubules lined with odontoblasts and fibrous tissue containing blood vessels in an arrangement similar to the dentin-pulp complex found in normal human teeth.

## ii. Stem Cells from Human Exfoliated Deciduous Teeth

These cells were isolated by Miura *et al*. They can differentiate into various cell types greater than DPSCs, including neural cells, adipocytes, osteoblasts-like and odontoblast-like cells. These cells form mineralised tissue, which can be used to enhance orofacial bone regeneration [11].

SHED for tissue engineering might be more advantageous than stem cells from adult human teeth; they were reported to have a higher proliferation rate than stem cells from permanent teeth. They are ideal for young patients at the mixed dentition stage who have suffered pulp necrosis in immature permanent teeth due to trauma.

## iii. Stem Cells from Apical Papillae

Stem cells residing in the apical papilla survive pulp necrosis because of their proximity to the vasculature of the periapical tissues.

## iv. Periodontal Ligament Stem Cells

Seo *et al*. described the presence of multipotent postnatal stem cells in the human PDL. Under defined culture conditions, PDLSCs differentiated into cementoblast-like cells, adipocytes, and collagen-forming cells. When transplanted into immunocompromised rodents, PDLSCs showed the capacity to generate a cementum/PDL-like structure and contributed to periodontal tissue repair.

# DNA PROBES AND PRIMERS IN DENTAL PRACTICE

## a. Methods

### Hybridization

Hybridisation involves the denaturation of double-stranded DNA into single strands and detecting single-stranded DNA (ssDNA) with a labelled, complementary ssDNA probe. Commercially available probe tests include a multitude of bacterial pathogens, such as Campylobacter species, Chlamydia trachomatis, Enterococcus species, Gardnerella vaginalis, Haemophilus influenza,

Legionella pneumophila, Listeria monocytogenes, Mycobacterium species, Neisseria gonorrhoeae, Streptococcus agalactia, and Streptococcus pyogenes, and pathogenic fungi protozoa, and some viruses.

Direct probe methods are much less sensitive (limited to 103 - 106 cells) when used without DNA amplification procedures because the number of target cells may fall below the sensitivity of the essay. This threshold is met by testing cell-rich oral specimens (*e.g.*, samples from mixed anaerobic infected periodontal pockets or plaque of initial carious lesions). Probes can be used for most cases directly, without preamplification. Thus, Additional targets for DNA probe identification can be found in the dental practice. They are the periodontopathogens Actinobacillus, actinomycetemcomitan,.

Bacteroides forsythias, Porphyromonas gingivalis, Prevetolla intermedia, Treponema denticola and caries agents-namely, Mutans streptococcus-group species. In fact, because of the high prevalence of periodontal diseases and caries. Oral infections are the main indication for DNA probe application.

**Polymerase Chain Reaction PCR**

PCR is a highly sensitive technique that can be enzymatically amplified by minute quantities of specific DNA (or RNA after reverse transcription). The technique can detect very small amounts of bacterial, fungal, or viral nucleic acid in clinical specimens. PCR-based tests are vital for research. They are commercially available to see the peri-odontopathogens as well as cariogenic agents.

**Application of DNA Probes and Primers in Periodontal Diseases**

• To monitor bacterial changes or shifts in the gingival sulcus or the periodontal pocket.
• PCR and combinatory molecular genetics techniques are used for the routine diagnosis of periodontal pathogens.
• Typing of S. mutans and S. sobrinus by arbitrarily primed PCR fingerprinting has been introduced. Routine screening for S. mutans by DNA probe hybridisation and glucosyltransferase directed PCR in saliva and plaque is now available for private practices.
• The DNA probes and PCR reactions are used for risk assessment in caries high-end medicine.

**FUTURE IN DENTAL PRACTICE**

1. Chairside test of saliva to identify salivary protein isoforms associated with increased dental caries risk.

2. Chairside test on DNA isolated from desquamated buccal epithelial cells to identify SNPs associated with increased risk for dental caries.
3. Implementation of dental caries prevention strategies linked to genetically established risk assessment.

## CONCLUSION

Advances in clinical sciences are everlasting; the quest for excellence should hold hands with technology and embrace newer techniques, methods, materials, and equipment with scientific validation of the same over-controlled trials.

## CONSENT FOR PUBLICATION

Not applicable.

## CONFLICT OF INTEREST

The authors declare no conflict of interest, financial or otherwise.

## ACKNOWLEDGEMENT

Declared none.

## REFERENCES

[1]     Kaur H, Singh H, Chaudhary S, Vinod KS, Singh B, Kinikar K. Ozone Therapy: An Update. J Res Adv Dent 2015; 4(2): 255-62.

[2]     Damle SG. Chapter 53, Advances in Pediatric Dentistry. In: Textbook of Pediatric Dentistry. 5th ed. New Delhi: Arya Medi Publishing House 2017; pp. 1170-202.

[3]     Srilatha A, Doshi D, Kulkarni S, Reddy MP, Bharathi V. Advanced diagnostic aids in dental caries – A Review. J Global Oral Health 2019; 2(2): 118-27.

[4]     dentistrytoday.com/k2/item/5977-early-caries-detection-using-the-ortek-ecd-lectronic-carie-
-detector-on-a-maxillary-first-molar

[5]     Tomer A, Raina A, Ayub F, Bhatt M. Recent advances in pulp vitality testing: A review. IJADS 2019; 5(3): 8-12.

[6]     Mythri H, Arun A, Chachapan D. Pulp vitality tests - an overview on comparison of sensitivity and vitality. Indian Journal of Oral Sciences 2015; 6(2): 41-6.
[http://dx.doi.org/10.4103/0976-6944.162622]

[7]     Shmueli A, Guelmann M, Tickotsky N, Ninio-Harush R, Noy AF, Moskovitz M. Blood Gas Tension and Acidity Level of Caries Exposed Vital Pulps in Primary Molars. J Clin Pediatr Dent 2020; 44(6): 418-22.
[http://dx.doi.org/10.17796/1053-4625-44.6.5] [PMID: 33378460]

[8]     Shiraguppi V, Deosarkar B, Das M, Gadge P, Malpani S. Root canal irrigation – review. Journal of Interdisciplinary Dental Sciences 2018; 7(2): 1-9.

[9]     Aniketh TN, Idris M, Geeta IB, *et al.* Root Canal Irrigants and Irrigation Techniques: A Review. J Evol Med Dent Sci 2015; 4(27): 4694-700.
[http://dx.doi.org/10.14260/jemds/2015/679]

[10]   Shah N, Choudhary D, Bansal A, Kukreja N. Regenerative endodontics: A road from dead to alive. Ind J Dent Sci 2014; 6(4): 86-91.

[11]   Seo BM, Sonoyama W, Yamaza T, *et al.* SHED repair critical-size calvarial defects in mice. Oral Dis 2008; 14(5): 428-34.
[http://dx.doi.org/10.1111/j.1601-0825.2007.01396.x] [PMID: 18938268]

# CHAPTER 11

# Management of Non-cavitated and Cavitated Carious Lesions

**Neeraj Gugnani**[1,*], **Naveen Manuja**[2] and **Parag D. Kasar**[3]

*¹ Department of Pediatric and Preventive Dentistry, DAV (C) Dental College, Yamuna Nagar, Haryana, India*

*² Department of Pediatric and Preventive Dentistry, Kothiwal Dental College, Moradabad, India*

*³ Deep Dental Clinic, Navi Mumbai, Maharashtra 400706, India*

**Abstract:** Carious lesions can range from early, non-detectable mineral loss, restricted to enamel, through to lesions that extend into dentine without any surface cavitation, to cavitated lesions, which destroy the tooth tissue and can be visible as cavities in the teeth. Cavitated caries lesions generally are non-cleansable and thus active; therefore, these lesions most commonly need to be restored. Selective removal of carious tissues is guided by the depth of the lesion, pulpal health, and choice of dental material. Fluoride is the cornerstone of the non-invasive management of non-cavitated caries lesions. Still, its ability to promote net remineralisation is limited by the availability of calcium and phosphate ions. Ideal remineralisation material should diffuse or deliver calcium and phosphate into the subsurface lesion or boost the remineralisation properties of saliva and oral reservoirs without increasing the risk of calculus formation. These options are often no longer feasible for carious lesions where the tooth tissue surface has become cavitated, as the biofilm is sheltered and cannot be easily removed or manipulated. In such situations, invasive (restorative) options are required. With the advent of adhesive restorations and facilitated by the described changing understanding of the pathogenesis of caries and carious lesions, a paradigm shift in restorative dentistry occurred. In asymptomatic, vital teeth with deep lesions, conservative carious tissue removal strategy,s that reduce tissue loss and pulp exposure risk must be balanced against removing adequate tissue to maximise restoration longevity. In two stages, the most recent inspiration for stepwise carious removal originates from the knowhow on Intra lesion changes in deep carious lesions. Natural enamel and dentin are still the best "dental materials" in existence; therefore, minimally invasive procedures that conserve a more significant part of the wild, healthy tooth structure must be considered desirable. Ultraconservative dentistry represents a significant step forward for the dentist, the profession, and especially the patient. A changing understanding of the disease of dental caries has initiated a paradigm shift in the management of carious lesions. Instead of merely removing the symptoms of the carious lesion, any treatment aims to manage the disease.

---

**\* Corresponding author Neeraj Gugnani:** Department of Pediatric and Preventive Dentistry, DAV (C) Dental College, Yamuna Nagar, Haryana, India; E-mail: Simran2871@Gmail.Com

**Satyawan Damle, Ritesh Kalaskar & Dhanashree Sakhare (Eds.)**

**Keywords:** Cavitated Lesion, Demineralisation, Dental Caries, Fluoride, Minimally Invasive Dentistry, Non-cavitated Lesion, Stepwise Excavation of Caries, Remineralisation, Restoration, The Death Spiral of Teeth, Ultraconservative Treatment.

## INTRODUCTION

Dental caries is the most prevalent disease worldwide, with billions of individuals affected by the resulting burden of pain, loss of function, impaired aesthetics, and speech. The oral microbiota is organised on dental hard tissues as biofilms; Under healthy conditions, these biofilms contain limited numbers of cariogenic bacteria (including streptococci and lactobacilli statendition of dental caries) caused by a shift in the oral microbiota composition towards increased proportions of cariogenic bacteria. The imbalance in the biofilm results in a discrepancy in the mineral loss and gain, with a resulting net mineral loss. If this continues over time, it can lead to the development of a carious lesion as the symptom of the caries disease process [1].

Carious lesions can range from early, non-detectable mineral loss, restricted to enamel, through to lesions that extend into dentine without any surface cavitation, to cavitated lesions, which destroy the tooth tissue and can be visible as holes in the teeth [1].

Traditionally, all carious lesions have been treated by removing all demineralised or affected and bacterially contaminated (infected) dentine and reputilising utilising restorations (for example, amalgam or composite), commonly known as a 'filling'. However, the pathophysiology of the disease process shows that carious lesions can be controlled by altering the factors leading to net mineral loss. This can be achieved by reducing carbohydrate intake; removing or controlling the biofilm activity, sealing the tooth surface from the environment; or rebalancing demineralisation and remineralisation, for example, by applying fluoride [1].

Caries lesions can be classified into two categories: non-cavitated and cavitated.

### Non-Cavitated Caries Lesions

A non-cavitated caries lesion (also sometimes referred to as an early lesion, an incipient lesion, or a white spot lesion) is a demineralised lesion without evidence of cavitation. As the lesion progresses, the outer surface, which is in contact with dental plaque and is protected by the salivary pellicle, is exposed to cycles of demineralisation and remineralisation, and it regains some minerals (including fluoride) and becomes less prone to further demineralisation. Non-cavitated lesions in pits and fissures may appear as a white, yellow, or brown discolouration (or a combination of these colours), which may be limited to the confines of the pits and fissures may extend from the pit-and-fissure system. Exceedingly early lesions are visible only after air drying. More advanced lesions are visible when the tooth is wet or dry [2].

## Cavitated Caries Lesions: (Fig. 1)

Cavitated lesions are lesions that have progressed to a more advanced stage. Cavitation usually occurs because of external forces that eventually lead to the collapse of the outer surface in a non-cavitated lesion, leading to a discontinuity or break in the surface. The gap in the surface may be limited to the enamel, or it may expose the dentin [2].

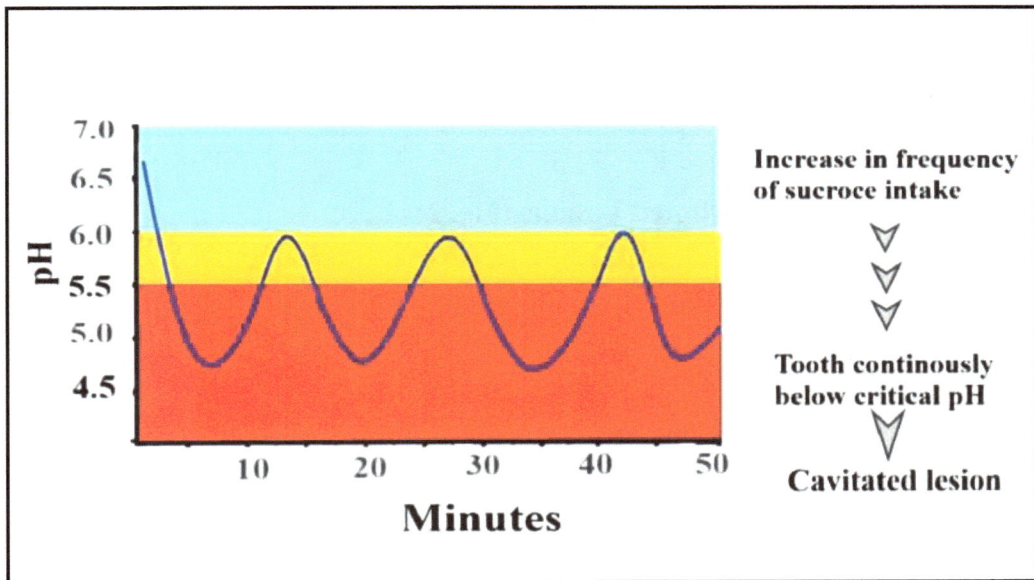

**Fig. (1).** Stephan Curve Showing Formation of a Cavitated Lesion.

**The International Caries Detection and Assessment System (ICDAS)** is a clinical scoring system used to detect and assess dental caries. This scoring system can be used on coronal surfaces and root surfaces. To detect and evaluate these lesions, it can be used for enamel caries, dentine caries, non-cavitated lesions, and cavitated lesions detect and estimate these lesions.

The international caries detection and assessment system (ICDAS) was developed to provide clinicians, epidemiologists, and researchers with an evidence-based approach to permit standardised caries detection and diagnosis in different environments and situations.

ICDAS measures carious lesions' surface changes and potential histological depth by relying on surface characteristics.

The ICDAS detection codes for coronal caries range from 0 to 6, depending on the severity of the lesion.

| Code | Description |
|------|-------------|
| 0 | Sound tooth surface: No evidence of caries after 5-sec air drying |
| 1 | The first visual change in enamel: Opacity or discolouration (white or brown) is visible at the entrance to the pit or fissure seen after prolonged air drying |
| 2 | The distinct visual change in enamel is visible when wet; the lesion must be visible when dry. |
| 3 | Localised enamel breakdown (without clinical visual signs of dentinal involvement) seen when wet and after prolonged drying |
| 4 | Underlying dark shadow from dentine |
| 5 | Distinct cavity with visible dentine |
| 6 | Extensive (more than half the surface) distinct cavity with visible dentine |

## Management of Non-cavitated Lesions (Fig. 2)

A recent expert-based consensus report recommended that a caries lesion's cavitation, cleanstability, and cleanability be considered for best management. The information also presented recommendations for thresholds between restorative and non-restorative interventions.

Arrested caries lesions do not need to be treated from a caries disease viewpoint (either restoratively or non-restoratively except when the goal is to address issues associated with esthetics, function, or risk for pulpal death. Non-cavitated active caries lesions should be treated using evidence-based non-restorative products or interventions. Some occlusal non-cavitated lesions might extend radiographically deep into dentin. These lesions can be treated non-restoratively (*e.g.*, using sealants), but it has been suggested that a trampoline effect (i.e., in which the surface of the lesion may cavitate because the body of the lesion is extensive and may undermine it) may result in the sealant failing, and thus treatment should be closely monitored.

Cavitated caries lesions generally are non-cleansable and thus active; therefore, these lesions most commonly need to be restored. Selective removal of carious tissues is guided by the depth of the lesion, pulpal health, and choice of dental material. Restoration of the existing cavity allows oral biofilms to be relocated to the tooth's surface and amenable to better control of the local disease process.

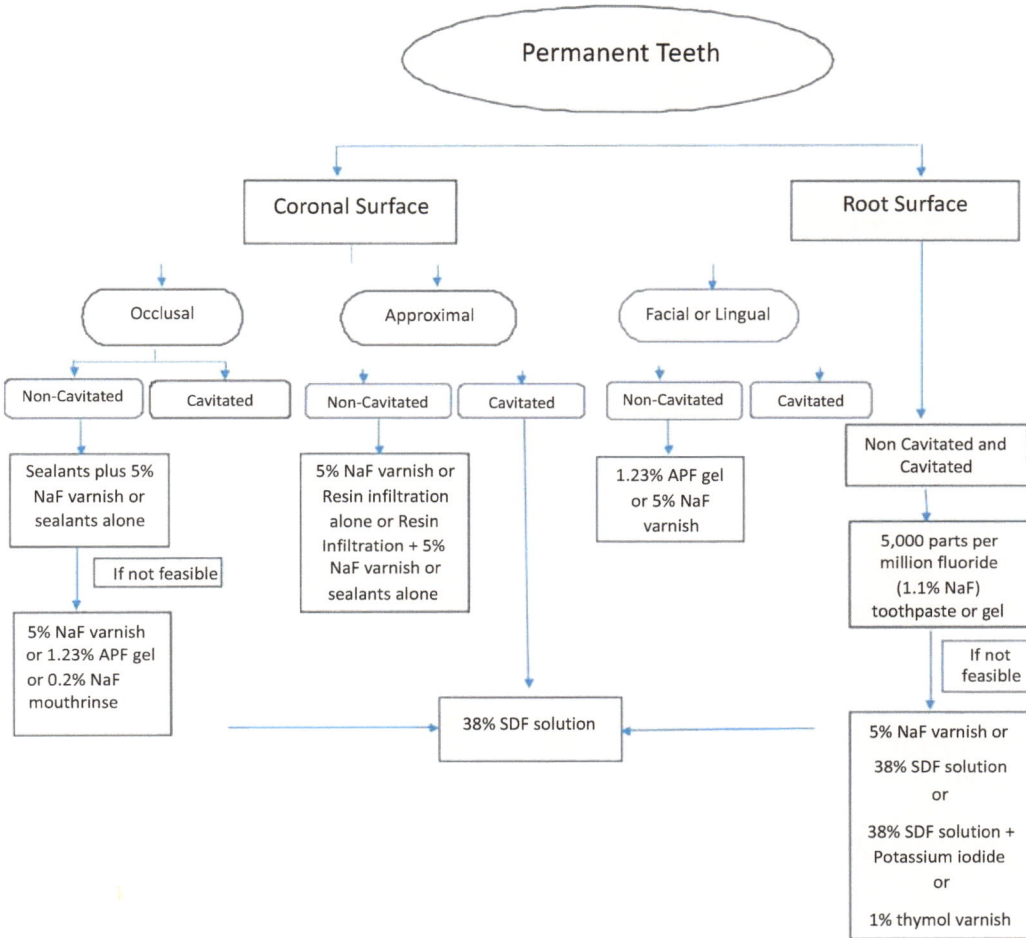

**Fig. (2).** Non-Invasive Management for Caries in Permanent Teeth [3].

In addition, restoring the cavity allows for the re-establishment of function and esthetics, which can be critical patient-level outcomes. Some cavitated lesions that are not palpably involved could be treated non-restoratively (*e.g.*, with silver diamine fluoride [SDF]), either temporarily or permanently, if the primary goal is to arrest the caries disease process, with the understanding that function and esthetics remain compromised because of the loss of tooth structure. Intended for some individuals, this compromise is the most appropriate person-centred approach to managing right cavitated lesions [3].

All non-cavitated lesions should receive preventive therapy to arrest remineralising the lesion. Modern dentistry aims to manage non-cavitated caries lesions non-invasively through remineralisation to prevent disease progression and improve aesthetics, strength, and function [4].

## REMINERALISATION

Remineralisation is when calcium and phosphate ions are provided from a source external to the tooth to promote ion deposition into crystal voids in demineralised enamel to produce net mineral gain. The utilised defines any accessible space in a crystal caused by ion loss from the demineralisation process. Therefore, this definition of remineralisation includes any crystal repair to bring about net mineral gain to an enamel subsurface lesion. Still, it does not extend to the precipitation of solid phases onto the enamel surface (Cochrane et al. 2010). At physiological pH, un-stimulated and stimulated parotid, submandibular, and whole saliva are supersaturated concerning most solid calcium phases. However, precipitation of calcium phosphate phases in saliva usually does not occur due to salivary proteins, particularly statherin and proline-rich phosphoproteins. The proposed mechanism of action is that the segments of the proteins containing phosphoseryl residues, particularly the statherin sequence, bind to calcium and phosphate ion clusters, preventing the growth of the ion cluster to the critical size required for precipitation and transformation into a crystalline phase. This necessary stabilisation of calcium and phosphate ions by salivary phosphoproteins ensures that the ions remain bioavailable to diffuse into mineral deficient lesions to allow for remineralisation of demineralised crystals while preventing surface deposition in the form of calculus.

### Role of Fluoride

Fluoride is the cornerstone of the non-invasive management of non-cavitated caries lesions. Still, its ability to promote net remineralisation is limited by calcium and phosphate ions [4]. Fluoride ions can push the remineralisation of non-cavitated caries lesions if adequate salivary or plaque calcium and phosphate ions are available when the fluoride is utilised. For fluorapatite or Fluorohydroxyapatite to form, calcium and phosphate ions are required and fluoride ions are.

When present in the liquid phase of remineralisation, fluoride will be incorporated into the enamel crystal, and the enamel will become more resistant to demineralisation. Once enamel is exposed to ionic fluoride, it may be taken up with Fluorohydroxyapatite or calcium fluoride formation. When fluoride is present in low concentrations in saliva and plaque fluid, fluoride ions are likely to be incorporated into the remineralising surface of the lesion, making the repaired section higher in fluoride than it originally was. The material formed on the lesion's character is more precisely called fluorohydroxyapatite.

## Formation of Fluorohydroxyapatite

Fluorohydroxyapatite is formed when the fluoride concentration in the solution is low, less than around 50 ppm, and in an acidic environment:

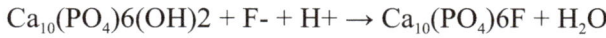

$$Ca_{10}(PO_4)6(OH)2 + F- + H+ \rightarrow Ca_{10}(PO_4)6F + H_2O$$

The fluorohydroxyapatite formed will be situated in the outermost layers of enamel and form an integral part of the tissue that is only lost if the entire mineral is worn away or dissolved entirely. Under neutral conditions, the formation of the Fluorohydroxyapatite is slow and unable to keep pace with normal wear of the tooth surface. Therefore, despite fluoride toothpaste, thorough daily tooth brushing reduces the fluoride content of buccal enamel surfaces over the years.

The necessary condition in the mouth for fluorapatite formation is that the oral fluids, saliva, and plaque fluid are supersaturated concerning fluorapatite. This is usually the case when the pH is above 4.5. Below pH 4.5, the oral fluids become increasingly unsaturated concerning fluorapatite, and Fluorohydroxyapatite dissolves increasingly with lower pH. The overall effect is reduced dental demineralisation because of the protective outer layer of Fluorohydroxyapatite. If fluoride is not available, the oral environment begins to favour demineralisation.

## Formation of Calcium Fluoride (Fig. 3)

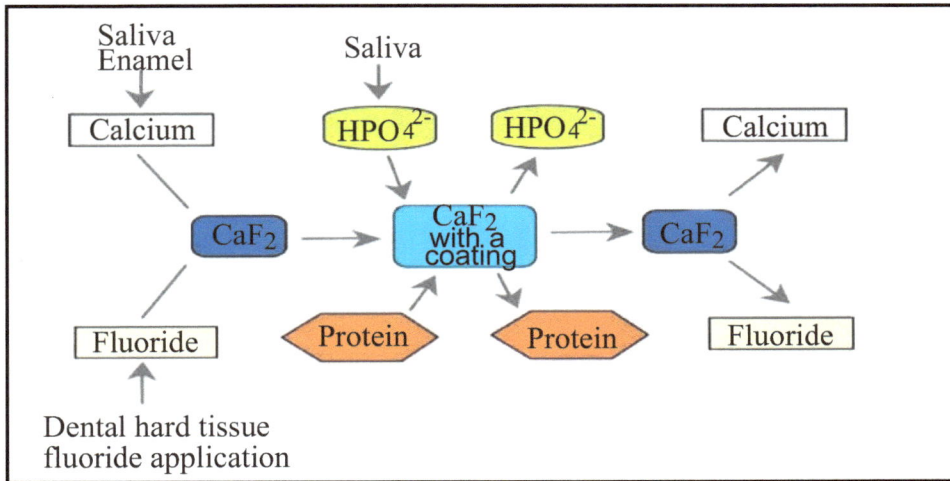

**Fig. (3).** Formation of Calcium Fluoride.

When the fluoride concentration in the solution bathing the enamel is above 100 ppm, calcium fluoride is formed as per following the chemical reaction:-

$$Ca_{10}(PO_4)_6(OH)_2 + {}_{20}F- + {}_8H+ \rightarrow {}_{10}CaF_2 + {}_6HPO_{42}- + {}_2H_2O .$$

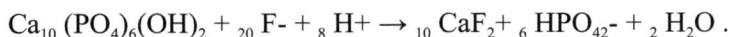

This reaction indicates what happens when the teeth are given a topical treatment or exposed to fluoride toothpaste containing NaF. The higher the fluoride concentration, the more calcium fluoride is formed. Further, a low pH in the solution has a powerful effect on calcium fluoride formation. The calcium fluoride is included in spherical globules scattered over the surface. Recent studies have shown a structure radiating from the centre outwards, indicating that the globules are formed from a central nidus where their mineralisation is released.

## Commercial Fluoride Varnish

Varnishes with up to 5% sodium fluoride are marketed for caries prevention. Calcium fluoride may also be incorporated into the product. After the varnish setting on the tooth or over the plaque, fluoride is released partly to the saliva and partly towards the underlying enamel surface with a caries lesion or into the underlying plaque. Locally, high fluoride concentrations can be obtained, and calcium fluoride formed. Eventually, the varnish is worn away, the calcium fluoride dissolves, and the preventive effect tapers off.

## Fluoride Toothpaste

Fluoride toothpaste contains 500–1500 ppm fluoride either in the form of sodium fluoride (NaF) or in the complexed form of monofluorophosphate (MFP, $Na_2PO_3F$), in which oxygen of the phosphate molecule has been replaced by fluoride, or in mixtures of the two salts, NaF and MFP. In NaF toothpaste, the sodium fluoride is dissociated, and the fluoride is present in free ionic form. The MFP molecule is hydrolysed by non-specific bacterial phosphatases when it meets the oral fluids and tissues and when it diffuses into plaque.

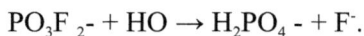

$$PO_3F_2- + HO \rightarrow H_2PO_4 - + F^-.$$

It is generally believed that the MFP molecule cannot diffuse through plaque to the enamel surface without being hydrolysed. Fluoride toothpaste is also formulated by including various amine fluorides. These are amphipathic compounds where amines substituted with long hydrocarbon chains are the cations for ionic fluoride. The amine parts are intended to improve fluoride delivery to the tooth surface and possess antimicrobial properties. Recently, toothpaste with fluoride contents of 2500 and 5000 ppm has been marketed for individuals with high-caries risk.

## Mineral or Ionic Technologies: Fluoride

Fluoride works primarily via topical mechanisms, which include:

1. Inhibition of demineralisation at the crystal surfaces inside the tooth.
2. Enhancement of remineralisation at the crystal surfaces (giving an acid-resistant surface to the reformed crystals.
3. Inhibition of bacterial enzymes. High levels of surface fluoride can increase resistance to carious lesion formation and dental erosion.

Numerous laboratory studies have shown that low fluoride levels, typical of those found after many hours in resting plaque and saliva and resulting from the regular use of fluoride dentifrices, can profoundly affect enamel demineralisation and remineralisation.

## Fluoride Effect on the Dynamics of the Caries Process (Fig. 4)

The predominant effect of fluoride (F) is not systemic, by pre-eruptive changing the enamel structure, but mainly locally, interfering with the caries process. Hence, F must be present in the right place (biofilm fluid or saliva) and at the right time (when biofilm is exposed to sugar or after biofilm removal) to interfere with de- and remineralisation events. The pH lowering dissolves enamel in dental plaque due to acid production every time sugar is ingested. However, if F is present in the biofilm fluid and the pH is not lower than 4.5, hydroxyapatite (HA) is dissolved whilefluorapatite (FA) is formed. The net result is a decrease in enamel dissolution since a certain amount of Ca and P, which was lost as HA, is recovered by enamel as FA. This mineral is FA (Fluropatite) during the pH drop.

Moreover, FA is deposited on the surface layer of enamel, while HA is dissolved from the subsurface. This indirect effect of F reducing enamel demineralisation when the pH drops is complemented by its natural impact on remineralisation when the pH rises.

Enhancing the redeposition of Ca and Pi present in the biofilm fluid on demineralised enamel is cleaned by brushing; saliva can remineralise it, but this effect is enhanced in the presence of F. As a result, small amounts of Ca and Pi lost my enamel during the pH drop can be more efficiently recovered if F is still present in the oral environment (biofilm fluid or saliva) after the cariogenic challenge. This effect should be considered natural, not induced, because it occurs irrespective of patient compliance or dentist intervention if, for example, an F-dentifrice is being used and F is made available to the oral cavity.

## Fluoride Effect on Caries Lesions

Since Fluoride enhances enamel remineralisation, its clinical use to repair early caries lesions was advocated ("fluoride therapy"). However, the effect of Fluoride in the dynamics of the caries process and its success in controlling caries should not be confused with its arrestment or reversal effect on caries lesions. Furthermore, it should be emphasised that shallow demineralised enamel areas remineralise faster than deep ones.

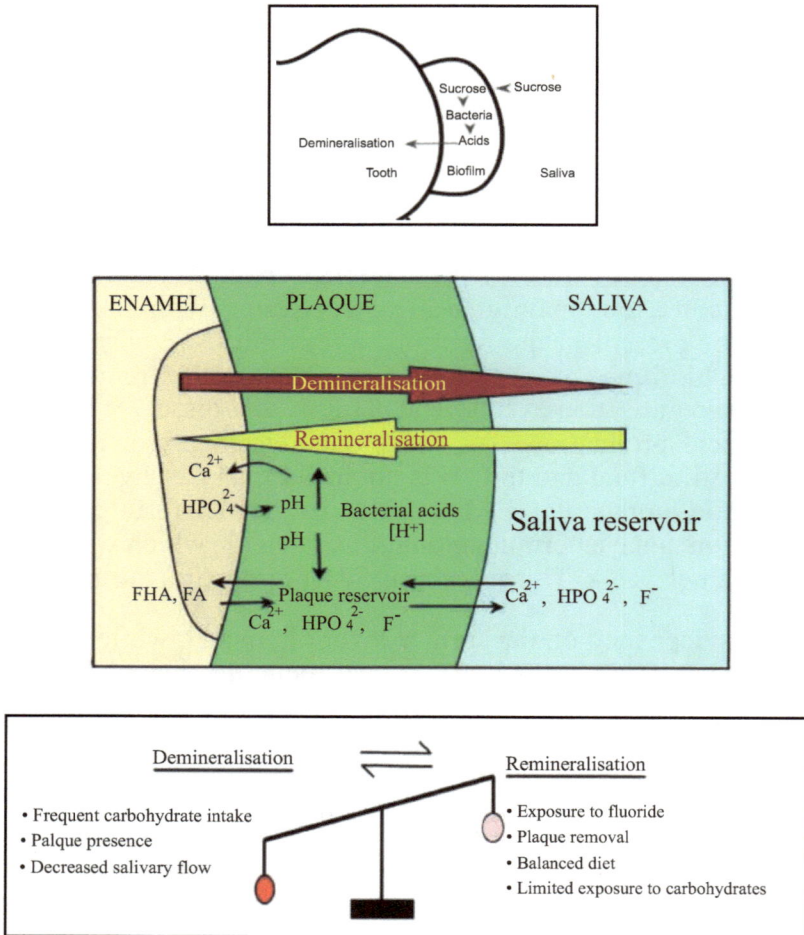

Fig. (4). Factors Affecting Demineralisation and emineralisation Inside and Outside Oral Cavity.

## 1) Non-Fluoride Enamel Remineralizing Systems

Ideal remineralisation material should diffuse or deliver calcium and phosphate into the subsurface lesion or boost the remineralisation properties of saliva and oral reservoirs without increasing the risk of calculus formation.

Several unique calcium phosphate remineralisation systems have been commercialised in recent years and can be categorised into three types: (I) stabilised amorphous calcium phosphate systems; (ii) crystalline calcium phosphate systems; and (iii) unstabilised amorphous calcium phosphate systems.

## Casein Phosphopeptide-Amorphous Calcium Phosphate

Casein is the predominant phosphoprotein in bovine milk and accounts for almost 80 per cent of its total protein, Casein phosphopeptides (CPP) contain the active sequence –Ser (P)-Ser (P)-Ser (P)-Glu-Glu and has a remarkable ability to stabilise calcium and phosphate as nanoclusters of ions in metastable solution. Through the active sequence, the CPP binds to form a nanocluster of calcium and phosphate ions to form nanocomplexes of around 1.5 nm radius, preventing the growth of the nanoclusters to the critical size required for nucleation and phase transformation.

The first technology involving casein phosphopeptide stabilised amorphous calcium phosphate, RecaldentTM (CPP-ACP), claimed that the casein phosphopeptides (CPP) stabilised high calcium and phosphate concentrations ions, together with fluoride ions, at the tooth surface by binding to the pellicle and plaque. The Recaldent technology was developed by Prof. Eric Reynolds of the University of Melbourne. (GC Tooth Mousse/Prospec MI Paste) (Fig. **5**) remineralisation system was created because the tryptic digestion of milk caseinate produced multiphosphorylated casein phosphopeptides (CPP), substantially increasing the milk protein's solubility and ability to stabilise calcium and phosphate ions. CPP-ACP has been shown to reduce demineralisation and enhance remineralisation of the enamel subsurface carious lesions. CPP is also believed to have an antibacterial and buffering effect on plaque and interfere in Streptococcus mutans' growth and adherence of Streptococcus mutants and Streptococcus sobrinus.

| Active Ingredients | Trademark (Manufacturer) | Commercial Preparation |
|---|---|---|
| CPP-ACP | MI Paste ™ (GC)/Tooth Mousse ™ (GC) | Topical Paste |
| | Trident XtraCare (Adams) | Chewing Gum |
| | Trident Total (Adams) | Chewing Gum |
| | Fuji VII™ EP(GC) | Glass ionomer cement |
| CPP-ACPF | MI Paste plus ™(GC)/Tooth Mousse plus™ (GC) | Topical Paste |
| | MI Varnish™ (GC) | Varnish |
| ACP | Nite White ™(Phillips) Day white ™(Phillips) | Tooth Bleaching Gel Tooth Bleaching Gel |
| | Aegis Ortho (Bosworth Co.) | Dental adhesive |
| | Aegis pit and fissure sealant (Bosworth Co.) | Pit and fissure sealant |
| | Relief ACP(Phillips) | Tooth desensitising gel |
| | Enamel on (Premier) | Toothpaste |

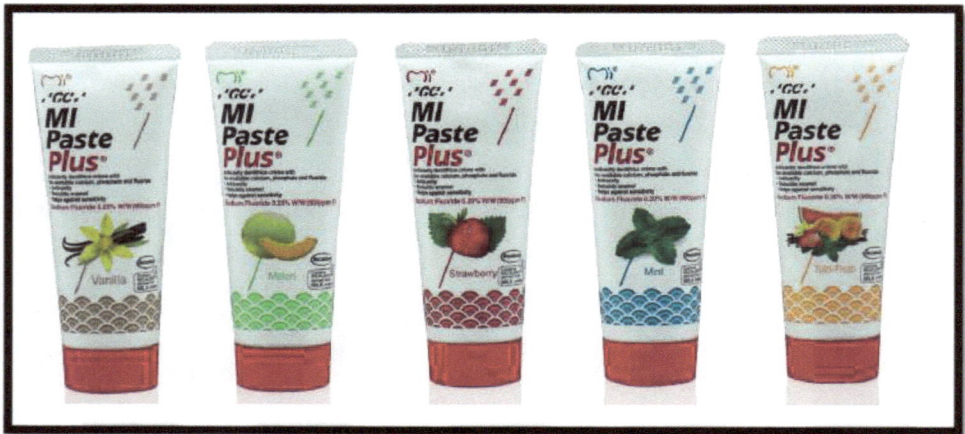

**Fig. (5).** Caesin phosphopeptides with amorphous calcium fluoride phosphate (CPP-ACFP).

## Bioactive Glass (Sodium Calciumphosphosilicate)- Novamin

Dr LenLitkowski and Dr Gary Hack developed this technology based on calcium sodium phosphosilicate bioactive glass, which is claimed to release calcium and phosphate ions intra-orally to help the self-repair process of teeth. When bioactive glass encounters saliva, it rapidly releases sodium, calcium, and phosphorous ions into the saliva available for remineralisation of the tooth surface. The ions are released from hydroxycarbonate apatite (HCA) directly. They also attach to the tooth surface and continue to remove ions and remineralise the tooth surface after the initial application. These articles have been shown to release ions and transform them into HCA for up to 2 weeks. Ultimately, these particles will completely transform into HCA. Novamin adheres to the exposed dentin surface and forms a mineralised layer that is mechanically strong and resistant to acid. There is a continuous release of calcium over time, which maintains the protective effects on dentin.

When introduced into the oral environment, the material releases sodium, calcium, and phosphate, which then interact with the oral fluids and form a crystalline hydroxycarbonate apatite layer that is structurally and chemically like natural tooth mineral. The calcium and *phosphate* ions are protected by glass, and the glass particles need to be trapped for the calcium and phosphate to be localised. While NovaMin alone and in combination with fluoride can enhance the remineralisation of enamel and dentin lesions and prevent demineralisation from acid challenges, the variety of therapeutic levels of fluoride with NovaMin increases the remineralisation of caries lesions more than either of them used alone.

## Amorphous Calcium Phosphate (ACP)

The ACP technology requires a two-phase delivery system to keep the calcium and phosphorous components from reacting with each other before use. The current sources of calcium and phosphorous are two salts, calcium sulfate and dipotassium phosphate. When the two salts are mixed, they rapidly form ACP that can precipitate onto the tooth surface. This precipitated ACP can readily dissolve into the saliva and be available for tooth remineralisation. Dr Ming S. Tung developed the ACP technology. In 1999, ACP was incorporated into toothpaste called Enamelon and later reintroduced in 2004 in Enamel Care toothpaste by Church and Dwight. It is also available as Discus Dental's Nite White Bleaching Gel and Premier Dental's Enamel Pro Polishing Paste. It is also used in the Aegis product line, such as Aegis Pit and Fissure Sealant, produced by Bosworth [5].

## Nano Hydroxyapatite (nHA)

Nanohydroxyapatite is both bioactive and biocompatible. It will lower the bioavailable F concentration in toothpaste, with NaF being slightly more of a concern than sodium monofluorophosphate. nHA functions by directly filling up micropores on demineralised tooth surfaces. When it penetrates the enamel pores, it also acts as a template in the remineralisation process by continuously attracting large amounts of calcium and phosphate ions from the remineralisation solution to the enamel tissue, thus promoting crystal integrity and growth [6].

## Dicalcium Phosphate Dihydrate

Dicalcium phosphate dihydrate is a precursor for apatite that readily turns into fluorapatite in fluoride. The inclusion of dicalcium phosphate dehydrate (DCPD) in a dentifrice increases the levels of free calcium ions in plaque fluid. These remain elevated for up to 12 hours after brushing, compared to conventional silica dentifrices [7].

## Tricalcium Phosphate (TCP) (Fig. 6)

Tricalcium phosphate has the chemical formula $Ca_3(PO_4)_2$ and exists in two forms, alpha and beta. Alpha TCP is formed when human enamel is heated to high temperatures. It is a relatively insoluble material in aqueous environments (2mg/100 mL in water). Crystalline beta TCP can be formed by combining calcium carbonate and calcium hydrogen phosphate and heating the mixture to over 1000 degrees Celsius for one day to give a flaky, stiff powder. The average size of the TCP particles can then be adjusted by milling them. Particle ranges from 0.01 to 5 microns in size. Beta TCP is less soluble than alpha TCP and thus in unmodified form is less likely to provide bio-available calcium. It is used in products such as Cerasorb®, Bio-Resorb® and Biovision.

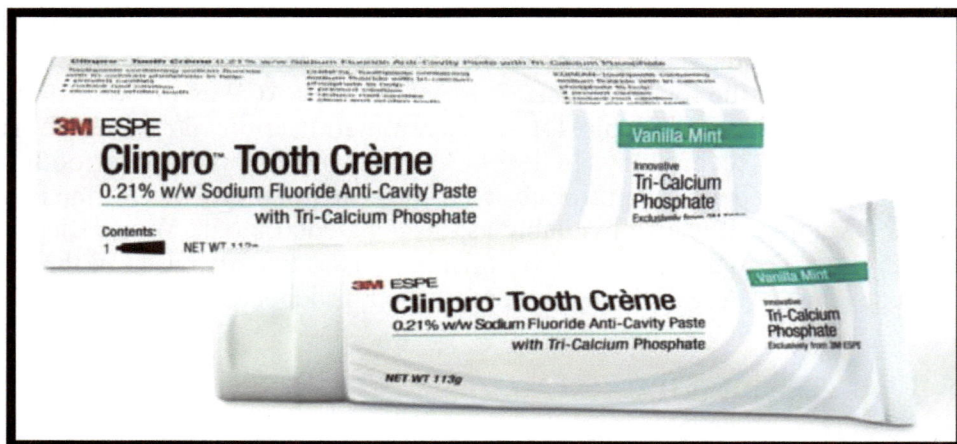

**Fig. (6).** TCP containing Clinpro Tooth crème.

TCP has also been considered one possible means for enhancing calcium levels in plaque and saliva. Some minor effects on free calcium and phosphate levels in plaque fluid and saliva have been found when an experimental gum with 2.5% alpha TCP by weight was chewed compared to a control gum without added TCP.

TCP technology should operate best as a remineralising agent at neutral or slightly alkaline pH. There is some laboratory evidence using bovine enamel models, which show increased surface microhardness and fluoride incorporation into the outer layers of the enamel [8].

## Calcium Carbonate Carrier – SensiStat

The SensiStat technology is made of arginine, bicarbonate, an amino acid complex, and calcium carbonate particles, a common abrasive in toothpaste. The arginine complex is responsible for adhering the calcium carbonate particles to the dentin or enamel surface and allowing the calcium carbonate to slowly dissolve and release calcium available to remineralise the tooth surface. Dr Israel Kleinberg of New York developed the SensiStat Technology. The technology was first incorporated into Ortek'sProclude desensitising prophy paste and later in Denclude.

## Theobromine

Theobromine is a member of the xanthine family, seen in cocoa [240 mg/cup] and chocolate [1.89%], and has been shown to enhance crystalline growth of the enamel. In a comparative evaluation of the remineralising potential of theobromine and sodium fluoride dentifrice, a significantly higher mineral gain was observed with theobromine and fluoride toothpaste relative to artificial saliva. Increased enamel microhardness after treatment with theobromine on the enamel surface has also been observed.

## Arginine Bicarbonate

Arginine bicarbonate is an amino acid with particles of calcium carbonate, which is capable of adhering to the mineral surface. When the calcium carbonate dissolves, the calcium is available to remineralise the mineral, while carbonate release may give a slight local pH rise. The studies on the demineralised bovine enamel blocks with arginine and fluoride formulations have shown that when used in combination with fluoride, arginine significantly increased fluoride uptake compared with fluoride alone, and lesions treated with arginine-containing toothpaste also showed superior fluoride uptake compared with those treated with conventional fluoride toothpaste.

## Eggshell Powder [ESP]

It is a natural source of calcium ions. ESP contains 94% calcium phosphate, 4% organic matter, 1% magnesium carbonate and a low concentration of strontium, fluoride, manganese, zinc, and copper ions. ESP has a vital role in bone and dental metabolism. Researchers proved that ESP could form high-quality hydroxyapatite. The minerals of ESP, when coming in contact with enamel caries-like lesions, diffuse into the superficial layer and obstruct the surface porosities.

## Caries Infiltration (Fig. 7)

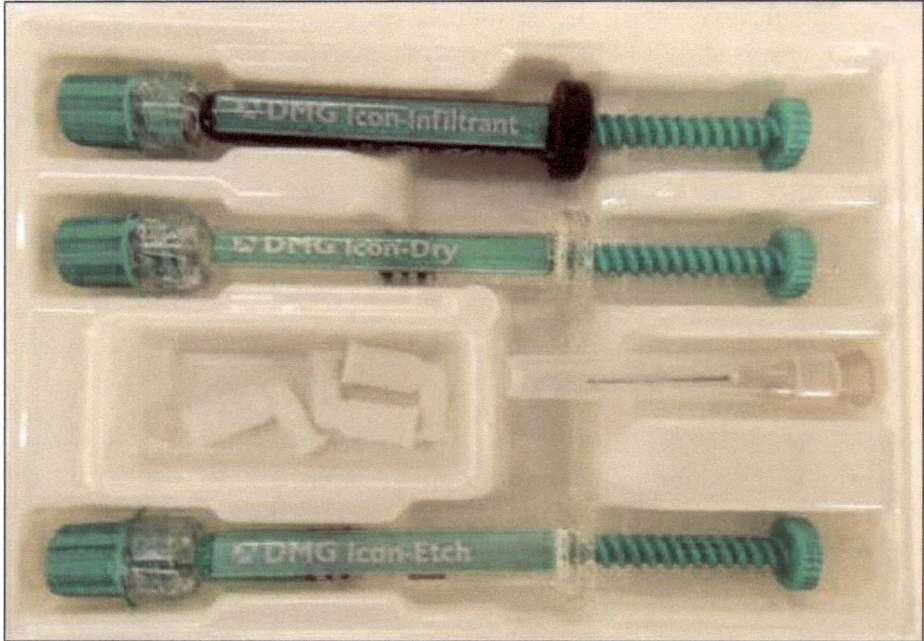

**Fig. (7).** Caries infritration system.

This is a new micro-invasive technique, which includes the resin infiltration up to the depth of the lesion. The infiltrant (ICON, DMG) can be used for both the vestibular and interproximal, non-cavitated lesion and is meant to stop lesion progression. The principle of masking enamel lesions by resin infiltration is based on changes in light scattering within the lesions. The novel technique involves the infiltration of the carious lesions with resin. This makes the difference in refractive indices between porosities and enamel negligible, and lesions appear like the surrounding sound enamel. It has a chameleon effect and requires no shade matching. Lesions lose their whitish opaque colour and blend reasonably well with surrounding natural tooth structure. Hence an immediate improvement in the esthetic appearance was observed.

The technique involves the application of etchant on the entire surface of the non-cavitated lesion with 15% hydrochloric acid (lcon-Etch-15%Hydrochloricacid, water, silica, and additives) for 2 minutes. After 2 minutes, the etchant is rinsed with water for 30 seconds, followed by the application of ethanol for drying (ICONDry), and a frosted chalky white appearance should be observed. The low viscosity infiltrant (tetrramethylene glycol dimethacrylate, additives and initiators) is applied and left for 3 minutes for its penetration and then light-cured [2].

## SEALANTS

Sealants are considered one of the most cost-effective evidence-based strategies available to prevent caries lesions on sound occlusal surfaces and have been advocated to arrest non-cavitated caries lesions.

Based on a 2018 ADA systematic review and subsequent evidence-based practice guidelines, sealants are recommended as an effective treatment for arresting the following caries lesions. Sealants effectively arrest non-cavitated lesions in occlusal and proximal coronal surfaces of primary and permanent teeth. Sealants can be used either alone or in combination with 5% NaF varnish (applied every 3–6 months).

However, a recent systematic review concluded that a combination of sealant plus 5% NaF varnish is the most effective strategy in arresting/reversing non-cavitated occlusal lesions. Because a recent systematic review concluded that is unclear which type of sealant material is more effective for caries control, the decision of which material to choose should consider the likelihood of loss of retention over time (i.e., resin-based materials have significantly higher retention rates than glass ionomer (GI materials) and the possibility of obtaining a dry field control during sealant placement (*i.e.*, GI materials are more hydrophilic). Limited data suggest that sealants may also be effective at arresting lesion progression when used on small cavitated or microcavitated lesions. However, a recent systematic review and meta-analysis concluded that when used on these types of lesions, current sealant materials require more repairs over time than minimally invasive restorations. Although sealants also are recommended to arrest non-cavitated lesions in interproximal surfaces, these lesions normally are not accessible. Thus, the procedure requires a second visit after tooth separation to be completed. Therefore, infiltration of non-cavitated lesions (*i.e.*, if not visible by direct observation, assessed based on radiographic depth as into enamel or outer third of dentin) has been developed as an alternative to be used in a single appointment.

Based on a 2018 ADA systematic review and subsequent evidence-based practice guidelines, infiltration is recommended as an effective treatment for arresting the following caries lesions. Using infiltration, whether alone or in combination with a 5% NaF varnish application every three months to 6 months, is effective at arresting interproximal coronal non-cavitated caries lesions. Because the infiltrated material currently is not radiopaque, the way to evaluate the success of lesion arrest is by monitoring the radiographic lack of lesion progression over time [3]. Sealants are discussed in detail in a separate chapter.

## Self-etch Sealants (Fig. 8)

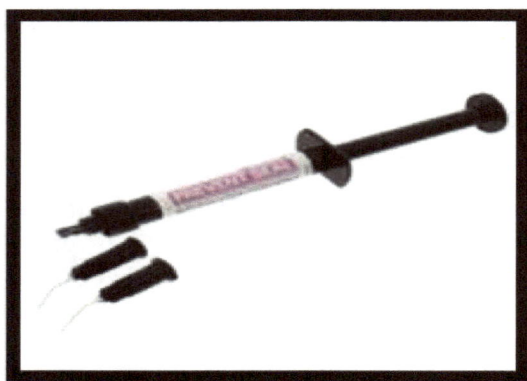

**Fig. (8).** Self-Etch Sealant.

Etching the tooth enamel with phosphoric acid is the conventional and critical step during any adhesive procedure to achieve a good bond. The bond strength between enamel and resin depends on obtaining an etching pattern that facilitates the formation of resin tags. Salivary contamination post etching of the enamel decreases the adhesion of the sealant due to the sealant's adhesion sealant's sticking to the shape of a surface coating, thus requiring the etching procedure to be repeated all over again. Achieving strict isolation for a longer duration is a difficult task while treating pediatric patients. Therefore, the process of application of sealant that is quick and simple is the need of the hour.

Prevent Seal (Itena) is one of the latest self-etching sealants that has been introduced in the dental market. The manufacturers claim the one-step application and fluoride-releasing properties of this sealant as claimed added advantages of preventing sealing (https://www.itena-clinical.com/en/care-prevention/-9-preventseal.html). However, it is important to study the physical properties of preventing seals, as they may differ from that of the conventional resin sealants. Nevertheless, the sealant's equivalence to the conventional techniques and sealants is yet to be explored.

## Antimicrobials

As dental caries result from a dysbiosis in the oral biofilm; they are restoring balance within that biofilm (with antimicrobials, prebiotics, probiotics, and so forth) has been advocated. Although chlorhexidine is one of the most investigated antimicrobial strategies for caries control and prevention, current evidence suggests that chlorhexidine rinses (0.2% or 0.12%) are ineffective at reducing dental caries. However, evidence supports the use of 1% chlorhexidine varnish to prevent root caries lesions [3].

Based on a **2018 ADA** systematic review and subsequent evidence-based practice guidelines, chlorhexidine is recommended as effective to arrest the resulting caries lesion. Professional application of 1% chlorhexidine plus 1% thymol varnish, applied every three months to 6 months, is practical to capture non-cavitated or cavitated root caries lesions. In addition, an alternative that has been suggested in the literature to enhance the control of oral biofilms and stop caries lesions is the so-called nonrestorative caries treatment approach. In this intervention, cavitated caries lesions with limited cleanability are opened (with either hand instruments or a handpiece) to enhance cleanability, access to saliva, and decrease food retention [3].

## Management of Cavitated Lesions

These options are often no longer feasible for carious lesions where the tooth tissue surface has become cavitated, as the biofilm is sheltered and cannot be easily removed or manipulated. In such situations, invasive (restorative) options are required in most cases, as indicated by a document published by the International Caries Consensus Conference Collaboration.

Cavitations that are clinically hard to detect (often called micro cavitation) may, upon radiographic assessment, be found to penetrate the dentine. These dentinal lesions have traditionally also been considered to require a restoration (Ricketts 1995), especially when the lesion has entered the middle third of the dentine and hence harbours large amounts of bacteria [1].

Even though it becomes increasingly clear that restoration is not necessary to stop the caries process in or on a tooth, placing restorations (sometimes also referred to as "fill-and-drill" practices) still occupies a central part within general dental procedures [9]. Though, logically, placing a restoration in a tooth should, at best, not result in additional loss of tooth structure, sacrificing healthy tooth tissue has long been the standard in operative and restorative dentistry. There were several reasons for this:

First, with conventional restorations, both direct and indirect, tooth preparation and the amount of removed tooth tissue were influenced by the material properties. Sufficient bulk was required to obtain adequate strength for non-adhesive restorations like amalgam fillings.

Second, the concept of "extension for prevention" prescribed extending the preparation margins in healthy and readily accessible areas.

Third, amalgam, which was used to restore cavities two decades ago, required micro-mechanical retention of the restoration material, again at the expense of sound tooth tissue [9].

With the advent of adhesive restorations and facilitated by the described changing understanding of the pathogenesis of caries and carious lesions, a paradigm shift in restorative dentistry occurred. With the increased awareness of the importance of sufficient healthy tooth tissue to prolong the oral lifetime of teeth, adhesive techniques allow minimal preparation. No additional sacrifice of healthy tooth tissue is required to place adhesive restorations, which helps avoid the placement of intra-canal endodontic posts to retain the repair. Adhesive dentistry, thus, assists in preserving tooth tissue and pulp vitality.

Even though the "dental countdown" cannot wholly be avoided, it can be delayed or stretched by:

a. Reducing the loss of healthy tissues as far as possible.
b. Avoiding the need for repetitive restorations by ensuring that placed restorations should be of the highest possible quality to guarantee good durability.

**The Function of Restoration will be Threefold**

1. Facilitating plaque control by providing a new, more easily cleanable surface. Even though a restoration will stop further progression of the carious lesion, it will not.
2. The caries process Moreover, when the biofilm on the restoration will be left undisturbed due to inadequate oral hygiene habits, the risk of secondary caries is high [9].
3. Protecting the pulp by stopping the carious lesion near the pulp. The biocompatibility of the restoration is important to avoid additional chemical trauma to the pulp.
4. Restoring the function, anatomy, and esthetics of the tooth. Whereas esthetics will be important in the visible teeth (maxillary incisors, canines, and

premolars), restoring the anatomy may prevent overeruption of affected teeth and the antagonistic tooth, and mesial tipping or drifting of adjacent teeth [9].

Provided that restorations remain necessary in tomorrow's dentistry, one important question that needs to be answered is: How much carious tissue do we need to remove before placing a restoration.

## Principles of Cavity Preparation

**Dr. G. V Black** published papers and texts on dental materials and preparation and restoration techniques between **1869** and **1915** [10].

**Dr. G.V. Black** wrote: "When a cavity has occurred in the occluding surface of a molar, the dentist prepares for filling with the idea that the fissures in this part of the enamel have favoured the occurrence of the cavity. For this reason, the fissures and grooves adjoining the cavity, even though not decayed, are cut away to such a point as seems to give an opportunity for a smooth, even finish of the margins of the filling. This is done as a prevention of future recurrence of decay…."

This led to the now-infamous term "extension for prevention ", which could be summarised as "the removal of the enamel margin by cutting from the point of greater liability to the point of lesser liability to recurrence of caries" [10].

Extension for prevention meant placing cavity margins at points or along lines that would be cleaned by the excursions of food in chewing. The aim was to prevent the recurrence of decay at the margins of fillings by positioning the margins to obtain this cleaning effect [11]. Black noted that in tooth preparations for smooth-surface caries, the restoration should be extended to normally self-cleaning areas to prevent caries' recurrence. This principle was known as extension for prevention and was broadened to include the extension necessary to remove remaining enamel defects such as pits and fissures.

Providing dental restorations could be the perfect therapy for all lesions-regardless of their surface status-if restorations fulfilled all the discussed aims: restoring form, function, and aesthetic for a lifetime. In such a case, restorations would be "better than tooth tissue". Such claims, however, are not supported by the clinical data. While the annual failure rates of restorations vary widely between studies and restoration types, it is inevitable that statistically, all restorations have a finite average lifetime-although called permanent restorations, restorations are not "permanent" [9].

The process of repeated and escalating re-interventions on dental restorations has been termed the "death spiral of restorations" or, as it eventually affects tooth survival, "the death spiral of teeth." This spiral is associated with repeated interventions, increasing treatment efforts and costs, and limited tooth survival.

**Death Spiral of The Tooth (Fig. 9)**

There are several ways to slow down this spiral: -

1) Placing long-lasting restorations.

2) Placed beneath near-ideal conditions by professionals with sufficient training and experience.

3) Repairing instead of replacing partially faulty restorations; lowering the risk of secondary caries by causally managing the disease caries.

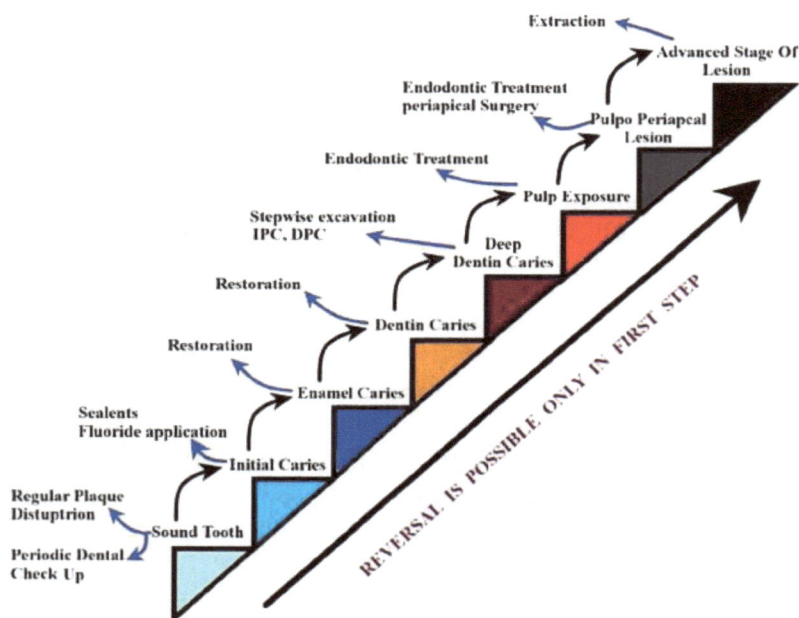

**Fig. (9).** Death Spiral of Tooth.

All these possibilities might allow slowing down the spiral and thus retaining teeth for longer, in elderly patients, even lifelong. However, in younger patients, they might well be insufficient to "stretch" the death spiral over a patient's lifetime. Avoiding entry into this spiral is therefore of absolute importance. Dentists should employ causal, non-invasive management options for preventing caries and carious lesions wherever possible. If required, they should strive to use sealants or other micro-invasive alternatives to manage early carious lesions. As a last resort, they should provide dental restorations, knowing that they place the tooth on a path of no return [9].

In asymptomatic, vital teeth with deep lesions, conservative carious tissue removal strategies that reduce tissue loss and pulp exposure risk must be balanced against removing adequate tissue to maximise restoration longevity. The criterion used to guide carious dentin tissue removal is hardness, judged by tactile feedback during the examination. The levels are described as Hard, Firm, Leathery, and Soft Dentin [9].

The four main strategies for carious tissue removal are:

1)Non-selective Removal to Hard Dentin (now considered overtreatment and too destructive and not recommended)

2)Selective Removal to Firm Dentin

3)Selective Removal to Soft Dentin

4)Stepwise Removal

Hardness will be one significant aspect to assess and describe carious tissue removal, which is why, though in some ways subjective, we will now describe what is meant when talking about soft, leathery, firm, and hard dentin.

**Soft dentin:** "Soft dentin will deform when a hard instrument is pressed onto it and can be easily scooped up (e.g., with a sharp hand excavator) with little force being required.".

**Leathery dentin:** "Although the dentin does not deform when an instrument is pressed onto it, leathery dentin can still be easily lifted without much force being required." The hardness of leathery dentin is between that of soft and firm dentin.

**Firm dentin:** "Firm dentin is physically resistant to hand excavation, and some pressure needs to be exerted through an instrument to lift it.".

**Hard dentin:** "A pushing force needs to be used with a hard instrument to engage the dentine, and only a sharp cutting edge or a bur will lift it. A scratchy sound or 'cri dentinaire' can be heard when a straight probe is taken across the dentin." [4].

**Non-Selective Removal to Hard Dentin (formerly also known as "complete removal")** aims to remove soft dentin, stopping the removal only when hard dentin (like healthy dentin) is reached. This is aimed at all areas of the cavity. The same criterion (the same endpoint) of carious tissue removal is used peripherally and palpably; it is termed non-selective.

Non-selective Removal of Hard Dentin includes the removal of demineralised dentin, which conflicts with modern aims and the guidelines stated above. It is overtreatment and not necessary. Moreover, in deep carious lesions with vital painless pulps, such removal bears significant risks for the pulp. While this approach was the standard in the past, it is now considered overtreatment and not recommended any longer, especially when dealing with deep lesions in teeth with vital pulp. It is not only not necessary but also not desirable.

## Selective Removal to Firm Dentin

In Selective Removal, not one but several different criteria (endpoints) are used to assess carious tissue removal in the periphery of the cavity and proximity to the pulp. One guiding principle during carious tissue removal is creating an environment that allows the best adhesive seal for restoration. This aim can be achieved when there is sound enamel and hard dentin at the periphery of the cavity. This approach also serves as another guiding principle, maximising restoration longevity. However, in the pulpal area of a cavity, another criterion (endpoint) is used, with firm dentin being left. Although removable, this firm dentin is physically resistant to hand excavation and requires effort to remove.

This approach is recommended for shallow or moderately deep lesions, but not deep lesions (i.e., those extending beyond the pulpal third or quarter of the dentineradiographically) in teeth with vital pulps, as even removal to firm dentin risks pulp exposure and harm. It is often required for shallow or moderately deep lesions because the cavity depth needs to be sufficient to allow enough sound enamel and dentin around the periphery for good quality bonding and a complete peripheral seal to be achieved.

## Selective Removal to Soft Dentin

Selective Removal to Soft Dentin is recommended for deep carious lesions in teeth with vital painless pulps. Here, avoiding pulp exposure and maintaining remaining dentin thickness are prioritised in the pulpal area. Consequently, it is expected that leathery or, if needed, soft carious dentin will remain in the pulpal aspect of the cavity, serving the guiding principle of maintaining pulp vitality. A sharp excavator or a probe can check the remaining carious dentin, which will deform and can be lifted under little force. In the periphery, achieving a good seal and maximising restoration survival are prioritised, with peripheral enamel and dentin being hard at the end of the removal process.

Selective Removal to Soft Dentin has been shown to reduce the risk of pulpal exposure compared with Non-Selective Removal to Hard or Selective Removal to.

Firm Dentin. Note that this removal technique has been previously known as partial or incomplete removal [12].

## Step Wise Excavation of Caries

Management of deep carious lesions in vital teeth is challenging. The traditional management of such lesions using non-selective (complete)carious tissue often leads to exposure to the pulp [12]. The most recent inspiration for stepwise carious removal in 2 stages originates from the knowhow on intralesional changes in deep carious lesions. The ecological plaque hypothesis provides the current platform for understanding the pathology of caries [13].

The stepwise excavation technique (Fig. **10a** to **f**) has been studied for over thirty years and was first proposed by **Magnusson and Sundell (1977)** and modified later by **Bjorndal** *et al*. **1997**.

A deep carious lesion has been defined as a "lesion where its penetration depth is in the range of three fourth of the entire thickness of the dentine or more when evaluated on a radiograph".

In the stepwise excavation technique, the first stage aims to convert the lesion activity into an arrested or slow-progressing environment. Leaving behind the carious dentine between 2 stages turns an active deep carious environment from a soft, discoloured, and wet tissue to carious dentin with a darker, harder, and drier appearance. The sealed period with a calcium hydroxide base material followed by a glass-ionomer restoration, for example, transforms carious dentine into a state where it is more clinically convenient to establish and finalise the final cavity for the permanent restoration. A gap between the temporary restoration and the retained carious dentine occurs due to shrinkage of active carious dentine that may take place during inactivation. The provisional restorative material allows the pulpal-dentinal complex to react by placing sclerotic dentine in dentinal tubules and producing tertiary dentine.

The current histological information of the inner pulpal quarter of carious dentine in deep lesions is that the infection has not yet reached the tertiary dentine and pulp. The pulp may be chronically inflamed but is typical without an infection within the pulp. The central part of a slow-progressing lesion with a total surface breakdown is noted with dark discoloured dentine and a healing pulp with evidence of reparative tertiary dentine. Pulp inflammation is not only a one-way route towards pulp cell impairment and subsequent necrosis and infection but as a "double-edged sword "where a so-called wanted inflammation, given the right balance, will cause healing, whereas an unstable inflammation will lead to necrosis [13].

FIRST STAGE IN STEP WISE CARIES EXCAVATION'

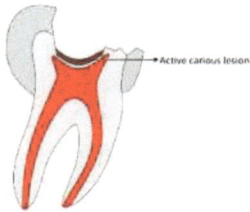

a) First stage of carious tissue
(removal non selective removal is done)

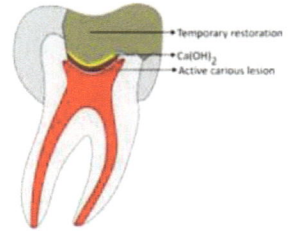

b) A coloring of the temporary restoration

AFTER A 6 MONTH INTERVAL

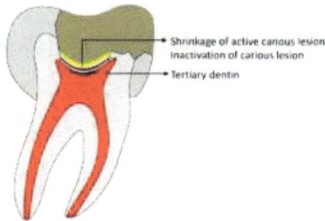

c) A darker, harder and dryer carious dentine. Marked region indicates the gap between restoration and the arrested carious dentine.

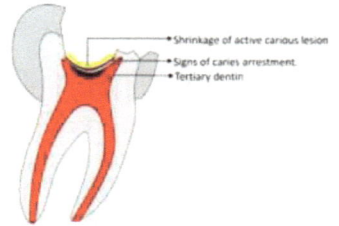

d) Removal of the temporary filling shows signs of lesion arrestment

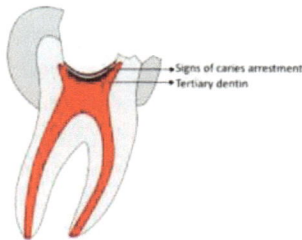

e) Hard excavators are used for the selective removal of arrested carious dentine.

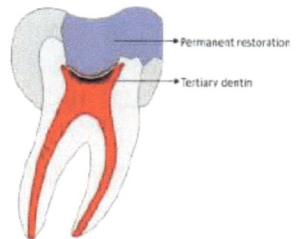

f) Final restoration done.
Tertiary dentine formed

**Fig. (10a to f).** Stepwise excavation of caries.

Moreover, if the carious-infected dentine is altered or removed, the pulp may eventually reach a threshold where a wanted inflammation can take over, ultimately guiding the healing phase [13].

Thus, the purpose of the stepwise excavation technique is:

1) To preserve pulp vitality.
2) Stimulate Re-mineralization and tubule sclerosis preserving affected dentin.

Natural enamel and dentin are still the best "dental materials" in existence; therefore, minimally invasive procedures that conserve a more significant part of the natural, healthy tooth structure must be considered desirable. Minimally invasive procedures are beneficial from a patient's standpoint as well. There is less discomfort and less need for local anaesthesia. Early detection and ultraconservative restoration prevent secondary caries. New instruments such as microabrasion devices and fistulotomy burs offer the dentist techniques that permit minimal preparation and maximum patient acceptance [12].

## Ultraconservative Preparation

The practitioner has several choices of ultraconservative treatment approaches.

**Small Round Burs:** While these familiar burs provide conservative preparation and good explorer access, they are slow and inefficient in cutting through the enamel [13].

**Air Abrasion:** Air abrasion is a powerful and focused narrow beam of 27 μm – 50 μm diameter aluminium oxide particles released at a pressure between 7 to 11 atm. The particles leave the jet nozzle at approximately 2,000 km/h. In doing so, 4,300,000 particles leave the machine every second. Air abrasion is particularly effective in removing hard material. At the same time, soft tissue slows the particles down and thus absorbs the kinetic energy. When directed against the tooth surface, these particles abrade it without producing heat, vibrations, and noise. It is a gentler and less painful procedure. There is no shattering of the enamel or microfractures as with the bur. Most systems can be performed without anaesthesia. The conservative preparations maintain the structural integrity of the tooth.

Air abrasion (Fig. **11**) is called micro dentistry or minimal invasion dentistry. Air abrasion saves the tooth structure and the treatment time. There is no tactile feeling because the handpiece tip does not touch the tooth. As the cutting particles exit straight at the information, it is an end–cutting device instead of the side–cutting bur or rotary handpiece. Air abrasion does not remove soft decay. To remove quiet decay, one needs to use a handpiece with a round bur at slow speed or a small, sharp spoon excavator. Air abrasion can be effective in the management of uncooperative children.

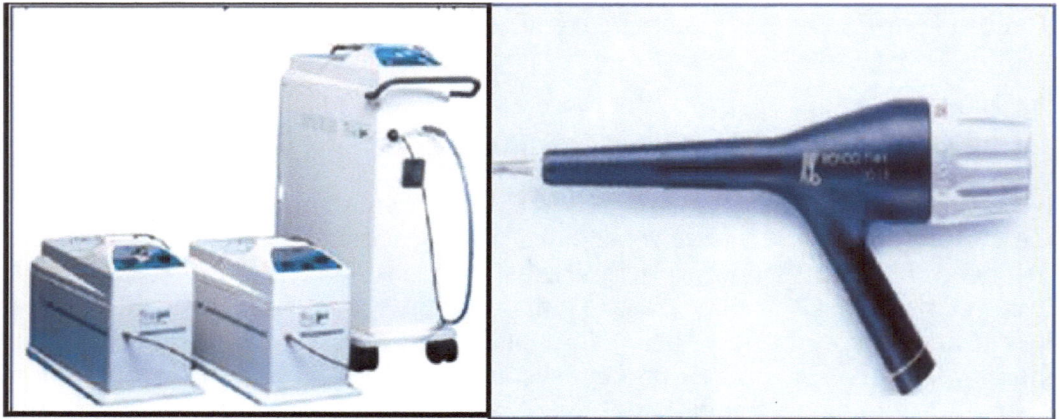

**Fig. (11).** Air Abrasion Unit, Air abrasion handpiece.

**Excisional Biopsy Burs:** These burs are fast-cutting, conservative, and inexpensive and are designed explicitly for recontouring the fissures and accessing decay with minimal enamel removal. These burs are limited to pits, fissures, and grooves.

**The Fistulotomy System:** A fissurotomy bur is a new approach to ultraconservative dental treatment. The shape and size of the bur are designed specifically to treat pit and fissure lesions. The head length is 2.5 mm, allowing the dentist to control the bur tip to cut just below the DEJ and no further. The cavity preparation must be matched with suitable restorative materials. The closest direct material to enamel is composite resin. Since the typical fistulotomy preparation is very narrow, long, and irregularly deep, the restorative material must flow easily into all the nooks and crannies. The dental material of choice is a flowable composite.

Ultraconservative dentistry represents a significant step forward for the dentist, the profession, and especially the patient. It involves the early detection and complete elimination of all accessible and non-accessible carious material from the tooth. Untreated caries can be highly and rapidly destructive. The earliest interception of decay maintains total dental health and increases the likelihood of the restored teeth lasting a lifetime [12].

A changing understanding of the disease dental caries has initiated a paradigm shift in the management of carious lesions. Instead of merely removing the symptoms of the carious lesion, any treatment aims to manage the disease. Up-t--date and evidence-based caries management will continue to involve restorations for the foreseeable future. Still, the limitations of the traditional and rather aggressive therapeutic approach should be acknowledged, and minimally invasive dentistry must be practised.

## Chemicomechanical Removal of Caries

An alternative to the conventional mechanical removal of caries is a chemomechanical method. The need for local anaesthesia is reduced or eliminated as there is little pain during the procedure. Chemicomechanical caries removal is a non-invasive technique eliminating infected dentin via a chemical agent. This process removes infected tissues and preserves the healthy dental structure, avoiding pulp irritation and patient discomfort. This is a method of caries removal based on dissolution. Instead of drilling, this method uses a chemical agent assisted by an atraumatic mechanical force to remove the soft carious structure. The chemicals used can be in the form of liquid (Caridex) or gel (Carisolv) [2].

## A) CARIDEX

CARIDEX consisted of two solutions; Solution I contain sodium hypochlorite, and Solution II contains glycine, aminobutyric acid, sodium chloride and sodium hydroxide. The two solutions should be mixed immediately before use to give the working reagent (pH ≈ 11), which is stable for one hour. Although the Caridex system initially proved to be quite popular, large volumes of solutions are needed (200-500ml), and the procedure is slow. Because of the time required for CMCR treatment, the large volumes of solution required, and the delivery system is no longer commercially available, the use of CMCR, despite its potential, became minimal.

## B) CARISOLV

Although this is like the Caridex and NMAB systems, it is in the form of a pink gel. They are applied to the carious lesion with specially designed hand instruments which did not require any delivery system or heating. This Gel consists of two carboxymethyl cellulose-based gels: a red gel containing 0.1 M amino acids (glutamic acid, leucine, and lysine), NaCl, NaOH, erythrosine (added to make the gel visible during use); and a second containing sodium hypochlorite (NaOCl – 0 w/v). The two are thoroughly mixed in equal parts at room temperature before use and then applied using a hand instrument onto the exposed carious dentin to leave a complex, caries-free cavity. The solution has a pH of around 11 (Figs. **12** & **13**).

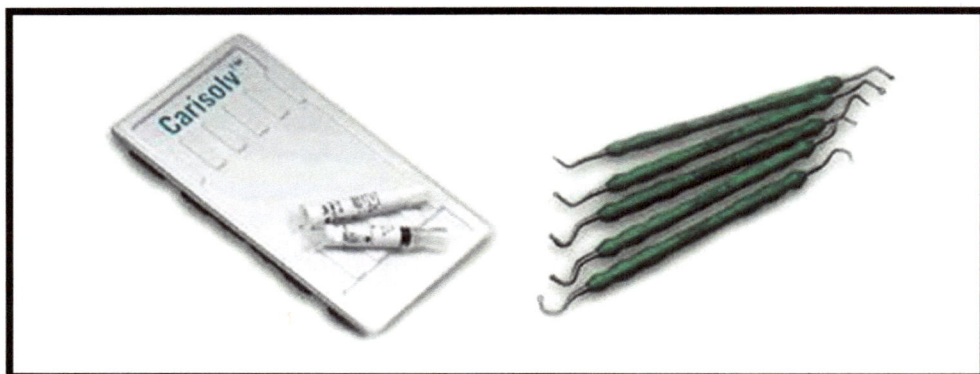

**Fig. (12).** Carisolv Gel and hand instrument.

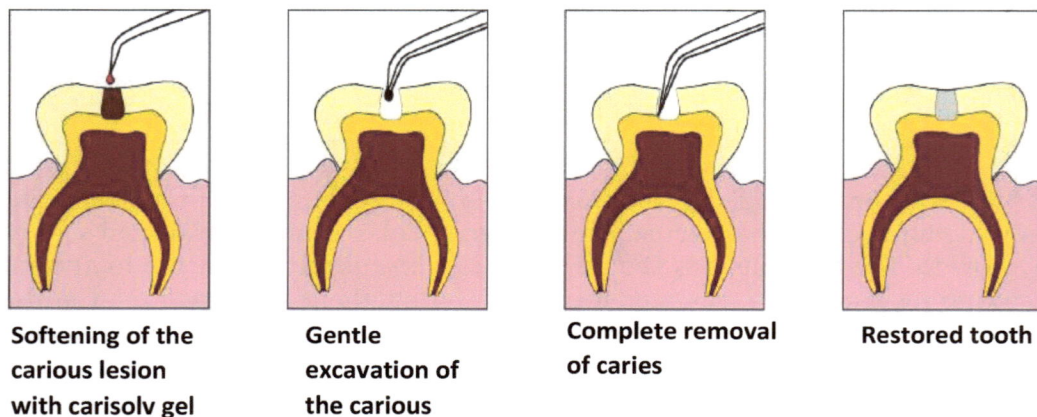

| | | | |
|---|---|---|---|
| **Softening of the carious lesion with carisolv gel** | **Gentle excavation of the carious** | **Complete removal of caries** | **Restored tooth** |

**Fig. (13).** Step-by-Step application of Carisolv.

The procedure of application:

- The gel is applied to the carious lesion with one of the hand instruments, and after 30 seconds, the carious dentin can be gently removed.
- More gel is then applied, and the procedure is repeated until no more carious dentin remains, a guide to this being when the gel removed from the tooth is clear.
- The time required for the procedure is about 9-12 minutes (range about 5-15 minutes), and the volume of gel is only 0.2 - 1.0 ml.

## *Advantages*

- Can be successfully used in uncooperative patients and special health care needs (SHCN) patients.
- It does not require local anaesthesia during the procedure since the gel softens the carious tissue.
- It allows minimally invasive techniques to be applied, considered to be less painful, noise and vibration-free, and patients are more comfortable than with the conventional method.
- Less perception of pain and more comfort. Able for the patient.
- Removes only infected layer and leads to more tissue preservation.
- No pulpal irritation.

## *C) PAPACARIE ®.*

To overcome the disadvantages of the cardiac and carisolv such as short shelf life, high corrosiveness, the requirement for specialised instruments, and high cost, a gel was developed in Brazil in 2003 by Bassadori *et al.,* which is commercially known as Papacarie®. Papacarie® is a gel containing papain and chloramine, which can be combined with manual tools for the minimally invasive removal of carious tissue. This method eliminates the need for local anaesthesia and a bur, thereby reducing the destruction caused to sound dental tissue (Fig. **14**).

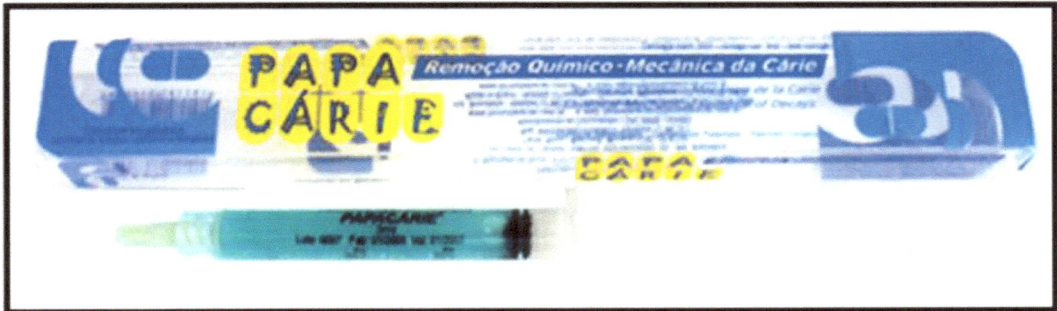

**Fig. (14).** Papacarie®.

## *Composition*

Papain is an end protein that acts only upon damaged tissue since plasma antiprotease is not present in the infected tissue, preventing papain's proteolytic action in tissues considered normal.

Chloramine is a compound containing chlorine and ammonia with antibiotic and disinfecting properties, used to irrigate root canals.

Toluidine blue is a photosensitive pigment that fixates on the bacterial membrane.

The new version of the product is denominated Papacarie Duo™, which was released in 2011 and had the same efficacy plus several additional properties, such as longer shelf life and no need for refrigerated storage. The gel also has greater viscosity, allowing more precise placement and less waste during the procedure.

### *Indication*

• Special health care needs patients.
• Efficient alternative for deproteinisation of the tooth enamel surface.

Before bonding orthodontic brackets with RMGIC.

### *Advantages*

1. Biocompatible gel with antibacterial properties.
2. The formation of a smear layer is not observed after using the gel.
3. Antimicrobial effectiveness, mainly regarding S. mutants and Lactobacillus.
4. Low cost and easy to apply.
5. Fast-acting.

### *D). CARIE CARE (Fig. 15)*

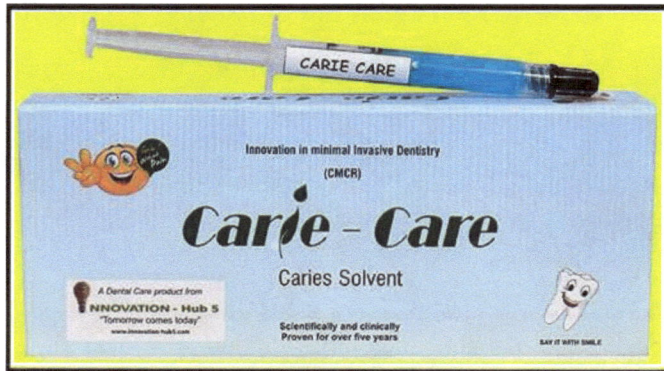

**Fig 15.** Carie-Care®.

Composition- Papaya extract (papain) 100mg, clove oil 2mg, coloured gel (blue), chloramines, sodium chloride and sodium methyl paraben.

Mechanism of action: Papain, a papaya extract, has antibacterial and anti-inflammatory properties and acts as a debris-removing agent. It does not harm healthy tissues and promotes tissue healing. It works only on carious tissue, which lacks plasmatic protease inhibitor alpha-1-antitrypsin; its proteolytic action is inhibited because healthy tissue contains this substance. Papaya extract breaks peptide bonds and involves deprotonation of Cys-25 by His-159. Cys-25 then performs a nucleophilic attack on carbonyl carbon which frees the amino terminal of the peptide; the enzyme is then deacylated by a water molecule and releases the carboxy-terminal portion of the peptide. Chloramines help in the healing process, shorten tissue repair time, and have the potential to dissolve carious dentin using chlorination of partially degraded collagen. This helps disrupt collagen structure, dissolves hydrogen bonds, and helps in tissue removal. Clove oil has an analgesic and antiseptic action. Sodium methylparaben is used as a preservative.

Procedure to use:

- Cariecare is applied directly onto the tooth having caries using a disposable applicator tip; soon, the gel changes the colour in the affected area.
- After 1 minute, the gel and dissolved caries are removed by a sharp spoon excavator.
- Cariecare is in the form of single preparation, which can be stored at four °C for more than six months.

## STAMP TECHNIQUE (Figs 16a and b)

One technique proposed by Dr Waseem Riaz, a London-based practitioner, is a 'Stamp technique' practised for direct composite resin restorations to obtain precise occlusal topography easily. It has also been reported for vertical bite reconstruction of worn-out dentitions. The stamp is like an index, which is the mini-impression made by putty before tooth preparation for a complete crown preparation. This stamp replicates the original anatomy of the tooth structure by copying the original unprepared tooth structure. This technique is used where the occlusal surface is almost intact before the restorative procedure. Or mild or moderate cavitated carious lesions, the cavitation is blocked with wax, and the occlusal pattern is sculpted on the wax [12 - 14].

The step-by-step procedure is illustrated in the figures.

Advantage of Stamp Technique:

- the reduced overall time once the skill is mastered as the post-restoration finishing time is decreased due to almost instantly desired good cusp-fossa relationship.
- reduced porosities present in the final restoration.

## Limitations

- This technique requires skill and clinical acumen to be perfectly performed.
- As flowable composite is usually preferred in this technique, decreased strength is expected.
- Time utilised for mastering and initially practising this technique is considerable. But this can be easily overcome with practice.

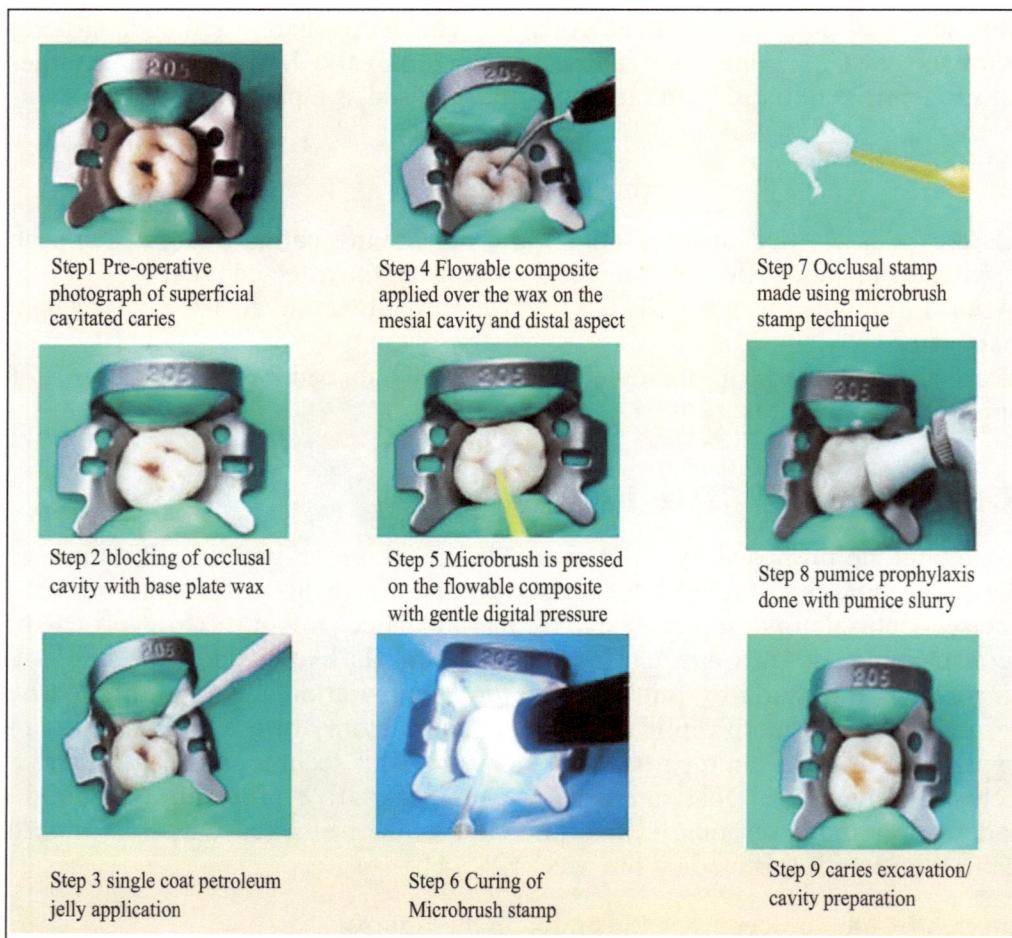

Step1 Pre-operative photograph of superficial cavitated caries

Step 4 Flowable composite applied over the wax on the mesial cavity and distal aspect

Step 7 Occlusal stamp made using microbrush stamp technique

Step 2 blocking of occlusal cavity with base plate wax

Step 5 Microbrush is pressed on the flowable composite with gentle digital pressure

Step 8 pumice prophylaxis done with pumice slurry

Step 3 single coat petroleum jelly application

Step 6 Curing of Microbrush stamp

Step 9 caries excavation/ cavity preparation

**Fig. (16a).** Stamp Technique.

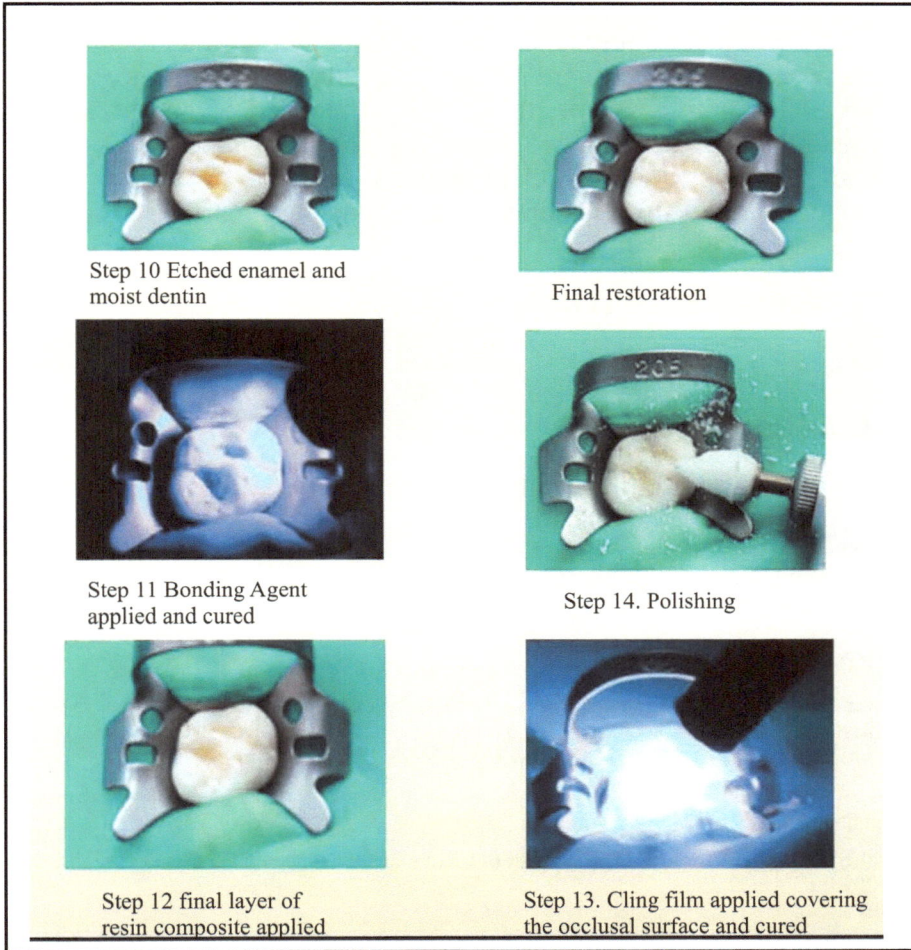

Step 10 Etched enamel and moist dentin

Final restoration

Step 11 Bonding Agent applied and cured

Step 14. Polishing

Step 12 final layer of resin composite applied

Step 13. Cling film applied covering the occlusal surface and cured

**Fig. (16b).** Stamp Technique.

It is imperative to mention that the correct and precise placement of the occlusal stamp is a prerequisite to obtaining an accurate cusp-fossa relationship. Without this, distortions may result, thus nullifying the prime objective of the technique.

## CONCLUSION

The objective is to facilitate clinicians to make suitable decisions regarding the nonrestorative management of caries lesions. In addition, in the decision-making process, clinicians must consider ceilings for restorative and nonrestorative care and strategies for nonrestorative management that are supported by the best available evidence. The judgement in proper evaluation and diagnosis must be considered for the patient's treatment needs. To maintain health and preserve tooth structure. The treatment approaches utilised by dental clinicians must evolve to integrate preventive and treatment solutions tailored to the care needs, which are straightforward to implement in the dental office and whose effectiveness is underpinned by scientific evidence. This chapter, Management of Non-cavitated and Cavitated Carious Lesions, elaborated in detail on the principles of non-invasive management of non-cavitated (initial) occlusal caries lesions, based on an evidence basis.

## CONSENT FOR PUBLICATION

Not applicable.

## CONFLICT OF INTEREST

The authors declare no conflict of interest, financial or otherwise.

## ACKNOWLEDGEMENT

Declared none.

## REFERENCES

[1]     Schwendicke F, Walsh T, *et al.* Interventions for treating cavitated or dentine carious lesions. Cochrane Database Syst Rev 2021; 7: CD013039.
        [http://dx.doi.org/10.1002/14651858.CD013039]

[2]     https://www.mchoralhealth.org/Dental-Sealant/.Anon-cavitated caries lesion, lesion without evidence of cavitation.

[3]     Margherita F. Nonrestorative Management of Cavitated and Noncavitated Caries Lesions. Dent Clin N Am 2019; 63(4): 695-703.
        [http://dx.doi.org/10.1016/j.cden.2019.06.001]

[4]     Schwendicke F. Management of Deep Carious Lesions. Springer Cham 2019; 130.

[5]     FJ Burke. From Extension for Prevention to Prevention of Extension: (Minimal Intervention Dentistry. Dent Update 2003; 30(9): 492-8, 500, 502.
        [http://dx.doi.org/10.12968/denu.2003.30.9.492]

[6]     Ole F, Nyvad B, Edwina K. Dental caries the disease and its clinical management. Wiley-Blackwell 2015; p. 480.

[7]     Freedman G, Goldstep F, Seif T, *et al.* Ultraconservative resin restorations. J Can Dent Assoc. Nov 65(10): 579-81.

[8]     Bjørndal L. Stepwise Excavation. Monogr Oral Sci 2018; 27; 68-81.
        [http://dx.doi.org/10.1159/000487834]

[9]     Labib ME, Hassanein OE, Moussa M, Yassen A, Falk Schwendicke. Selective *versus* stepwise removal of deep carious lesions in permanent teeth: a randomised controlled trial from Egypt—an interim analysis. BMJ Open 2019; 9(9): e030957.

[10]    Llena C, Leyda AM, Forner L. Non-Cavitated Caries Lesions: A New Approach to Medical Treatment. In: Li MY (Ed.) Contemporary Approach to Dental Caries. InTech; 2012.

[11]   Tung MS, Eichmiller FC. Dental applications of amorphous calcium phosphates. J Clin Dent 1999; 10(1 Spec No): 1-6.
[PMID: 10686850]

[12]   Huang SB, Gao SS, Yu HY. Effect of nano-hydroxyapatite concentration on remineralization of initial enamel lesion *in vitro*. Biomed Mater 2009; 4(3): 034104.
[http://dx.doi.org/10.1088/1748-6041/4/3/034104.]

[13]   Gaffar A, Blake-Haskins J, Mellberg J. In vivo studies with a dicalcium phosphate dihydrate/MFP system for caries prevention. Int Dent J 1993; 43(1) (Suppl. 1): 81-8.
[PMID: 8478133]

[14]   Walsh LJ. Contemporary technologies for remineralization therapies: A review. Int Dentistry SA 2009; 11: 6-16.

# Lasers in Pediatric Dentistry

**Gholam Hossein Ramezani[1,*], Alireza Mirzaei[2] and Anahita Bagheri[2]**

[1] *Department of Pediatric Dentistry, Dental Faculty, Tehran University of Medical Science, Tehran, Iran*

[2] *RWTH Aachen University, 52062 Aachen, Germany*

**Abstract:** In recent years, the desire of Dental Clinicians and patients to use lasers for the treatment of Dental conditions has increased. Knowledge of laser functions and biological features of oral tissues is crucial for understanding the effect of dental lasers. Choosing a suitable dental laser for different tissues effectively reduces tissue damage. Other types of lasers are used in dentistry, which effectively treats lesions by providing innovative and minimally invasive treatments that also have biostimulation, anti-inflammatory, and analgesic effects. Among lasers, erbium lasers, being less invasive and having caries removal properties, have been optimally considered in pediatric dentistry. Lasers in children can also have efficient antiseptic effects on vital and non-vital pulp therapies of primary teeth.

One of the most common oral problems in children is dental trauma. Laser-based therapies can significantly reduce pain and surgical problems. Laser therapy is a suitable and valuable treatment strategy in children despite surgery problems and provides practical health solutions. Findings have shown that different lasers, based on their wavelength, can cause incisions on the soft and hard tissues of the mouth and teeth in the form of various mechanisms such as vaporisation or ablation, and these effects vary according to the wavelength used; however, choosing an infrared laser allows the dentist to better interact with specific targets such as gums, mucous membranes, and mouth injuries. This chapter examines the critical effects of lasers in pediatric dentistry.

**Keywords:** Erbium Laser, Lasers , Treatment of Caries, YAG Lasers.

--------------------------------------------------------------------------------
\* **Corresponding author Gholam Hossein Ramezani:** Department of Pediatric Dentistry, Dental Faculty, Tehran University of Medical Science, Tehran, Iran; E-mail: gh.h.ramezani@gmail.com

# INTRODUCTION

## Pediatric Laser Dentistry

Since dental caries and untreated dental problems can severely affect children's general health and well-being, dental care and treatment are crucial. However, there is ample evidence that the children and adolescents suffer from various oral diseases, such as oral mucosal lesions. Many physicians confront children who are afraid of the unknown and do not cooperate with the physician and Dental clinicians, which can create challenges for dental professionals in providing therapeutic care. Therefore, familiarity with children's psychological, behavioural, and physical needs is necessary. In this case, the role of modern and new technologies such as lasers cannot be denied. Light has been used as a therapeutic agent for many years. Nowadays, lasers are used in many cases in various fields of medicine and surgery and can replace knives in dental surgery. The word LASER stands for light amplification by stimulated emission of radiation. A laser is a one-way, single-colour electromagnetic energy that allows high-energy light beams to be transmitted and focused in one place. This energetic beam of light can have chemical, mechanical, or thermal effects on the body. Lasers have been introduced to the medical field to meet patients' diagnostic and therapeutic needs faster and more effectively. Since contemporary dentistry is based on the use of minimally invasive methods, the laser can be an excellent alternative to drilling due to less pain, noise, and vibration (Figs. **1a - c**) and can be used to diagnose and prevent dental diseases and can also help maintain the remaining healthy structures by removing diseased tissues (decayed tissues).

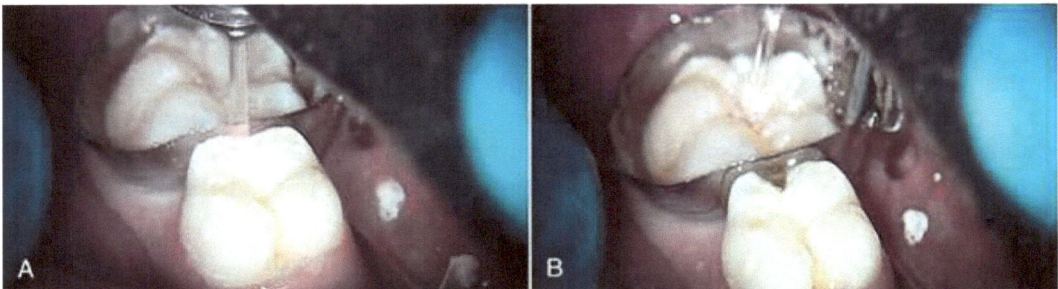

**Fig. (1a). A,** Class II caries. Matrix band is placed on the adjacent tooth to prevent accidental removal of its structure. **B,** Class II caries removal with Er: YAG laser.

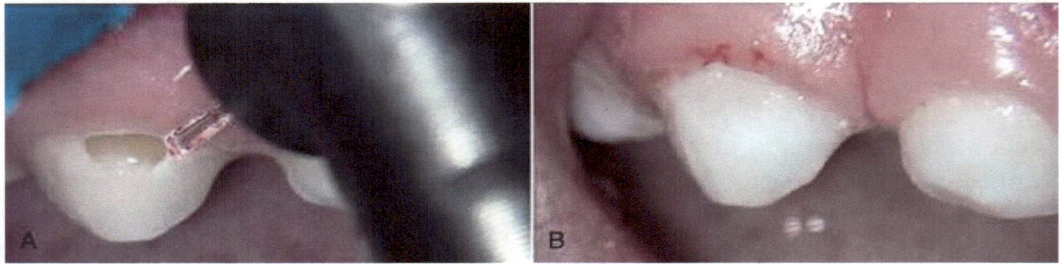

**Fig. (1b). A,** Class V caries removal combined with access gingivectomy. Both procedures were completed with an erbium laser: **B,** Immediate postoperative view of restoration.

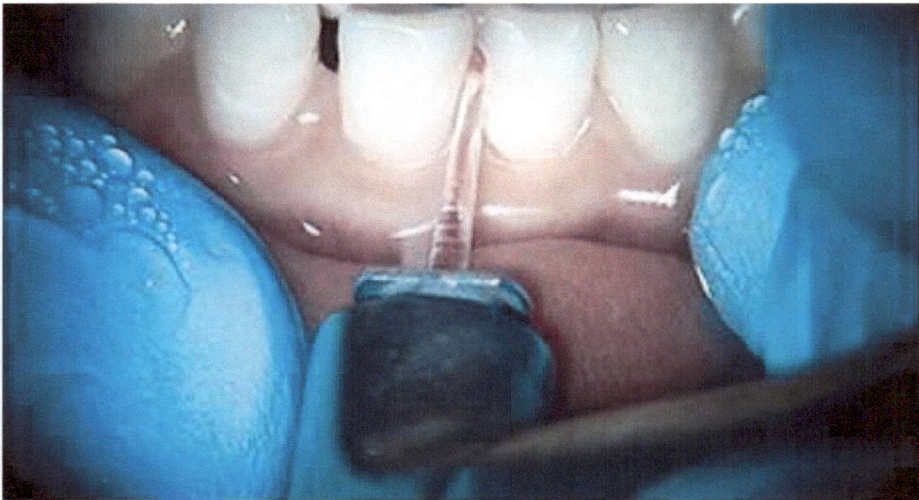

**Fig. (1c).** Class III caries removal on permanent central incisors with erbium laser.

Maintaining a dry mouth increases the doctor's vision and induces better results. In addition, the replacement of sharp tools with lasers attracts more patients to dental clinics. The American Academy of Pediatric Dentistry (AAPD) recommends using lasers in restorative dentistry and soft tissue therapy for infants and children, including patients with special health needs. Other benefits of using a laser in dentistry are listed in Table **1**.

**Table 1. Other clinical benefits of laser.**

| Minimal invasiveness | Useable for carious tissues |
|---|---|
| Antiseptic effects | Useable in carious and root canal lesions |
| It has a Micro retentive surface. | Useable in rough, clean, and deformed surface without smear layer |
| Application in soft tissues | Useable in carious gums near the proximal surface, evaporating and thickening the pulp. |

When a laser is applied to a tissue, the laser energy is absorbed into the target tissue. Different laser wavelengths have different absorption coefficients depending on the components in dental tissue, such as water, pigment, blood, and mineral content (hydroxyapatite) (Fig **2**). Laser energy can be absorbed or transmitted based on the composition of the target tissue. Fig. (**3**) shows the types of laser and tissue interactions.

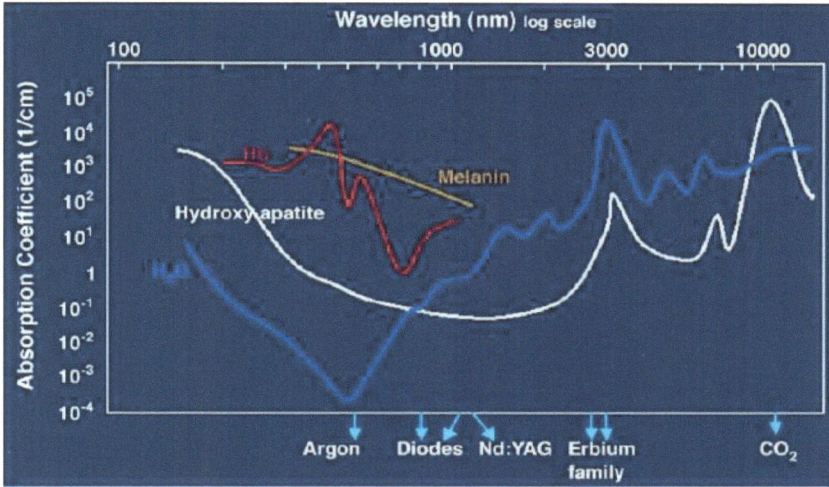

**Fig. (2).** Curves of different tooth compositions' approximate absorption of varying laser wavelengths.

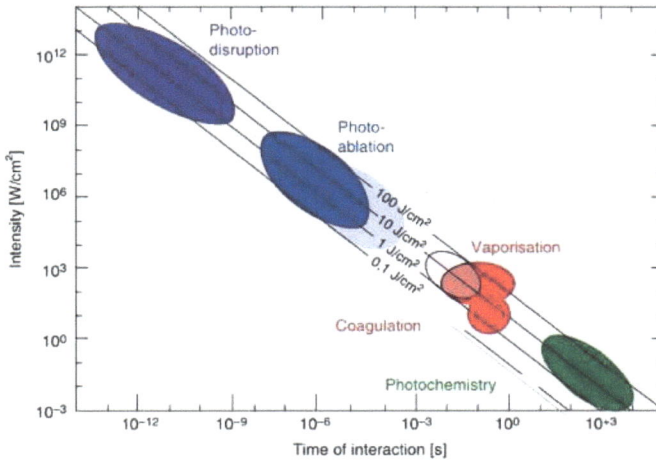

**Fig. (3).** Mechanisms of laser and tissue interaction over time.

Lasers are divided into four main groups based on their specific applications: solid-state lasers, liquid lasers, gas lasers, and semiconductor lasers. Gas lasers have a more straightforward design in comparison with other types. The relative dispersion of the emitting atoms in the gases creates a relatively homogeneous environment; this group is continuous-wave lasers. The essential characteristic of liquid lasers is their ability to change their frequency. Lightness and high optical power output are among the features of semiconductor lasers that make them famous. In another classification, based on the clinical use of lasers in dentistry, they are divided into types used only for soft tissues, soft and hard tissues, Low-Level laser Therapy treatments, photopolymerisation, and caries diagnosis. The main types of lasers used as surgical treatment tools in the oral cavity include neodymium (Nd: YAG) lasers, erbiums (Er: YAG, Er, Cr: YSGG), argon (Ar) lasers, carbon dioxide ($CO_2$) lasers, and diodes (Fig. **4**). Pediatric dentists can use the family of erbium lasers as safe and efficient lasers for treating hard and soft tissues of the oral cavity. The low penetration depth of erbium lasers, high affinity for water, lack of heat damage, and minimal reflective properties make them an ideal laser for pediatric dentistry.

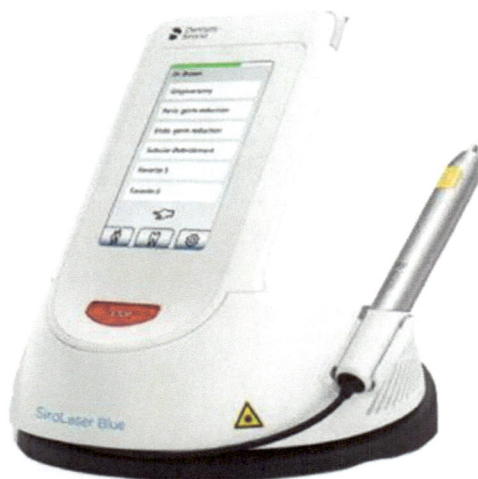

**Fig. (4).** Image of a diode laser device.

## Pediatric Laser Dentistry: Hard Tissue Laser Application

### *Application of Laser for the Diagnosis, Prevention, and Treatment of Caries*

There are several uses for lasers in pediatric dentistry. A laser is a valuable tool for diagnosing and monitoring carious lesions. Tooth decay, the most common infectious disease, may affect the health and development of the pediatric population. Therefore, appropriate dental treatments are necessary to restore children's oral and general health. Clinical benefits of different types of lasers in the treatment of hard tooth tissue (such as other lasers to eliminate caries and prepare teeth by creating cavities in the tooth for restoration) have increased the interest of dentists and researchers in the application of lasers. Diagnodent diagnostic technology uses a 655-nanometer diode laser to diagnose primary caries, also called laser-induced fluorescence (Fig. **5**).

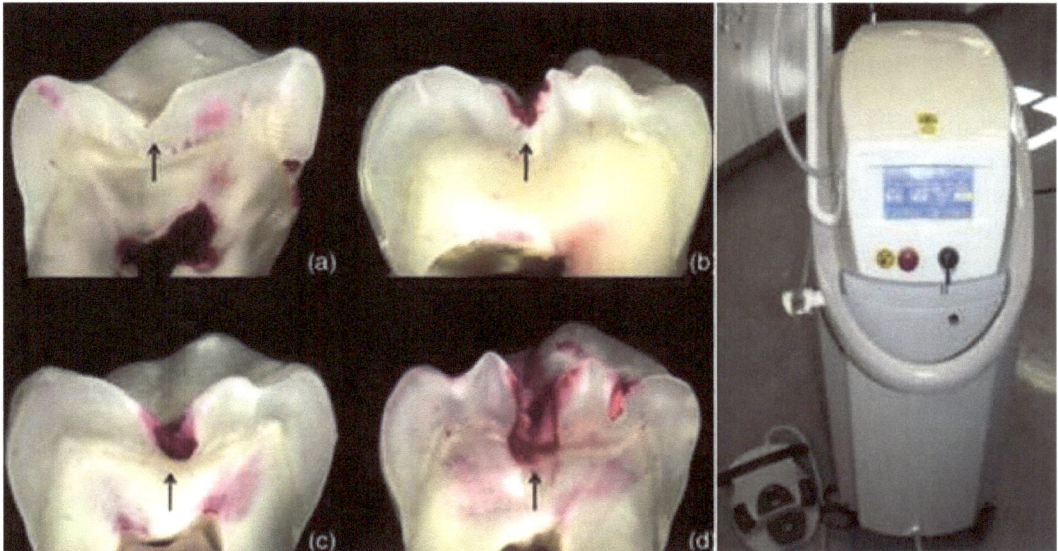

**Fig. (5).** Right: Image of laser fluorescence device, KEY3 laser model. She left: Histological examination. **a)** No caries. **b)** Caries that have spread to half of the enamel. **c)** Caries that have spread to the inner half of the enamel. **d)** Caries in dentine.

When the laser irradiates the tooth, light is absorbed by organic and inorganic substances in dental tissues and metabolites such as bacterial porphyrins. These porphyrins show fluorescence after stimulation with red light. Diagnodent offers the degree of demineralisation and tooth decay through fluorescence emitted from the surface of occlusal or proximal teeth. On the right side of Fig. (**5**), you can see the image of the Laser fluorescence device. You can see the tooth's histological examination on the left side after using the Light-Emitting Diode-Based device.

The application of this tool is very effective in diagnosing caries in children. Due to children's fear of dentists and lack of cooperation, preparing radiographs to diagnose various lesions is problematic. If their head moves, it changes the position of the film, and therefore the process should be repeated. In an *in vitro* comparative experiment with Er, Cr: YSGG laser irradiation on a normal dentition in deciduous teeth, it was found that laser irradiation had minor heat damage to surrounding tissues, minimal heat-induced changes in tooth challenging tissue composition, and desired level of protection. The laser removes the minimum amount of hard tissue and allows teeth to be prepared with less risk of pulp exposure. In caries prevention, lasers are used to increase the resistance of the enamel surface against acid attack and to adapt the tooth surface to place sealants and preventive resin repairs. Another application in hard tissue is tooth restoration and pulp treatment. Er: YAG lasers are safe and effective in eliminating caries and preparing cavities in children and adults without significant damage to tooth structure or causing discomfort to patients. In a study by Al-Batayneh et al., the effectiveness of the Er: YAG laser in eliminating caries in children and its safety for the primary and permanent dental pulp was evaluated. By comparing different dentin extraction methods for deciduous teeth, a lower level of over-preparation was found in the erbium laser group than the milling group, which confirms that the use of erbium lasers is a minimally invasive laser approach [1]. In another study, the effects of Er: YAG on dentin structure and bond strength of deciduous teeth before treatment were investigated. SEM observations showed that the surface morphology of dentin incisions changed after etching and after Er: YAG laser treatment with different amounts of energy and frequency (Fig. **6**) [2].

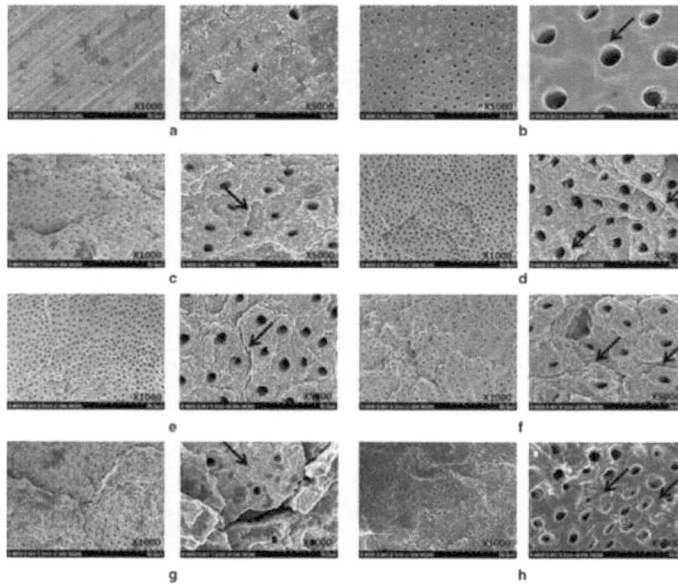

**Fig. (6).** SEM images showing dentin surface morphology after various energy treatments. **a)** control group, **b)** etching group, the arrow represents open dentinal tubules. **c)** 50 mJ laser group, arrow indicates protrusion of dentin around the tube. **d)** 100 mJ laser group, arrows indicate fish-scale and lamellar dentin. **e)** 150 mJ laser group, arrow indicates dentinal cracking. **f)** 200 mJ laser group, arrow indicates deep dentin cracking around the tube. **g)** 250 mJ laser group, arrow indicates fish-scale disappearance and lamellar morphology. **h)** 300 mJ laser group, arrow indicates collapsed tissues between dentin tubes, coking or carbonisation.

## *Application of Laser in Fissure Sealant*

Dental pit and fissure sealant are non-invasive practical approaches to prevent tooth decay in children and adolescents. Sealants are composed of different materials and enter the tooth using other techniques. Resin, one of the most commonly used materials for dental sealants, helps maintain the integrity of the occlusal surface of the tooth and acts as an effective mechanical barrier against plaque formation, which in turn reduces the incidence of cleft caries (Fig. **7**) [3].

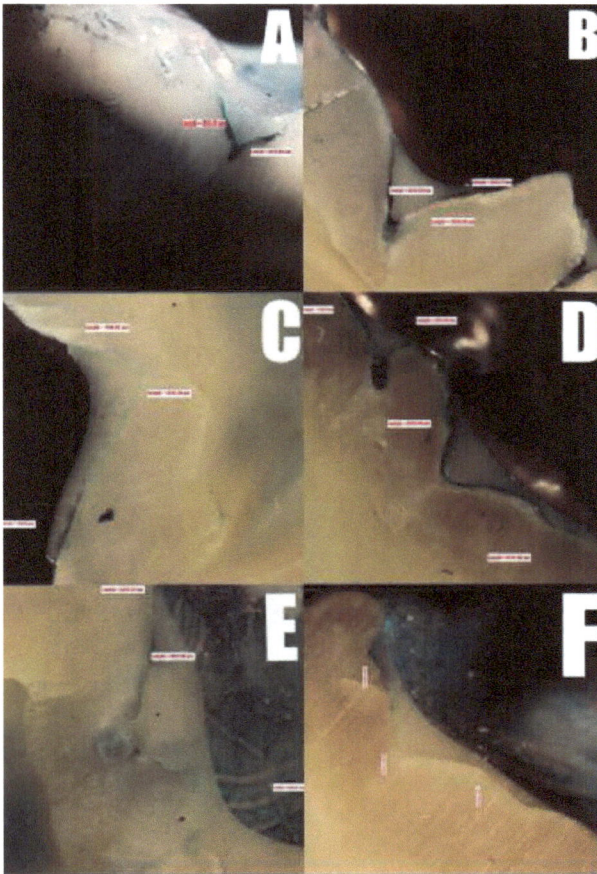

**Fig. (7).** Image of different groups tested. **A)** Mechanical preparation of Bur and application of sealant. **B)** Mechanical preparation of Bur, etching, and sealant. **C)** Mechanical preparation of Bur, etching, bonding, and sealant. **D)** Mechanical preparation of laser and sealant. **E)** Mechanical laser preparation, use of etching and sealant. F) Mechanical preparation of laser, etching, bonding, and sealant.

Various methods adequately prepare the tooth surface for fissure sealants, such as rotary drilling, blasting, phosphoric acid etching, or laser technology [4]. Laser irradiation does not require etching acid in the enamel before placing the sealant or composite. On the other hand, using lasers for this purpose has other benefits such as minimally invasive treatment, noise reduction during treatment, no contact or vibration on the tooth surface, and reducing the need for anaesthesia. In addition, preventing rotating tools increases treatment safety when treating young children and makes it more acceptable to patients [4]. Before using dental pits and fissure sealants, lasers can be used to prepare the tooth surface. The laser can also be used for conditioning, cleaning, and disinfecting pits and fissures.

## Application of Laser for the Treatment of Molar-Incisor Hypomineralisation (MIH)

The MIH, pictured in Fig. (**8**), was first described in 2001 by Weerheijm *et al.* [5]. MIH is defined as a growth-induced dental defect that involves the Hypomineralisation of 1 to 4 permanent molars and is often affected by similar permanent Incisors. MIH prevalence worldwide is between 3 and 44%, and four of every five children have MIH. Children are more likely to be sensitive to MIH than others [5]. Laser is a treatment in the most severe cases with the least amount of invasion and can also effectively protect the existing dental structure; since the use of lasers possibly increases fluoride absorption and resistance of enamel, its application for the treatment MIH should be considered. In addition, the erbium laser preparation can be used in treating severe MIH lesions due to low and favourable changes in dental tissues and minor discomfort. It can be considered a treatment for MIH in children [6].

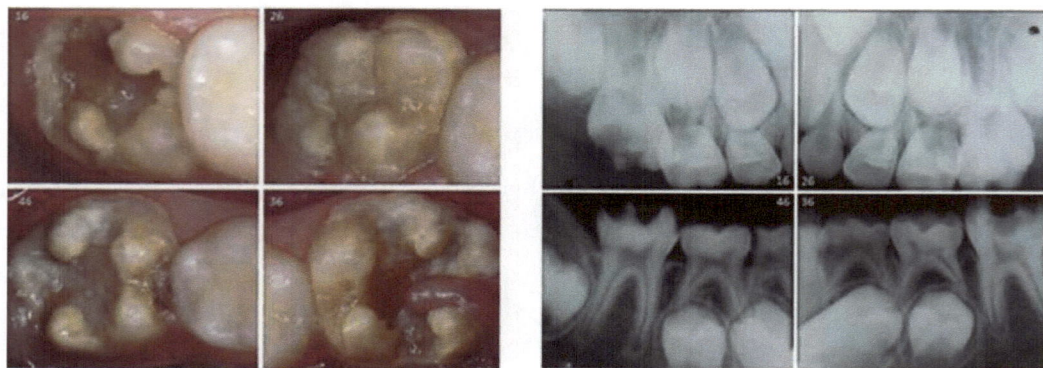

**Fig. (8).** Clinical view and Radiographic aspects of first permanent molars with Hypomineralisation.

## Erbium Lasers and Composite Adhesion

The use of orthophosphoric acid is a critical step in bonding. Self-etch bonding agents can be improved by using a chemical pretreatment with sodium hypochlorite. Glass ionomers produced with erbium lasers show greater microleakage than samples prepared with diamond bur [6]. Some researchers believe that acid etching should be performed after using erbium lasers to eliminate decay. In addition to reducing microleakage in the enamel restoration, it eliminates the transmuted surface area of dentin induced by these lasers [7]. In a study by Nahas *et al.*, the results showed that Er: YAG and Er, Cr: YSGG lasers increased the self-adhesion values of the resin stream and improved its lifespan by removing the smear layer, opening the dentin tubes, and increasing the penetration of the resin into the microstructure [8].

## *Application of Laser in Endodontics*

Protecting primary teeth from pulp changes due to caries or trauma is a major therapeutic challenge in pediatric dentistry and poses severe emotional problems for patients and parents. Lasers can be used to treat live and non-living pulp, such as pulp capping, pulpotomy, and pulpectomy. Pulpotomy is a general procedure in deciduous teeth, and lasers are suggested as an alternative to Formocresol and ferric sulfate [6]. Laser-Doppler flowmetry, developed to assess blood flow in the vascular system, can also be used to detect blood flow in the dental pulp. The laser technique requires less time to complete cleaning and shaping than rotary or hand tools, has similar results in cleanliness compared to rotary tools, and is better than hand tools. Er: YAG, Er, Cr: YSGG, and $CO_2$ lasers for pulp coagulation showed better than calcium hydroxide after two years (Fig. **9**) shows the use of lasers in endodontics.

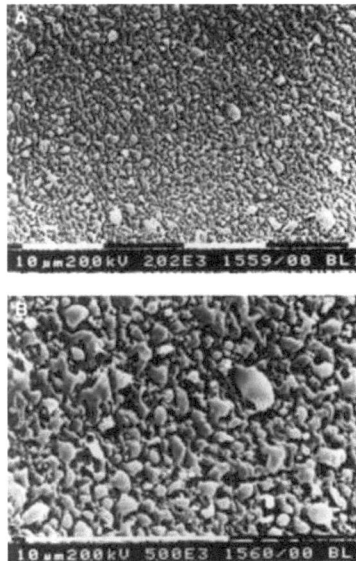

**Fig. (9).** Photomicrograph of the lasered area with an intensity of 0.5 J / $cm^2$. **A)** The surface is composed of more refined grains of molten material evenly distributed on the surface (original magnification x2000). **B)** The same area at x5000 magnification. The central location of the pipe openings is not visible.

## Pediatric Laser Dentistry: Soft Tissue Laser Application

### *Application of Laser for Periodontics and Pathology*

Lasers can be used in pediatric soft tissue treatments such as a frenectomy, surgery, and some oral pathologies such as pyogenic granuloma, mucocele, fibroma, hemangioma, cold sores, and aphthous ulcers. Lasers can also remove excess gums to accurately place stainless steel crowns, widely used in repairing damaged molar teeth. The laser provides an opportunity for the safe treatment of periodontal disease in children without causing allergic reactions or bacterial resistance. All laser wavelengths perform gingival surgery, plastic surgery, and surgical procedures with minimal need for local anaesthesia without bleeding. Of all the lasers used in dentistry, the Er: YAG laser is the most promising for periodontal treatment. The antiseptic effect of different laser wavelengths has been used to treat adults. For them, both the thermal impact of near and medium infrared lasers and the photochemical effect of PDT is effective in managing invasive periodontitis. However, the treatment of young patients with periodontitis has been less studied [9].

### *Application of Laser in Orthodontics*

The use of lasers for orthodontics began about twenty years ago. It rapidly took its place in solving various problems related to orthodontic treatment, such as opening ceramic brackets and etching the enamel surface and gingival mucosal surgery. The forces used in orthodontics cause the tooth to move in the periodontal ligament space and subsequently cause the alveolar bone to regenerate through bone resorption and placement. These mechanical forces used during orthodontic treatment lead to acute inflammations that cause pain and discomfort in the teeth and their supporting tissues. Low-level laser therapy has been reported to help control the pain caused by orthodontic arch placement. The exact mechanism of pain control of lasers is not well understood. Since chemical mediators such as prostaglandin E2 and interleukin-1-$\beta$ are significantly expressed in the periodontium after orthodontic treatment, and these factors cause pain and allergies, it is thought that the laser reduces pain by inhibiting the secretion of inflammatory mediators. Fig. (**10**) shows the application of laser in orthodontics.

## Pediatric Laser Dentistry: Dental Trauma

Trauma is a lesion that occurs in supporting structures, especially the alveolar bone, gums, ligaments, and lips. Traumatic dental injuries are a public health problem worldwide, with one in two children aged 8 and 12 suffering from tooth damage [10]. Trauma can have short-term and long-term negative consequences and may impair pulp stability. Different interventions and treatment options are available depending on the type of injury. Treatments for children and adolescents may be other than adults, mainly due to primary teeth and facial growth during puberty. Therefore, managing damaged teeth and minimising the effects of trauma in this age group is very important (Fig. **11**). Lasers can be used to treat traumatic injuries without using sutures, with a good and fast recovery rate, and with minimal discomfort for patients.

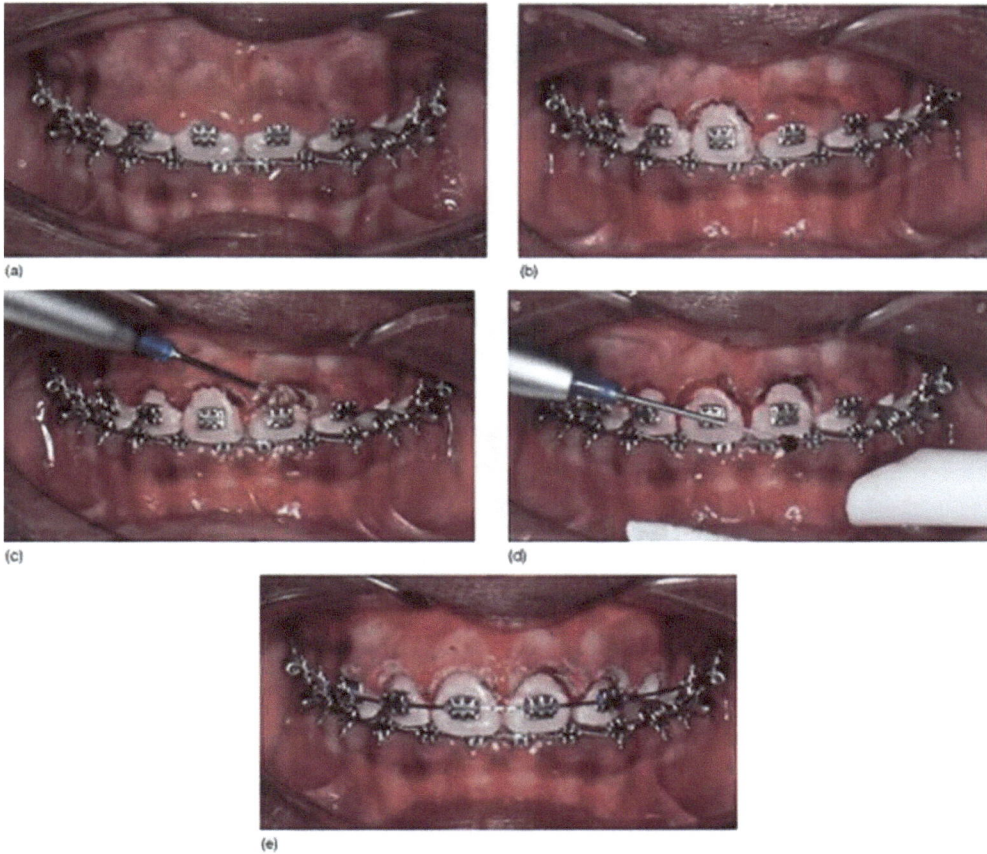

(a)     (b)     (c)     (d)     (e)

**Fig. (10). a-e)** Removal of excess tissue due to poor oral hygiene. **d)** Pulling the fiberoptic tip to the side can lead to tissue accumulation that must be removed with a 2x2 gauze. High-speed suction is significant to remove the mass using a laser.

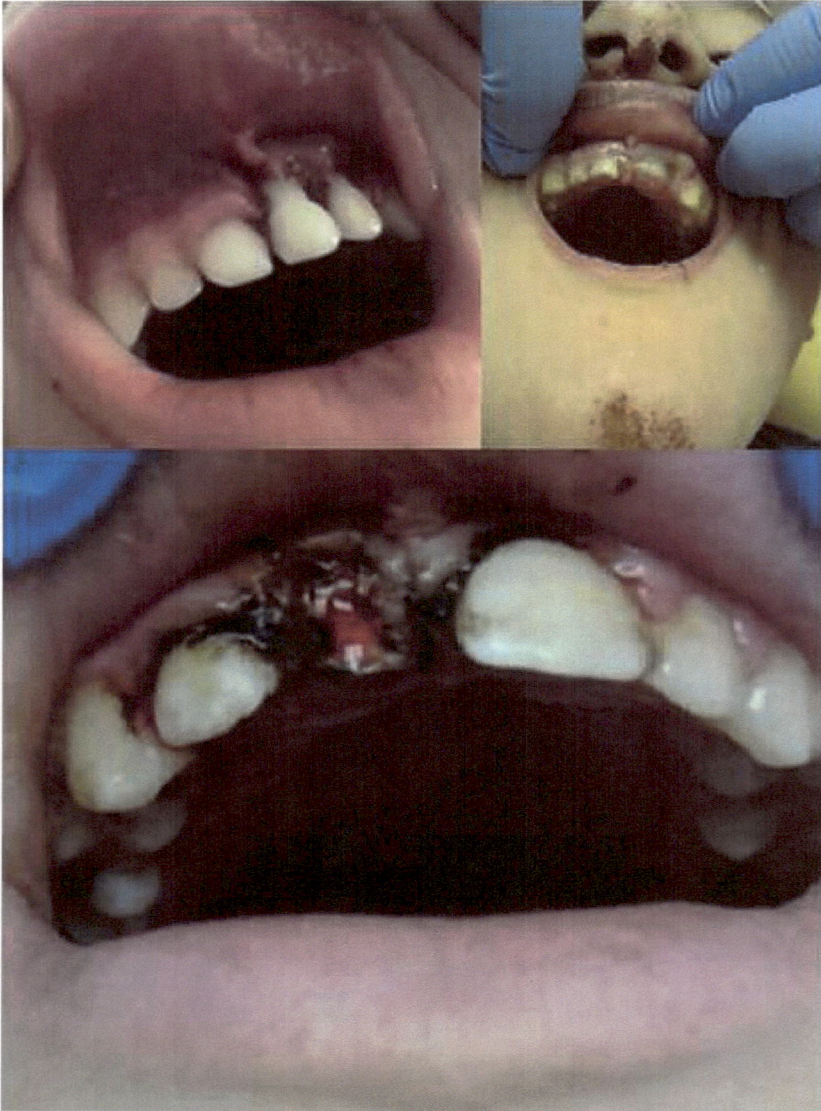

**Fig. (11).**  Images of trauma in children.

## *Application of Laser in Dental Traumatology: Hard Tissues and Pulp*

Crown fractures may involve the enamel and dentin and, if complicated, sometimes destroy the pulp. Therefore, traumatic lesions can cause damage to dental tissues and pulp, resulting in pulp necrosis, and clinical interventions require the use of specific protocols. Therefore, accurate and timely diagnosis is necessary to increase tooth survival. Lasers can be used as a replacement for rotary instruments in pediatric restorative dentistry, allowing safe and minimally invasive interventions. Among the lasers used, erbium wavelengths can produce good results in the dental cavity, reduce postoperative discomfort and sensitivity, and provide minimally invasive methods in dentistry. These lasers can perform all procedures such as preparation and finishing the tooth margin, pulp coagulation, pulpotomy, or even pulpectomy [11]. Also, Doppler flowmetry using lasers and ultrasound are new technologies for monitoring pulp stability. Doppler flowmetry shows pulp blood flow and can be used to assess pulp freshness. This method is non-invasive, reliable, and painless and is well tolerated by children. This treatment can also help monitor removable teeth.

## *Application of Lasers in Traumatic Injuries of Soft Tissue*

Trauma to the alveolar bone, gums, periodontal ligament, frenum, and lips causes damage to hard and soft tissues [11]. Lasers are now a viable option for treating oral benign tissue obstruction. They provide good clotting combined with effective disinfection, pain relief for treating traumatic injuries, do not require suturing, and have a rapid recovery. Helium-neon lasers were initially used for treatment, but today semiconductor diode lasers of 830 nm or 635 nm are more commonly used (Fig. **12**). In all types of luxation injuries, lasers have not only antibacterial and detoxifying effects (Er: YAG, Nd: YAG, and diodes) but also provide favourable conditions for the bonding of periodontal tissue especially in permanent teeth. After using lasers, rapid healing of wounds and traumatic pain in soft tissues has also been reported [12, 13].

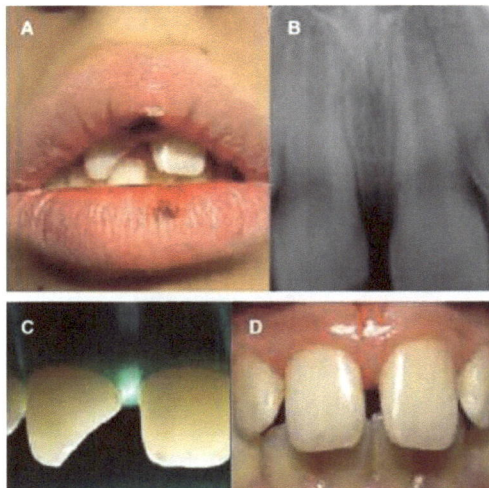

**Fig. (12).** Deep but uncomplicated fracture of the tooth crown 2. **A)** Initial condition. **B)** Radiographic examination. **C)** Minimally invasive treatment with erbium laser. **D)** Clinical appearance after repair with composite resin.

## Photobiomodulation in Pediatric Dentistry

Photobiomodulation (PBM), also known as low-level laser therapy (LLLT), has become a method of interest for many researchers due to its anti-inflammatory function, ability to increase collagen production, reduce inflammatory secretions, and increase blood vessels. Due to PBM's ability to heal both soft tissues such as mucosa and skin and mineral and hard tissues such as bones and teeth, PBM is widely used in various treatments. This treatment uses ionising light sources in the visible and near-infrared spectrum and enhances non-thermal biological processes on the tissues [14]. Low-level lasers work through photochemical and photobiological effects on target tissues. Bioactive responses activated in PBM therapy are related to three cellular mechanisms: cytochrome c oxidase in mitochondria, light-sensitive receptors in cell membranes, and a set of extracellular growth factors (TGF-b1). The light radiation used for PBM can scatter in the tissues and heal the wound. PBM also enlarges blood vessels and modulates inflammatory processes, the proliferation of fibroblasts, keratinocytes, chondrocytes, osteoblasts, and improves bone restoration [14]. Low-level lasers produce between 50 and 500 mW of power and have stimulus and inhibitory effects. Their application in pediatric dentistry includes anaesthesia, treatment of damaged anterior teeth, muscle spasm and cellulite treatment, temporomandibular joint problems, weakening of the gag reflex, and reduction of postoperative complications. Various studies show that PBM therapy is a safe and effective treatment and has different clinical applications such as primary molar teeth treatment, removal of general pain intensity, and treatment of minor recurrent aphthous stomatitis in pediatric dentistry (Fig. **13**).

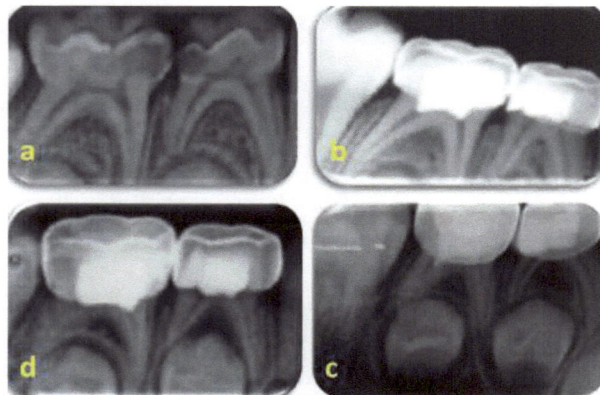

**Fig. (13).** Periapical radiography shows the success of low-level lasers in pulpotomy treatment in # 84 and # 85 teeth. **a)** Preoperative radiography. **b)** Postoperative radiography. **c)** Radiography at 3-month follow-up. **d)** Radiography at 9-month follow-up.

## CONCLUSION

Since dental problems can seriously affect children's general health and well-being, dental care and treatment are essential health services for children. On the other hand, children cannot tolerate every treatment due to fear of the unknown. Therefore, treatment of dental problems in this age group can create challenges for dentists in providing medical services. Among the existing treatments, modern and new technologies such as lasers have an influential role in making treatments tolerable for children. Laser treatment can be a less invasive method to treat dental problems in children due to less pain, noise, and vibration. On the other hand, in this treatment method, the remaining healthy structures can be preserved while removing the diseased tissues. Therefore, lasers can be incredibly efficient in pediatric dentistry and provides many benefits for the patient and the dentist. This method can treat hard and soft tissues and traumatic injuries. Of course, it is necessary to mention that choosing the correct wavelength for each treatment and applying suitable parameters such as energy level, proper radiation time, *etc.*, play an essential role in the success of treatment.

## CONSENT FOR PUBLICATION

Not applicable.

## CONFLICT OF INTEREST

The authors declare no conflict of interest, financial or otherwise.

## ACKNOWLEDGEMENT

Declared none.

## REFERENCES

[1]    Al-Batayneh OB, Seow WK, Walsh LJ. Assessment of Er:YAG laser for cavity preparation in primary and permanent teeth: a scanning electron microscopy and thermographic study. Pediatr Dent 2014; 36(3): 90-4.
[PMID: 24960377]

[2]    Wang J, Yang K, Zhang B, *et al.* Effects of Er:YAG laser pre-treatment on dentin structure and bonding strength of primary teeth: an *in vitro* study. BMC Oral Health 2020; 20(1): 316.
[http://dx.doi.org/10.1186/s12903-020-01315-z] [PMID: 33172456]

[3]    Schwimmer Y, Beyth N, Ram D, Mijiritsky E, Davidovich E. Laser Tooth Preparation for Pit and Fissure Sealing. Int J Environ Res Public Health 2020; 17(21): 7813.
[http://dx.doi.org/10.3390/ijerph17217813] [PMID: 33114507]

[4]    Bortolotto T, Mast P, Krejci I. Laser-prepared and bonding-filled fissure sealing: SEM and OCT analysis of marginal and internal adaptation. Dent Mater J 2017; 36(5): 622-9.

[5]    Davidovich E, Dagon S, Tamari I, Etinger M, Mijiritsky E. An Innovative Treatment Approach Using Digital Workflow and CAD-CAM Part 2: The Restoration of Molar Incisor Hypomineralization in

Children. Int J Environ Res Public Health 2020; 17(5): 1499.
[http://dx.doi.org/10.3390/ijerph17051499] [PMID: 32110963]

[6]    Olivi G. Caprioglio, C. Olivi, M. Genovese, M. Paediatric laser dentistry. Part 2: Hard tissue laser applications. Eur J Paediatr Dent 2017; 18(2):163-6.

[7]    Mallishery S. Dedhia, S. Sawant, K. An Era of Lasers- Application of Erbium Lasers in Pediatric Dentistry. IOSR J Dent Med Sci 2019; 18(10): 1-7.

[8]    Nahas P, Nammour S, Gerges E, Zeinoun T. Comparison between Shear Bond Strength of Er:YAG and Er,Cr:YSGG Lasers-Assisted Dentinal Adhesion of Self-Adhering Resin Composite: An Ex *vivo* Study. Dent J 2020; 8(3): 66.
[http://dx.doi.org/10.3390/dj8030066]

[9]    Olivi G, Caprioglio C, Olivi M, Genovese MD. Paediatric laser dentistry. Part 4: Soft tissue laser applications. Eur J Paediatr Dent 2017; 18(4): 332-4.
[PMID: 29380621]

[10]   Ak A. Oner Ozdas, D. Zorlu, S. Karataban PK. Dental Traumatology in Pediatric Dentistry. In: Gözler S (Ed.) Trauma in Dentistry. IntechOpen; 2019.
[http://dx.doi.org/10.5772/intechopen.84150]

[11]   Soliman MM, Alzahrani F, Arora P.. Lasers Use in Different Dental Pediatric Aspects. EC Dental Science 2018; 17(3): 150-9.

[12]   Calazans T, de Campos P, Melo A, *et al.* Protocol for Low-level laser therapy in traumatic ulcer after troncular anesthesia: Case report in pediatric dentistry. J Clin Exp Dent 2020; 12(2): e201-3.
[http://dx.doi.org/10.4317/jced.56176] [PMID: 32071703]

[13]   Görür I, Orhan K, Can-Karabulut DC, Orhan AI, Öztürk A. Low-level laser therapy effects in traumatized permanent teeth with extrusive luxation in an orthodontic patient. Angle Orthod 2010; 80(5): 968-74.
[http://dx.doi.org/10.2319/110109-612.1] [PMID: 20578871]

[14]   Marañón-Vásquez GA, Lagravère MO, Borsatto MC, *et al.* Effect of photobiomodulation on the stability and displacement of orthodontic mini-implants submitted to immediate and delayed loading: a clinical study. Lasers Med Sci 2019; 34(8): 1705-15.
[http://dx.doi.org/10.1007/s10103-019-02818-0] [PMID: 31154599]

# CHAPTER 13

# Genetic Aspect of Dental Diseases

**Abi M. Thomas**[1,*], **Niraja Gupta**[2], **Madulika Kabra**[2] and **Prachi Goyal**[3]

[1] *Christian Dental College Ludhiana, Ludhiana, Punjab 141008, India*

[2] *Division of Medical Genetics, Department of Pediatrics, AIIMS, New Delhi, India*

[3] *M.M. College of Dental Sciences & Research, MMU, Mullana, Haryana, India*

**Abstract:** Genetics is the study of genes at all levels from molecules to populations. Common dental diseases such as dental caries, periodontal disease and malocclusion are influenced by environmental factors. However, even in these diseases, the genetic aspects that influence the degree of susceptibility should not be overlooked. Dental practitioners would find value in understanding the genetic contribution to caries risk as they would be able to explain to patients that some forms of decay are more strongly associated with inherited risk and these patients could be monitored more closely and provided with more aggressive preventive programs.

**Keywords:** Chromosome, Dental diseases, Genetic counselling, Genetics, Syndromes.

## INTRODUCTION

Genetics is the study of genes at all levels from molecules to population. The term gene is referred to as a basic unit of heredity lying in chromosomes. Each gene is responsible for a specific trait or character of an individual. There are hundreds and thousands of genes responsible for specific functions in an individual.

The transmission of characters through generations is determined by genes located on the chromosomes. The genotype of an individual indicates the characters transmitted through the genes. The physical expression of these characters is designated as phenotype. Autosomal characters are borne by autosomes (22 pairs of chromosomes) and sex-linked chromosomes. Genes are located at chromosome loci as alleles. Two different alleles at a particular locus of a chromosome indicate heterozygosity, whereas identical alleles at a locus indicate homozygosity. Males with the expression of X-linked characters

---

* **Corresponding author Abi M. Thomas:** Christian Dental College Ludhiana, Ludhiana, Punjab 141008, India;
E-mail: abithomas@gmail.com

**Satyawan Damle, Ritesh Kalaskar & Dhanashree Sakhare (Eds.)**

(unpaired alleles) are termed hemizygous. A dominant character is defined as one whose phenotypic expression is possible in the heterozygous state. A recessive character manifests only in the homozygous state. A disorder caused by a gene on any of the 22 pairs of autosomes has autosomal inheritance, while a disorder caused by any gene on one of the sex chromosomes shows sex-linked inheritance. Drawing and interpreting H a pedigree is an integral part of the diagnosis of single-gene disorders.

Four major patterns of genetic transmission are possible:

1. Autosomal dominant (AD)

2. Autosomal recessive (AR)

3. X-linked dominant (X-L-D)

4. X-linked recessive (X-L-R)

## Genetics and Dentistry

The successful completion of the Human Genome Project in 2000 led to the development of new tools for human genetic studies. These tools have been widely applied to many human traits of complex etiology. The three most common problems in dentistry are dental caries, periodontal problems, and malocclusion, all of which have a multifactorial etiology. But the role of hereditary factors in these diseases has been better understood with the help of these tools. Also, understanding the role of human traits in orofacial clefts, growth and development disorders and syndromes is important in the management of such disorders. In the past, lack of evidence of any clear-cut single gene defects has been met with many difficulties in managing many of these disorders. Despite this, twin studies, molecular genetic technology, gene mapping techniques, *etc*. are now providing approaches for locating various genes associated with various diseases and disorders. Pursuing oral health in childhood, the clinician can observe various abnormalities and intervene early to remedy the situation and in more complex cases, refer patients to specialists in medical genetics and or genetic counsellors. For this purpose, the clinician must have a thorough knowledge of basic genetics [1].

## Chromosomal Aberrations – Classification

The basic structure of a chromosome includes a short arm "p," a long arm "q" and the centromere separating the two arms.

Numerical abnormalities of chromosomes include either a complete loss or gain of a chromosome so that the total number is less or more than 46. Such a defect is called aneuploidy. Aneuploidy involving autosomes is incompatible with life and most fetuses carrying them abort spontaneously. Babies alive have a variable degree of malformations and neurodevelopmental abnormalities. These are sporadic events with low recurrence risk. If a complete set of chromosomes is duplicated, then it is known as polyploidy. Being euploid (2n) is the normal state. Structural rearrangements are balanced, *i.e.*, there is no loss of genetic material. Sometimes, during meiotic rearrangements, unbalanced gametes may be produced. Embryos from such gametes are either aborted or have postnatal anomalies and malformations.

## Structural Abnormalities

Such structural abnormalities (Fig. **1**) include:

- **Inversions** may occur around the centromere (pericentric) or involve one arm only (paracentric).
- **Translocation** between 2 non-homologous chromosomes is either reciprocal involving a mutual exchange or Robertsonian which is a special translocation involving chromosomes 13, 14, 15, 21 and 22.
- **Deletion:** Breaking away from the loss of a portion of a chromosome e.g., Cri-du-chat syndrome.
- **Duplication:** An over-representation of the specific chromosomal region.
- **Isochromosome** is formed when there is a loss of one arm with duplication of the other arm of the chromosome.
- **Mosaicism** is the occurrence of two distinct cell lines arising from a single zygote due to early mitotic errors of replication.

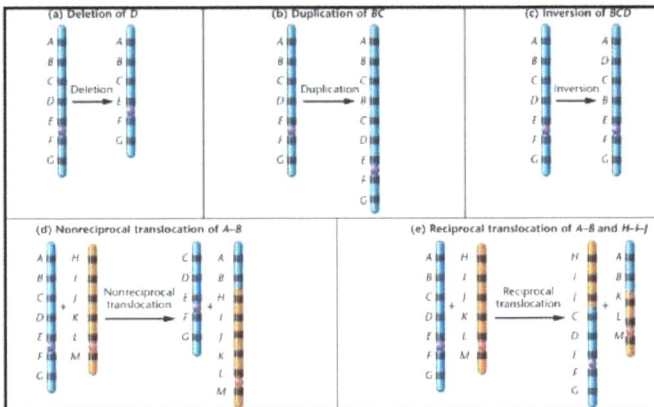

**Fig. (1).** Structural abnormalities in the chromosomes.

## Down 'S Syndrome (Fig 2)

Down's syndrome or trisomy 21, is a chromosomal condition caused by the presence of all or part of an extra 21st chromosome. It is named after John Langdon Down, the British physician who described the syndrome in 1866. The effects and extent of the extra copy vary greatly among people, depending on genetic history, and pure chance. The incidence of Down syndrome is estimated at 1 per 733 births, although it is statistically more common with older parents (both mothers and fathers) due to increased mutagenic exposures to some older parents' reproductive cells. Other factors may also play a role. Often Down syndrome is associated with some impairment of cognitive ability and physical growth, and a particular set of facial characteristics. The average IQ of children with Down syndrome (Fig **2**) (is around 50, compared to normal children with an IQ of 100.

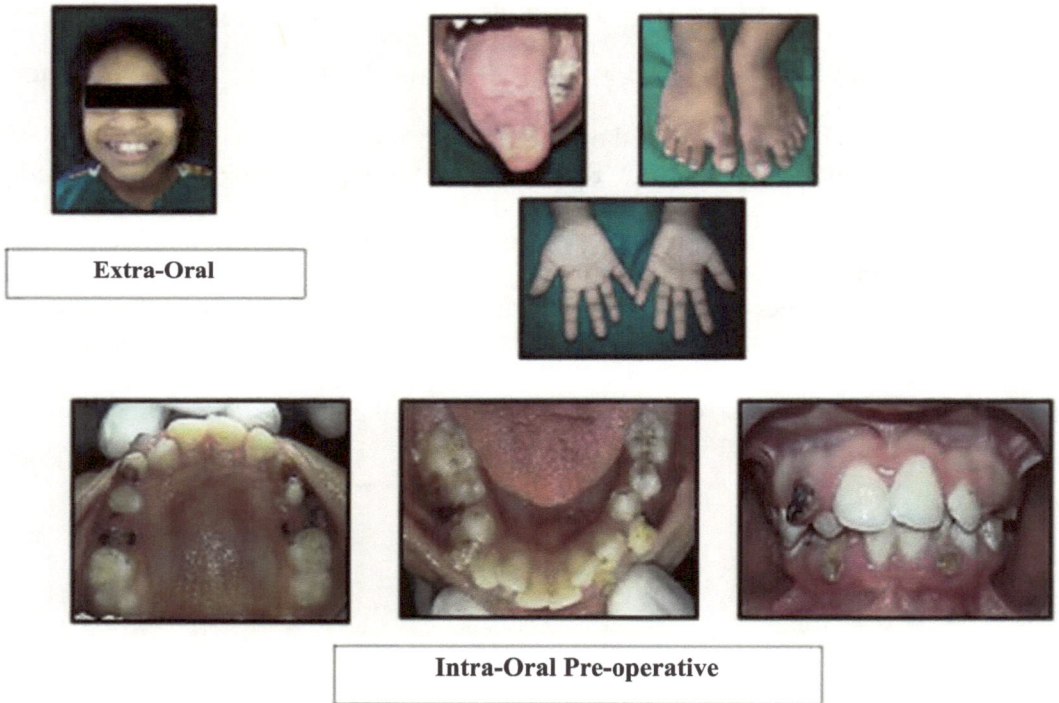

**Extra-Oral**

**Intra-Oral Pre-operative**

**Fig. (2).** Clinical photographs of a case of Down's syndrome.

Individuals with Down syndrome may have microgenia (an abnormally small chin), an unusually round face, macroglossia (protruding or oversized tongue), an almond shape to the eyes caused by an epicanthic fold of the eyelid, up slanting palpebral fissures (the separation between the upper and lower eyelids), shorter limbs, a single transverse palmar crease (a single instead of a double crease across one or both palms), poor muscle tone, and a larger than normal space between the big and second toes. Health concerns for individuals with Down syndrome include a higher risk for congenital heart defects, gastroesophageal reflux disease, recurrent ear infections that may lead to hearing loss, obstructive sleep apnea, and thyroid dysfunctions.

## Molecular Mechanism of Dentinogenesis

Studies using mouse embryos and birds as experimental animals revealed a strict genetic control of odontogenesis, which determines the position, number, size, and shape of the teeth. The cytodifferentiation of dental epithelium occurs during the bell stage; cells near the mesenchyme are differentiated into ameloblasts, which produce enamel. The adjacent mesenchymal cell differentiates into odontoblasts and is involved in dentin formation. Mesenchyme surrounding the tooth bud will develop forming the supporting structure of the tooth, for example, the periodontal ligament that anchors the tooth to the alveolar bone.

Morphogenesis and differentiation of teeth are the results of complex interactions at the molecular level between the ectoderm and the mesenchyme. A crucial role was attributed to transcription factors that have a homeodomain, which consists of 60 amino acids with a helix–turn–helix DNA binding motif and is encoded by a homeobox sequence: short chains of 180 bp, located in the vicinity of the gene's 3' end. The homeodomain transcription factors are involved in the regulation of homeobox gene expression sites, thus activating gene expression in multicellular organisms during embryonic development.

Important factors in tooth morphogenesis are the family of fibroblast growth factors (FGE) and transforming growth factors (TGF, including BMP–4–bone morphogenetic protein 4), the family of Wnt (wingless) and morphogenesis molecule shh (sonic hedgehog).

Different genes involved in the formation of teeth belong to signaling pathways with functions in regulating the morphogenesis of other organs. Mutations in these genes have pleiotropic effects in addition to causing non-syndromic dental abnormalities and anomalies associated with different genetic syndromes.

## Dental Agenesis

Congenital lack of one or more teeth is the most frequent anomaly in humans. In hypodontia 1-6 teeth (excluding molar 3) are missing; in oligodontia – more than 6 teeth are missing (excluding molar 3). Anodontia is the complete absence of teeth which is rare, reported in a family in China and the mode of inheritance is believed to be autosomal recessive.

The frequency of cases of non-syndromic hypodontia/oligodontia is 80% when missing a tooth, less than 10% when missing several teeth and less than 1% when missing many teeth. Four genes have been identified so far to be associated with non-syndromic hypodontia/oligodontia. The identified genes are:

a. MSX1 – hypodontia NS
b. PAX9 – oligodontia NS
c. AX1N2 – oligodontia associated with colorectal cancer
d. EDA1 - oligodontia NS

Cases of hypodontia/oligodontia may or may not be associated with syndromes like hypohidrotic ectodermal dysplasia, Ankyloblepharon-ectodermal defects-cleft lip/palate (AEC) syndrome.

## Genetics And Dental Caries

Dental caries is a complex, chronic, multifactorial disease and one of the most prevalent diseases. Caries appears to concentrate on specific groups of individuals. The phenomenon is termed polarization, and its cause remains obscure, representing one of the epidemiological disease aspects in which a portion of the population is in most need of treatment. The Vipeholm study provided evidence of an individual's resistance to caries despite being on a highly cariogenic diet. This suggests that susceptibility or resistance to caries could be a result of one or more genotypic, phenotypic, and environmental influences [2]. Heredity has been linked with dental caries incidence in the scientific literature for many years.

The pathogenesis of the caries process is better understood today, but it is quite more complex than was believed in the early days of dental research. The salivary gland's secretion and density and structural integrity of enamel are directly under genetic control [3].

Some of the genes found to be associated with caries are as follows [4]-

1. Ameloblastin (AMBN) – mainly responsible for Enamel matrix formation, found to be associated with caries, dental fluorosis.

2. Amelogenin (AMELX) - mainly responsible for tooth mineralization, is associated with caries.

3. Aquaporin 5(AQPS) - regulates saliva production and is associated with caries.

4. Carbonic Anhydrase VI (CA6) - regulates the pH of saliva and is associated with caries [5].

5. Enamelin (ENAM) - responsible for enamel matrix formation, is associated with molar incisor hypomineralization and dental caries [6].

6. Estrogen-related receptor (ESRRB) - plays a role in enamel hardness, found to be associated with caries.

7. Matrix metalloproteinase 16 (MMP16) - responsible for the degradation of extracellular protein is associated with caries [7].

8. Tuftelin 1(TUFT1) - responsible for enamel matrix formation, is associated with caries.

**9.** Tuftelin –interacting protein 11 (TFIP11) - responsible for enamel matrix formation- has been found to have a relation to causing dental caries.

## Genetics and Periodontal Diseases

The hereditary basis for susceptibility to periodontal diseases is less understood as compared to dental caries. This has been due to the relative complexity of the disease, continually emerging new knowledge about its pathogenesis, and lack of clarity in diagnosis and classifying these diseases [8].

Evidence for a genetic contribution to individual differences in risk of periodontal disease is clearest for early-onset periodontitis [9]. Some of the pioneering initial studies of the mode of inheritance of susceptibility to early-onset periodontitis concluded that the increased prevalence in women, as well as the lack of father-t--son transmission in families, indicated that susceptibility is inherited as an X-linked dominant trait.

In one of the largest studies (100 families), Marazitta and colleagues (1994) found the strongest evidence for an autosomal-dominant susceptibility gene, with 70% penetrance. Kozak et al. have reviewed the role of selected cytokines including interleukins (IL-1, IL-2, IL-6, IL-8, IL-10, IL-13, IL-16, IL-17, IL-18, IL-23, IL-35), matrix metalloproteinases (MMPs) and tumour necrosis factor-α (TNF-α) and their gene polymorphisms in the pathogenesis of the periodontal disease.

The following are the genes found to be associated with periodontal diseases-

1. Interleukin -1 – plays a role in the pro-inflammatory response, found to be associated with Periodontitis.

2. Interleukin -6 – responsible for pro-inflammatory response and bone resorption, found to be associated with periodontitis, and apical periodontitis.

3. Interleukin 8- responsible for immune response in the body and found to be associated with apical and chronic periodontitis [10].

4. Interleukin -37- responsible for immune response in the body, found to be associated with severe periodontitis, and tooth loss.

5. Matrix metalloproteinase 2 – responsible for degradation of extracellular matrix during development, and tissue repair in the body, found to be associated with periodontitis.

6. Matrix metalloproteinase 3- found to be associated with chronic periodontitis.

7. Meta-analysis demonstrated that polymorphisms in the IL-1A, IL-1B, IL-6, IL-10, MMP-3 (chronic form), and MMP-9 (chronic form) polymorphisms were significantly associated with the risk of developing periodontitis, whereas other polymorphisms in the IL-4, IL-8, IL-18, Fc$\gamma$, COX-2, MMP-2, MMP-3 (aggressive), MMP-8, and MMP-9 (aggressive) polymorphisms had no significant association with risk of developing periodontitis.

**Papillon Lefevre Syndrome (Fig. 3)**

Papillon Lefevre syndrome is an autosomal recessive trait characterized by palmoplantar hyperkeratosis and early-onset periodontitis affecting both primary and permanent dentitions. This syndrome was first described by Papillon MM and Lefevre P in two siblings in 1924. Most of the cases (nearly 50%) are the result of consanguineous marriages. Cathepsin C gene mutations are the underlying causes of this syndrome. There is rapid periodontal destruction by age of 4 to 5 years followed by complete exfoliation. This pathological breakdown is identically followed in the permanent dentition. The severity of alveolar bone loss results in atrophic jaws. Whether these conditions are monogenic or multifactorial, the cells, biochemical processes and host defense processes are affected to varying degrees in all of them, leading to increased susceptibility to developing periodontal disease. Significantly, the genes responsible for these conditions do not appear to cluster on one chromosome and this further highlights the multifactorial and diverse nature of periodontal diseases. (Fig 3I, II.III).

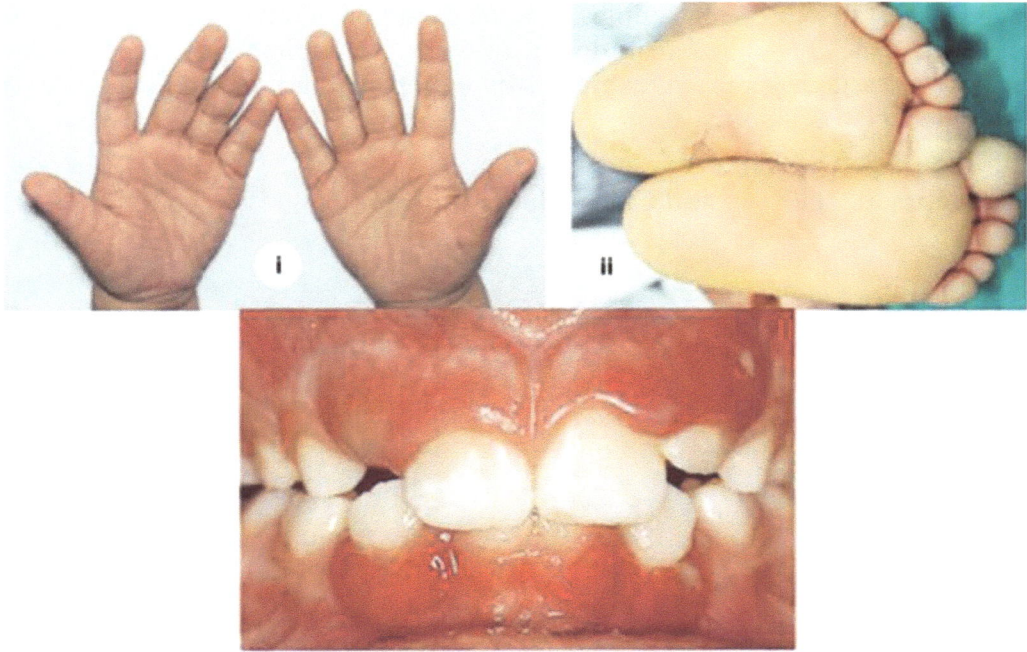

**Fig. (3).** Keratosis affecting i. the palms of the hand ii. The soles of the feet iii. Severe gingival inflammation in a child with Papillon lefevre syndrome.

**Clinical implications:** The major clinical implications of studying the role of the host genome in various periodontal diseases lie in a better understanding of the variability in disease manifestation as well as having some diagnostic value. By recognizing that some forms of periodontal disease may have a strong genetic component, it has become necessary to identify susceptible individuals, and screen their immediate relatives for signs of developing periodontal problems. In addition, by recognizing that some periodontal diseases may be a part of syndromic conditions, early recognition of these signs can help in the identification of such syndromes.

Genetic and environmental factors play an important role in the etiology of malocclusion. The bulk of the evidence for genetic factors of various types of malocclusion arises from family and twin studies.

Studies about Class II division 1malocclusion, showed a higher correlation between the patients and their immediate family and data from random pairings of unrelated siblings, thus supporting the concept of polygenic inheritance for class II division 1 malocclusion. Also, there is strong support for Class II division 2 malocclusion, for familial occurrence based on several published reports including twin and triplet studies. Familial studies of mandibular prognathism are suggestive of heredity in the etiology of this condition. Various models have been suggested, such as autosomal dominant with incomplete penetrance simple recessive, variable both in expressivity and penetrance with differences in different racial populations.

- **Genetics of Cleft Lip and Cleft Palate (Fig. 4)**

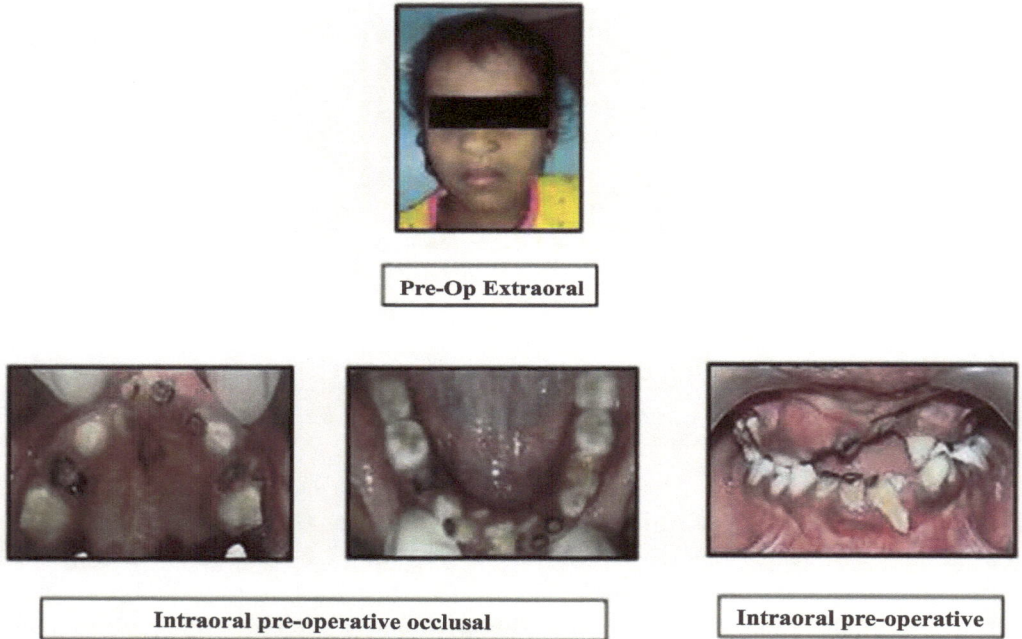

Pre-Op Extraoral

Intraoral pre-operative occlusal

Intraoral pre-operative

**Fig. (4).** Clinical photographs of a cleft lip and palate patient.

Orofacial clefts can have variable severity and manifest as cleft lip alone (CL), cleft palate alone (CP), and a combination of the two (CLP). These could be either syndromic or nonsyndromic (70% CLP and CL; 50%CP only), the latter being commoner than syndromic forms. The genetic causes of nonsyndromic OFC are being explored extensively. Various studies have shown genetic basis in cleft lip and palate where they found siblings of patients with cleft lip (with or without cleft palate) have an increased frequency of cleft lip (with or without cleft palate) and not isolated cleft palate and siblings of patients with isolated cleft palate have an increased frequency of isolated cleft palate and no cleft lip. The concordance rate of cleft or palate is expected to be higher in monozygotic twins than in dizygotic pairs. A large multi-ethnic study on 12000 patients showed a variable association for 9 genes *PAX7, IRF6, FAM49A, DCAF4L2*, 8q24.21, *NTN1,*

*WNT3-WNT9B, TANC2*, and *RHPN2* in US and Europe, Asians, mixed Native American/Caucasians, and Africans.

• **Genetics and Oral Cancer**

It is due to mutations in protoncogene (polymorphism in GST gene) or CYP (Cytochrome P450) or mutations in tumour suppressor gene (p16, 9p 21, APC5q 21-22 and p53). The common cancer predisposition syndromes are Werner's syndrome, Bloom syndrome, Fanconi's anaemia and Ataxia telangiectasia.

There is a wide spectrum of syndromes that include dental, oral, and craniofacial abnormalities (https://www.omim.org/search/advanced/geneMap). Generally, the majority of patients with craniofacial syndromes have associated dental abnormalities. In our experience, the most common disorders include cleft lip/palate or cleft lip only, Pierre Robin sequence, Ectodermal dysplasia, hemifacial microsomia, and 22q deletion syndrome that have characteristic diagnostic features. Dental, oral, and craniofacial features of some of these syndromes are mentioned as follows-

• **Syndromes Involving Oro-Facial Clefts**

*22q11.2 Deletion Syndrome*

It is one of the most frequent microdeletion syndromes with an incidence of 2 to 5 in 10000 live births.

*Craniofacial Features*

Cleft palate, palatal anomalies and hypertelorism are seen in more than 75% of patients. Other features include short philtrum, thick lips, long asymmetric face, microcephaly, malar flattening, bulbous nose, thin alae nasi, micrognathia and retrognathia.

*Oral and Dental Features*

These patients show a high prevalence of missing permanent teeth especially mandibular incisors, maxillary second premolars and maxillary lateral incisors. The development and eruption of permanent teeth are often delayed with enamel opacities. Other features are hypo-mineralization of permanent dentition and impaired salivary flow.

### Ectrodactyly, Ectodermal Dysplasia and Clefting (EEC) Syndrome

It is an autosomal dominant disorder characterized by a triad of ectrodactyly (claw-like hands & feet), ectodermal dysplasia and orofacial clefts. Ectrodactyly has been reported in 68 – 84% and ectodermal dysplasia in 50 – 77% cases.

### *Craniofacial Features*

Orofacial cleft has been described in 40 – 70% of patients. 1-5% of patients have zygomatic, mid-facial, maxillary, and mandibular hypoplasia; however, these features are not typical of EEC syndrome.

### *Oral and Dental Features*

Primary and permanent dentitions are affected in patients with EEC. The common dental features are hypodontia, enamel hypoplasia, and poorly developed and peg-shaped teeth. The dental age and tooth eruption are late.

### *Kabuki Syndrome (Ks)(Fig. 5)*

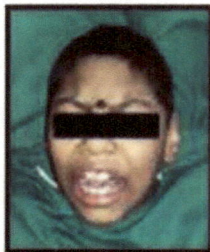

**Extra-Oral Photograph**

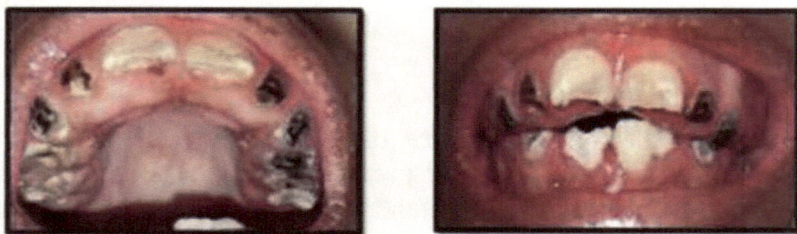

**Intra-Oral Pre-operative Photographs**

**Fig. (5).** Microcephaly in a patient with Kabuki syndrome.

Two types of Kabuki syndrome have been identified: Kabuki 1 with autosomal dominant inheritance and Kabuki 2 with X-linked dominant inheritance.

KS patients have developmental delay, early puberty, scoliosis, clinodactyly of the fifth fingers or hypermobility and dislocation of hip and knee joints, seizures, and muscle hypotonia.

### *Craniofacial Features*

It includes microcephaly (Fig. **5**), arched eyebrows, long eyelashes, long palpebral fissures with everted lower eyelids and large protruding ear lobes. Cleft palate and high arched palate are common findings in KS syndrome.

### *Oral and Dental Features*

The common manifestations include hypodontia with agenesis of incisors and or premolars. Other features are microdontia, peg-shaped incisors supernumerary and widely spaced teeth, and retention of primary and permanent teeth. Malocclusions such as open bites and the unilateral posterior crossbite are commonly observed in KS syndrome.

### *Van Der Woude Syndrome (Vws) (Fig 6)*

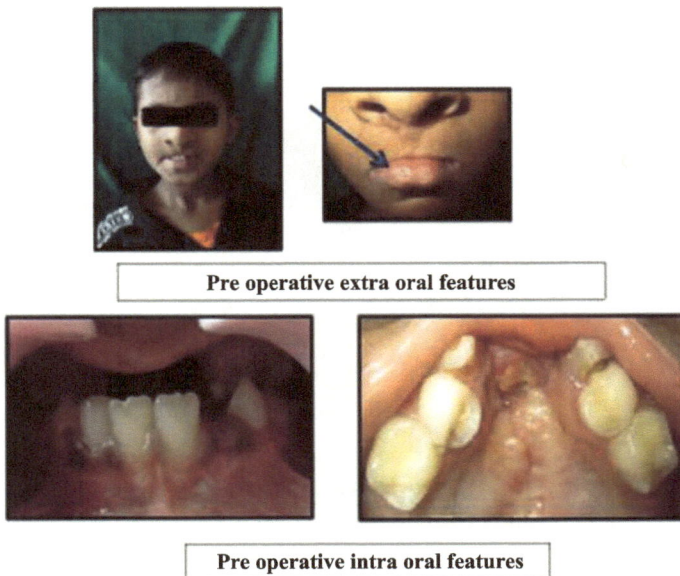

Pre operative extra oral features

Pre operative intra oral features

**Fig. (6).** Clinical photographs of a patient with Van Der Woude syndrome.

It is the most frequent form of syndromic clefting and accounts for 2% of all cleft lip and palate patients. It is characterized by paramedian lip pits and sinuses and orofacial clefting.

### *Craniofacial Features*

Clefts are reported in 21 – 100% of VWS patients.Patients usually show underdeveloped maxillary sagittal length and maxillary height.

### *Oral and Dental Features*

Paramedian lower lip pits have been reported in 88% of patients with VWS. Hypodontia and dental hypoplasia are considered cardinal features in VWS patients.

Tooth agenesis is reported in up to 80% of cases. The most affected teeth are the maxillary second premolars, followed by the maxillary lateral incisors.

### *Pierre Robin Syndrome (PRS) (Fig. 7)*

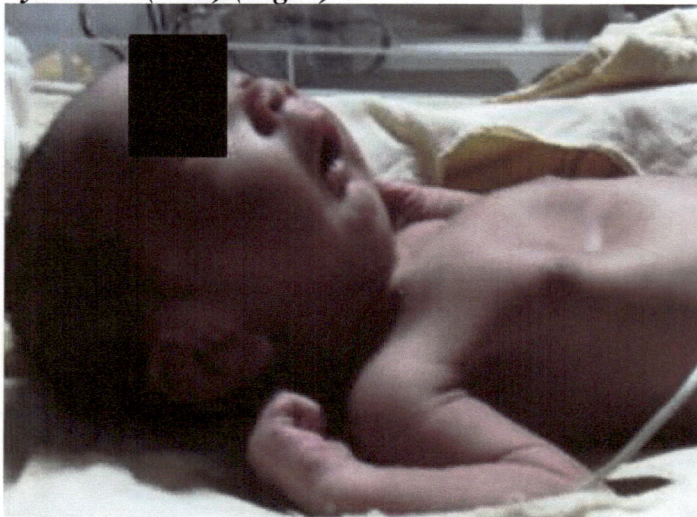

**Fig. (7).** Child with Pierre Robin Syndrome.

It is first described by Pierre Robin a French surgeon, but it is now called Pierre Robin Sequence. The exact etiology is unknown. A growth defect of the embryonic mandible due to mutation in the SOX 9 gene could be the primary cause.

## *Craniofacial Features*

The cleft palate is a common finding in PRS in 75 – 100% of patients. PRS patients have a variable mandibular morphology; the mandibular length is significantly smaller and the ratio between ramous height and mandibular body is higher as also is the gonial angle.

## *Oral and dental features*

Glossoptosis (abnormal dorsal position of the tongue) result in respiratory obstruction, vagal syncope and feeding problems. The prevalence of tooth agenesis in the permanent dentition is reported to be 30 – 50%. The most affected teeth are mandibular $2^{nd}$ premolars.

## Disorders Related to Dental Abnormalities

### *Hypodontia*

### *Hypohidrotic Ectodermal Dysplasia Fig. (8) -*

It is associated with reduced sweating, sparse hair and hypodontia or congenital absence of teeth. It is inherited in an autosomal dominant/ autosomal recessive or X-linked recessive manner. *The* ectodysplasin (EDA), *EDAR* gene, encoding the EDA receptor, or in the *EDARADD* gene encoding the domain associated with *EDAR, WNT10A, TRAF6* are the causative genes.

## *Craniofacial Feature*

Depressed nasal bridge, mid-face hypoplasia, periorbital and perioral hyperpigmentation (Fig. **8a**).

## *Oral and Dental Features*

Teeth are peg-shaped (Fig. **8b**), less in number with around nine permanent teeth and smaller than usual (Fig. **8C**).

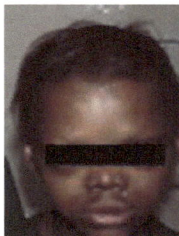

(a).

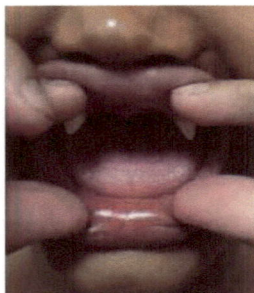

(b).

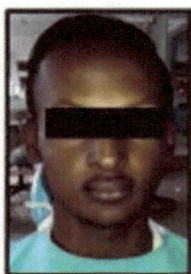

| Extra oral photograph | OPG |

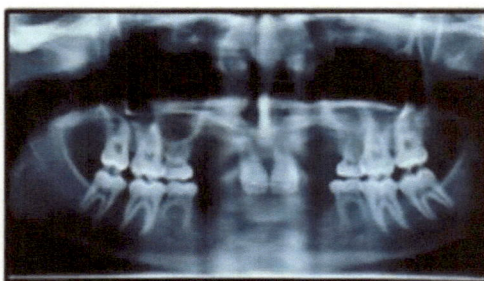

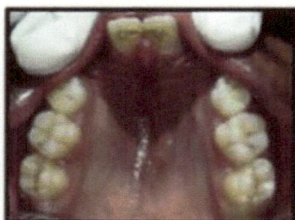

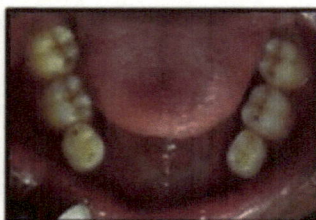

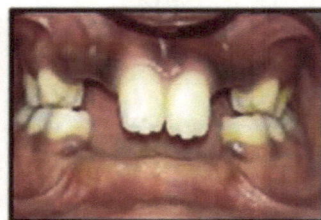

| Intraoral pre-operative Occlusal | Intraoral pre-operative |

**Fig. (8a-c).** Clinical photographs of a patient with Hypohidrotic Ectodermal Dysplasia.

## Supernumerary Teeth

Cleidocranial dysplasia is an autosomal dominant skeletal dysplasia characterized by absent to hypoplastic clavicles (Fig. **9a**), dental abnormalities and delayed closure of sutures. It is caused by heterozygous pathogenic variants in RUNX2 causing halo insufficiency of the protein.

**Craniofacial features** include large anterior fontanelle with frontal and parietal bossing and narrow sloping shoulders.

**Oral and dental features** include the presence of supernumerary teeth and dental **crowding** (Fig. **9b**).

### • Syndromes involving Gingivo-Dental Tissues

#### *Chediak-Higashi Syndrome*

This is an autosomal recessive condition which occurs due to pathogenic variations in the LYST gene that encodes for a lysosomal trafficking regulator protein. The phagocytic function of immune cells is drastically affected in these patients, making them significantly prone to infections.

#### *Oral and Dental Features*

As a result, severe forms of periodontitis and early exfoliation of both deciduous and permanent teeth are common findings in these patients.

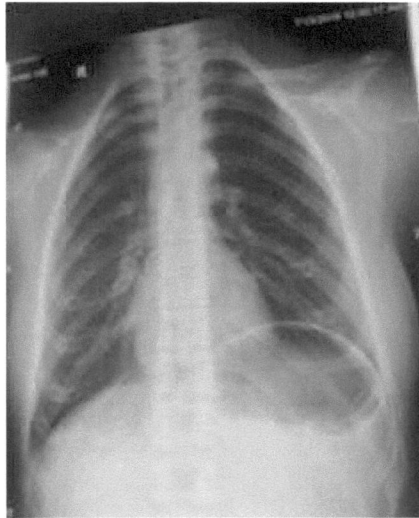

**Fig. (9a).** Hypoplastic clavicles.

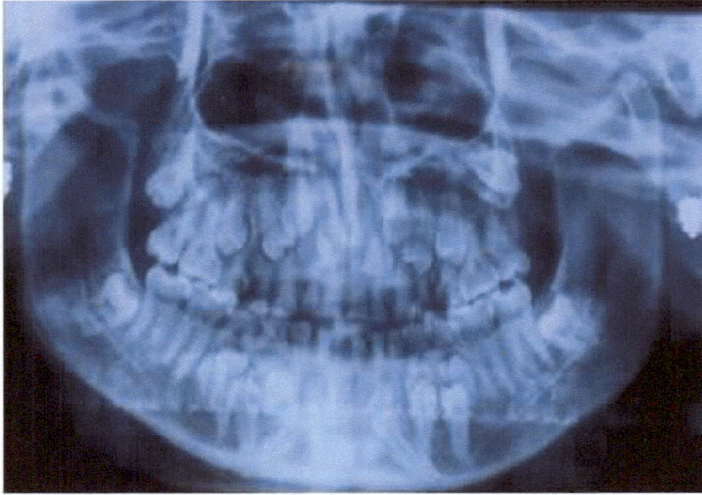

**Fig. (9b).** Supernumerary teeth and dental crowding.

## Ehlers–Danlos Syndromes

Ehlers–Danlos syndromes (EDSs) are connective tissue disorders characterized by joint laxity and skin hyperextensibility, scarring, and bruising. Periodontal EDS (EDSPD; previously EDS VIII) is a subtype with autosomal dominant inheritance with severe periodontal inflammation. Genes C1r and C1s encode serine proteases that are major constituents of human complement subcomponent C1. Complement is part of the innate immune system and is involved in inflammation. Serious complications including arterial or gastrointestinal ruptures have also been reported [11].

### Oral and Dental Features

Common dental abnormalities observed in vascular EDS were pulp shape modifications (52.2%), exceeding root length (34.8%), and molar root fusion (47.8%). Dentinogenesis imperfecta is a consistent finding in osteogenesis imperfecta/EDS overlap syndrome.

## Neurofibromatosis Type I (Nfi)

It is a tumour predisposing syndrome which is clinically heterogeneous. It is caused by heterozygous mutations in the neurofibromin gene (NF1) on chromosome 17q11. The incidence is 1 in 2000 – 3000 live births. Neurofibromas are benign tumors which may occur along nerves and in the proximity of the spinal cord. The hallmark features of NF1 are café-au–lait spots, iris lisch nodules, multiple neurofibromas and facial dysmorphologies.

## Cranio-facial Features

Patients affected with NF1 commonly show macrocephaly, short mandible, maxilla, and low set face. In approximately 20% of patients, enlargement of the mandibular canal has been described.

## Oral and Dental Features

Intra orally patients with NF1 usually show unilateral swelling of the gingiva. This may manifest with diffuse enlargement of the attached and in some cases – the interproximal gingiva. These are caused by plexiform neurofibromas consisting of hypertrophic nerves. In rare cases, the melanin pigmentation of gingiva is seen.

Dental phenotype often comprises impacted, supernumerary, missing or displaced teeth and in some cases periapical cementum dysplasia is apparent.

### • Syndromes Involving Branchial Arches:

The branchial arch syndrome affects the first and second branchial arch derivatives and the frequent syndromes are Hemi facial Microsomia (HFM), Treacher–Collins (TCS) – 3 types and Mobius syndrome (MBS).

## Hemifacial Microsomia (HFM)

It is the most frequent craniofacial condition after cleft lip palate and affects 1 in 4000 – 5600 live births. Although in a small number of cases it is inherited in an autosomal dominant way, most cases are sporadic. The etiology is complex as there are several mechanisms involved in the normal development of the first and second pharyngeal arches and the exact genetic etiology is not known. This can be a feature of many syndromes.

## Cranio-Facial Features

Hypoplasia of the zygomatic, mandibular, and maxillary bones and facial muscle hypoplasia. Colobomas of the upper eyelids are common. Patients with HFM tend to have large and steep gonial angles, a retrognathic mandible and a mildly convex face. Despite their shorter mandibles, the mandibular growth rate is normal.

## Oral and Dental Features

In deciduous and permanent dentition the mesiodistal dimensions of all molars are smaller and are most pronounced in the mandibular permanent first molar on the affected side. The canines and the incisors have normal size both in the deciduous and in the permanent dentition, although deviating development of the mandibular canines has also been reported. The prevalence of tooth agenesis is seen in approximately 25% of patients and the mandibular second premolar and second molars are the ones most affected. Tooth development is delayed in patients with HFM with an absent mandibular ramus and glenoid fossa in the most severe cases.

### *Treacher Collins Syndrome (TCS)*

It is an autosomal dominant condition with 90% penetrance and variable expressivity, affecting 1:50000 live births. There are three types - TCS1 and TCS2 show AD inheritance while TCS3 is an AR condition. TCS1 is caused by mutations in the Treacle Ribosome Biogenesis factor 1 (TCOF1) gene which encodes a nucleolar phosphoprotein involved in g RNA transcription. TCS2 and TCS3 are caused by mutations in the RNA polymerase 1 subunit D (POLRID) gene at 13 q 12.2 and RNA polymerase 1 subunit C (POLRIC) gene at 6 p 21.1, respectively.

### *Cranio-Facial Features*

The common features of TCS are downward slanting palpebral fissures, malar hypoplasia, atresia of the external ear canal, microtia, and coloboma of the lower eyelid and facial asymmetry. The rare features include cleft palate and choanal stenosis or atresia. A large proportion of children with TCS are reported to have a narrow-arched palate, hypoplasia of the maxilla and a retrognathic mandible.

### *Oral and Dental Features*

Dental anomalies are reported in 60% of children with TCS and tooth agenesis is the most frequent and it commonly affects mandibular second premolars followed by maxillary second premolars, lateral incisors, and maxillary canines. Other features that are reported include impacted maxillary supernumerary teeth, hypoplastic and mispositioned maxillary central incisors and ectopic eruption of maxillary first molars.

### *Moebius Syndrome*

It is a rare disorder with congenital facial and abducent nerve palsy with impaired ocular abduction. The exact etiology is not known, and most cases are sporadic through few AD families have been reported. Monogenic etiology is not proven but some genes have been implicated.

## *Cranio-Facial Features*

The earliest manifestation is sucking impairment and excessive drooling with respiratory difficulty. Other anomalies are Orofacial dysmorphology and jaw abnormalities, micrognathia, microstomia, narrow and high arched maxilla and cleft palate.

## *Oral and Dental Features*

The common features include hypoplastic upper lip and a frontal open bite seen in 50% of patients. Other features are agenesis of lower second premolars, enamel hypoplasia, crowding, short-fissured tongue *etc*.

## *Rothmund Thomson Syndrome*

It is an autosomal recessive inherited disorder characterized by a rash that progresses to poikiloderma, sparse hair, eyelashes and or eyebrows, skeletal and dental abnormalities, and an increased risk for cancer, especially osteosarcoma. It is caused by pathogenic variations in the *RECQL4* helicase gene, detected in 60-65% of cases.

## *Craniofacial Features*

Acute phase starts in infancy between 3-6 months, with erythema on the cheeks and face. Other features include sparse scalp hair, eyelashes and or eyebrows.

## *Oral and Dental Features*

Common findings are rudimentary or hypoplastic teeth, enamel defects, delayed tooth eruption, microdontia, congenitally missing teeth and increased incidence of caries.

## GENETIC COUNSELLING

As most craniofacial syndromes have an underlying genetic basis, it is imperative to provide adequate genetic counselling for adequate management and for preventing recurrences. It is a process of communication and education that addresses the concerns relating to the development and/or transmission of a hereditary disorder. It is provided to couples with a family of genetically inherited disorders or a history of earlier childbirth with any such condition. The steps involved in genetic counselling include the establishment of the diagnosis, assessment of the risk of recurrence, communication with the couple, discussion of the options, and long-term contact and support. Couples should be explained the mode of inheritance of the disease, the possibility of the proportion of children affected, the risk of transmission to the next generations through asymptomatic female carriers, grades of severity of the disorder in subsequent generations, and the prognosis of the disorder if an affected child has already been born. It is important to evaluate the parents for subtle abnormalities especially when an autosomal dominant mode of inheritance is non-suspected.

Prenatal diagnosis is possible for a specific genetic disorder running in the family. Prenatal ultrasound also helps us in diagnosing major craniofacial and mandibular abnormalities.

## CONCLUSION

Genetics plays a major role in the growth and development of the craniofacial region including teeth and tooth-supporting structures. Mutations in genes involved in these functions predispose an individual to diseases affecting oral health. Significant advances in human genetics that are now taking place should soon enable screening of those individuals at risk and the implementation of targeted preventive measures to protect them from various oral diseases.

## CONSENT FOR PUBLICATION

Not applicable.

## CONFLICT OF INTEREST

The authors declares no conflict of interest, financial or otherwise.

## ACKNOWLEDGEMENT

Declared none.

## REFERENCES

[1]   Azzaldeen A, Mai A, Muhamad A. Genetics and Dental Disorders – A Clinical Concept. Part; 1. IOSR Journal of Dental and Medical Sciences (IOSR-JDMS). 2017; 16(11): 35-42.

[2]   Opal S, Garg S, Jain J, Walia I. Genetic factors affecting dental caries risk. Aust Dent J 2015; 60(1): 2-11.
[http://dx.doi.org/10.1111/adj.12262] [PMID: 25721273]

[3]   Küchler EC, Pecharki GD, Castro ML, *et al.* Genes Involved in the Enamel Development Are Associated with Calcium and Phosphorus Level in Saliva. Caries Res 2017; 51(3): 225-30.
[http://dx.doi.org/10.1159/000450764] [PMID: 28395292]

[4]   Li X, Liu D, Sun Y, Yang J, Yu Y. Association of genetic variants in enamel-formation genes with dental caries: A meta- and gene-cluster analysis. Saudi J Biol Sci 2021; 28(3): 1645-53.
[http://dx.doi.org/10.1016/j.sjbs.2020.11.071] [PMID: 33732050]

[5]   Esberg A, Haworth S, Brunius C, Lif Holgerson P, Johansson I. Carbonic Anhydrase 6 Gene Variation influences Oral Microbiota Composition and Caries Risk in Swedish adolescents. Sci Rep 2019; 9(1):

452.
[http://dx.doi.org/10.1038/s41598-018-36832-z] [PMID: 30679524]

[6]     Devang Divakar D, Alanazi SAS, Assiri MYA, *et al.* Association between ENAM polymorphisms and dental caries in children. Saudi J Biol Sci 2019; 26(4): 730-5.
[http://dx.doi.org/10.1016/j.sjbs.2018.01.010] [PMID: 31048997]

[7]     Lewis DD, Shaffer JR, Feingold E, *et al.* Genetic Association of *MMP10*, *MMP14*, and *MMP16* with Dental Caries. Int J Dent 2017; 2017: 1-7.
[http://dx.doi.org/10.1155/2017/8465125] [PMID: 28348596]

[8]     da Silva MK, de Carvalho ACG, Alves EHP, da Silva FRP, Pessoa LS, Vasconcelos DFP. Genetic Factors and the Risk of Periodontitis Development: Findings from a Systematic Review Composed of 13 Studies of Meta-Analysis with 71,531 Participants. Int J Dent 2017; 2017: 1-9.
[http://dx.doi.org/10.1155/2017/1914073] [PMID: 28529526]

[9]     Salles AG, Antunes LAA, Küchler EC, Antunes LS. Association between Apical Periodontitis and Interleukin Gene Polymorphisms: A Systematic Review and Meta-analysis. J Endod 2018; 44(3): 355-62.
[http://dx.doi.org/10.1016/j.joen.2017.11.001] [PMID: 29306532]

[10]    Finoti LS, Nepomuceno R, Pigossi SC, Corbi SCT, Secolin R, Scarel-Caminaga RM. Association between interleukin-8 levels and chronic periodontal disease. A PRISMA-compliant systematic review and meta-analysis. Medicine 2017; 96(22): e6932.
[http://dx.doi.org/10.1097/MD.0000000000006932] [PMID: 28562542]

[11]    Kapferer-Seebacher I, Schnabl D, Zschocke J, Pope F. Dental Manifestations of Ehlers-Danlos Syndromes: A Systematic Review. Acta Derm Venereol 2020; 100(7): adv00092.
[http://dx.doi.org/10.2340/00015555-3428] [PMID: 32147746]

# CHAPTER 14

# Probiotics and Oral Health

## N. Venugopal Reddy[1,*], Dhanashree Sakhare[2] and Parag D. Kasar[3]

[1] *Mamata Dental College & Hospital, Khammam, Telangana 507002, India*

[2] *Lavanika Dental Academy, Melbourne, Australia*

[3] *Deep Dental Clinic, Navi Mumbai, Maharashtra 400706, India*

**Abstract:** Humans are host to oral microbiomes in a positive relationship which is a critical determinant for regulating oral symbiosis. When the balanced condition is transformed into an acidic environment, the percentage. mutans streptococci and Lactobacillus species increase. However, to be beneficial in the oral cavity, probiotics must first aggregate and attach to the oral tissue, creating a protective barrier to prevent the colonisation of the pathogenic microorganisms. The growth and activity of probiotics are enhanced by nondigestive oligosaccharides, namely, prebiotics, which cannot be digested by the host but enhance the beneficial effects of probiotics by selectively stimulating the growth and activities of the probiotics.

**Keywords:** Oral diseases, Oral Health, Probiotics.

## INTRODUCTION

Humans are a unique reservoir of a heterogeneous and vivacious group of microbes, forming the human-microbiome superorganism.

The emergence of microbiota with resistance and tolerance to existing conventional drugs and antibiotics has decreased the drug efficacies. Health professionals are aware of the rapid pace of changing health care.

Furthermore, the modern ergonomics-med nano-encapsulated multiplex supplements appear to be high cost and problematic. Henceforth, a simple, low-cost, responsive, and intrinsic approach to achieving health benefits is vital in the present era, which is imparted by probiotics and prebiotics as well as synbiotics and have been the subject of extensive research in the past few decades [1].

---
* **Corresponding author N. Venugopal Reddy:** Mamata Dental College & Hospital, Khammam, Telangana 507002, India; E-mail: drnvenugopalreddy@gmail.com

**Satyawan Damle, Ritesh Kalaskar & Dhanashree Sakhare (Eds.)**

Probiotics, live microbial food supplements that beneficially affect the host by improving its intestinal microbial balance, are quickly gaining interest as functional foods in the current self-care and complementary medicine [2].

## Terminologies

PREBIOTICS Glenn R. Gibson, in 2017 introduced the concept of prebiotics. Prebiotics are primarily fibers that are non-digestible food ingredients and beneficially affect the host's health by selectively stimulating the growth or activity of some genera of microorganisms in the colon, generally lactobacilli and Bifidobacterium [3].

WHO defines prebiotics as a non-viable food component that confers health benefits on the host associated with microbiota modulation [1].

## PROBIOTICS

Ferdinand Virgin probably used the term probiotics. He invented the term "probiotic" in 1954, in his article entitled "Anti-und Probiotics", comparing the harmful effects of antibiotics and other antibacterial agents on the intestinal microbiota with the beneficial effects ("probiotics") of some beneficial bacteria. When he studied the detrimental effects of antibiotics and other microbial substances on the gut microbial population, it was first used by Lilly and Stillwell in 1965 to describe "substances secreted by one microorganism which stimulates the growth of another" and thus was analogised with the term antibiotic [3].

Parker (2008) defined probiotics as "organisms and substances contributing to intestinal microbial balance." Retaining the word substances in his definition of probiotics resulted in a wide association that included antibiotics.

According to Salminen (1998), a probiotic is "a live microbial culture or cultured dairy product that beneficially influences the host's health and nutrition." According to Schaafsma (1998), "Oral probiotics are living microorganisms that exert health effects beyond inherent basic nutrition upon ingestion in certain numbers".

The currently used definition approved by WHO and FAO in June 2014 is "Probiotics are living microorganism which, when administered in adequate amounts, confer a health benefit for the host" [3].

## Postbiotics

In the absence of viable organisms, bacterial products may have similar effects on signalling pathways and barrier function. These bacterial products are broadly characterised as postbiotics. They can be defined as non-viable bacterial products or metabolic by-products from probiotic microorganisms with biological activity in the host. For practical reasons, probiotics and prebiotics have been described as conbiotics by specific authors and symbiotic by others.

## Synbiotics

It is the interaction between probiotics and prebiotic effects in the Gastrointestinal tract. It has a more beneficial impact on human health than alone. It recovers the intestinal microbial environment and activates the host immune function, preventing bacterial translocation. It is safe, convenient & straightforward as a food supplement.

## History of Probiotics

Probiotics are microorganisms, mainly bacteria, which benefit the host's health. Many studies support the role of probiotics as a contributor to gastrointestinal health, and nowadays, many authors are trying to prove their influence in oral health maintenance. To review the published literature to know the importance of using probiotics as a preventive and therapeutic method for oral infectious diseases management.

Before the existence of microorganisms, it was believed that bacteria played a pivotal role in dairy products such as kefir, koumiss, lin, en and yoghurt; sacred milk was often used therapeutically. The concept of 'probiotics' evolved in the 20th century from the ideas of Russian Nobel Prize laureate Elie Metchnikoff, professor at Pasteur Institute in Paris, that the bacteria in fermented products could compete with microbes detrimental to the host and thus can be beneficial for health [3]. Elie Metchnikoff reported that Bulgarians lived longer than other nations and supposed that this was because they consumed fermented milk products containing viable bacteria. Lactic acid lowers gut pH and inhibits the growth of some pathogenic bacteria. Later in 1950, a probiotic was trailed for scouring treatment among pigs, which led to a successful result. In 1974 another turning point about the probiotics was found by Mann and Spoering. They discovered that blood serum cholesterol could be reduced by fermented probiotics [4].

The first probiotic species introduced were *Lactobacillus acidophilus* by Hull in 1984 and Bifidobacterium bifidum by Holcomb 1991. Henry Tissier at Pasteur Institute identified a bacteria common in breastfed infant stool Bifidobacterium. More than 100 years ago, W.D. Miller gave the first accurate understanding of the dental caries process by demonstrating that it was a bacterially-mediated process. WHO described probiotics in 1994 as the next most important in the immune

Defence system, followed by antibiotic resistance. These concepts made a new field for probiotics in dentistry and medicine [3].

## Microbiota in Probiotics

Presently at least 700 different bacterial species are known that can colonise the different surfaces of the oral cavity. Every human being is roughly inhabited by about 100 to 200 of these 700 species. There is thus a substantial diversity between different people [4]. Oral commensals thrive at a pH range between 6.0 and 7.0, the typical pH of resting biofilms colonising healthy tooth surfaces [5]. Many harmless bacteria have been changed into potential pathogens. Resistant genes have been passed among the bacteria by gene transfer. Lactobacillus rhamnoses GG, ATCC 53103 produces a growth inhibitory substance against Streptococcus sobrinus, and it is also proposed to reduce the risk for caries [4]. Streptococcus salivarius strains appear to be excellent candidates for an oral probiotic since they are early colonisers orally and are numerically predominant members of the tongue microflora of healthy individuals. The most used probiotic bacterial strains belong to the genera Lactobacillus and Bifidobacteria. In the oral cavity, lactobacilli usually comprise 1% of the total cultivable bacteria; commonly isolated species include L. paracaseie, L. Plantarum, L. rhamnosus, L. salivarius. Bifidobacteria species isolated from oral samples include B. bifidum, B. dentium and B. longum. Species of Lactobacillus and Bifidobacteria may benefit the oral cavity by inhibiting cariogenic Streptococci and Candida. Probiotics for the oral cavity need to contain many different bacteria to compete with potential pathogens in the oral cavity (Figs. **1** - **3**).

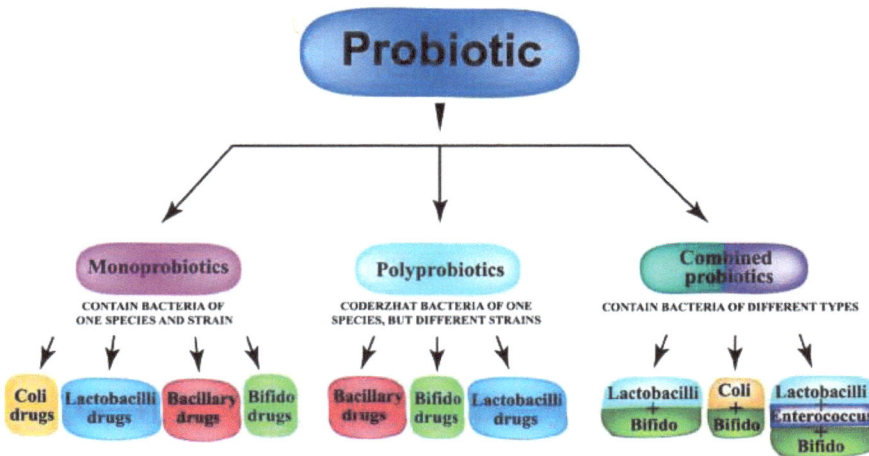

**Fig. (1).** Classification of probiotics.

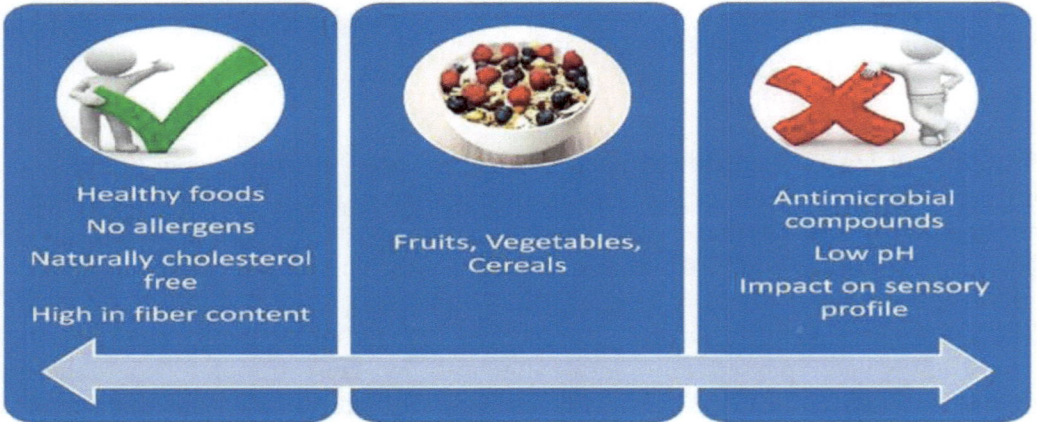

**Fig. (2).** Advantages and disadvantages of probiotics.

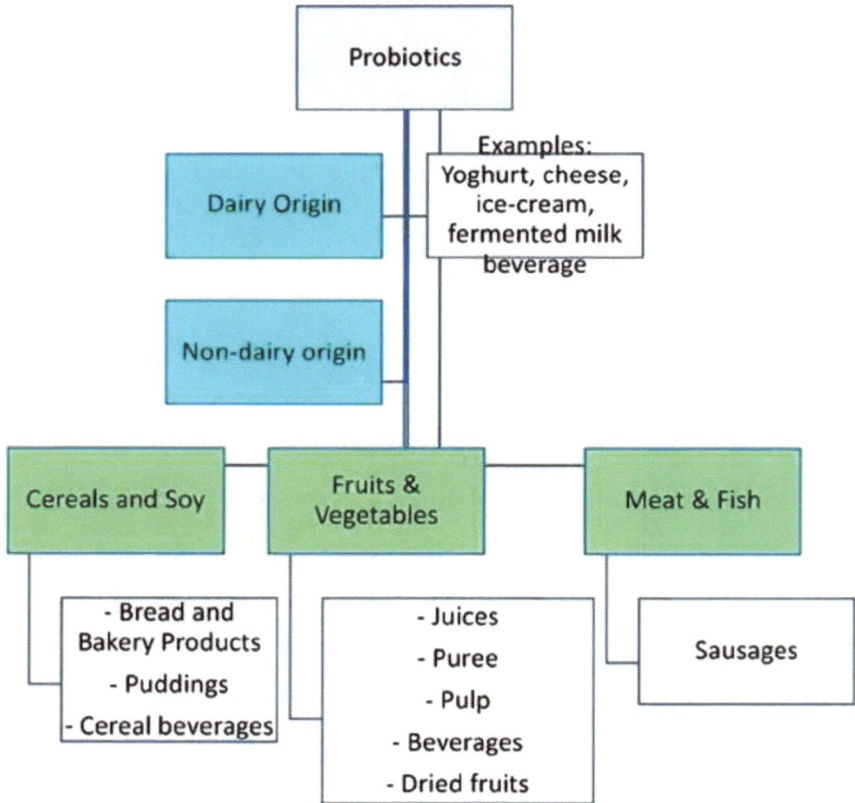

**Fig. (3).** Classification of probiotic foods.

## Properties of Probiotics

An ideal probiotic preparation should have the following properties:

1. High cell viability.
2. Ability to persist in the intestine even if the probiotic strain cannot colonise the gut.
3. Adhesion to the gut epithelium to cancel the flushing effects of peristalsis.
4. They should be able to interactor to send signals to the immune cells.
5. They should be non-pathogenic.
6. Resistant to processing.
7. Must have the capacity to influence local metabolic activity [6].

## Introducing Probiotics in the Oral Cavity

At this point, ideal vehicles of probiotic installation should be determined. Probiotics should adhere to dental tissue for a longer duration to establish a cariostatic effect and thus should be a part of the biofilm to fight cariogenic bacteria. An essential requirement of an organism to be an 'oral probiotic' is the ability to adhere to and colonise surfaces in the oral cavity. The most commonly studied organism in the oral cavity is *Lactobacilli*. Various studies have concluded that permanent colonisation in the oral cavity was unlikely and suggested the probiotic be used regularly (Fig. **4**).

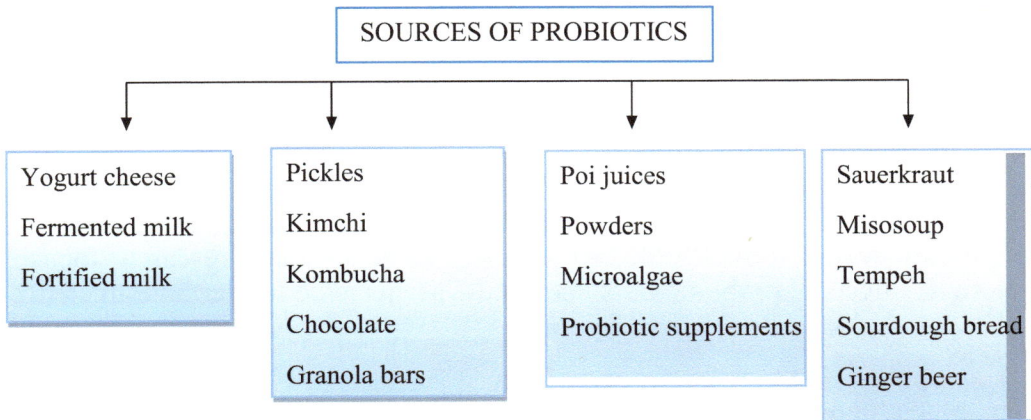

```
                    ┌─────────────────────────┐
                    │   SOURCES OF PROBIOTICS  │
                    └─────────────────────────┘
```

| Yogurt cheese | Pickles | Poi juices | Sauerkraut |
|---|---|---|---|
| Fermented milk | Kimchi | Powders | Misosoup |
| Fortified milk | Kombucha | Microalgae | Tempeh |
| | Chocolate | Probiotic supplements | Sourdough bread |
| | Granola bars | | Ginger beer |

**Fig. (4).** Probiotic sources.

Regular consumption of probiotics can decrease the numbers of salivary mutans Streptococcus and lactobacilli; dairy products like Bio-yoghurt with L rhamnosus harboured this microorganism in saliva up to 2 weeks after discontinuing consumption of probiotics. It is still questionable if probiotics can colonise in the mouth (Table **1**).

Table 1. Vehicle, strain & outcome pertains to probiotics.

| Vehicle | Strain | Outcome |
|---|---|---|
| Lozenges | *S. salivarious* | Reduces oral VSC levels |
| **Straw, tablet** | *L. reuteri* ATCC 55 730 | S. mutans level reduction |
| **Cheese** | *L.rhamnosus* GG. *Propionibacterium JS* | Reduced risk of high yeast counts and Hypo salivation |
| **Rinse solution** | *W. cibaria* | Reduction of VSC |
| **Capsule, liquid** | *L.sporogenes, L. bifidum, L.bulgaricus, L. acidophilus, L. casei, L.rhamnosus* | Increased salivary counts of lactobacilli without significant decrease in S. mutans counts |
| **Yoghurt drink** | *L. rhamnosus* GG | Temporary oral cavity colonization |
| **Probiotic toothpaste** | *Lactobacillus paracasei* | significant reduction in streptococcus mutans and lactobacilli bacterial counts |

Milk and cheese are known to contain compounds that reduce the risk of dental caries. In a recent study, it was found that milk containing probiotic Lactobacilli minimises the risk of caries significantly. Thus, probiotic LGG bacteria may benefit children's oral health and reduce the risk of the highest level of Streptococcus mutans.

However, there is no evidence of the long-term effects of the selected strain on oral tissue. Probiotics are used as passive local immunisation vehicles against dental caries in oral immunology.

Regarding milk and cheese, one should also recognise the large body of evidence relating to casein phosphopeptides and other milk-derived materials and their role in biomineralisation and other processes. At this point, research focusing beneficial effects of probiotic milk and cheese seems to be further investigated.

## Dosage

The French food safety agency reported that

1. The dose of probiotics ingested is an essential factor in obtaining high concentrations in the various compartments of the gastrointestinal tract
2. It is often said that probiotic concentrations must be greater than or equal to $10^6$ CFU/mL in the small intestine (ileum) and $10^8$ CFU/g in the colon, but the

scientific basis for these statements is relatively weak.
3. The concentrations in the colon have been proposed because they correspond to less than 1/1000 of the autochthonous flora present.

This quantity is not easy to determine as it is strain-specific, and it probably depends upon the type of benefit sought with the administration of probiotics [1].

## Dynamics of Probiotics

The general mechanisms of action of probiotics can be divided into three categories.

1. Modulation of immune response
2. Normalisation of intestinal microbiota
3. Metabolic effects.

The mechanisms of probiotic action in the oral cavity could be analogous to those portrayed for the intestine. Thus, oral colonisation by probiotic bacteria has often been considered essential for exerting oral effects. However, the possibility of systemic effects cannot be excluded, although the total IgA (immunoglobulin) levels in saliva seem unaffected by probiotic use. The ecological plaque hypothesis supports the normalisation of intestinal/oral microbiota, suggesting that the selective pressure present in environmental conditions can alter the balance between disease and oral health. As bacteria can influence their environment, and both antagonistic and synergistic interactions are suggested for bacteria in dental plaque, the environmental pressure described in the ecological plaque hypothesis could be introduced partly by bacteria. As there are bacterial species associated with oral diseases, some species seem to be related to oral health; however, it is still questionable that bacteria administered in food could be used as probiotics to normalise oral microbiota. There are many possible mechanisms for how pathogen exclusion may take place.

First: several probiotics alter the ability of pathogens to adhere to or invade colonic epithelial cells *in vitro.*

Second: probiotics could sequester essential nutrients from invading pathogens and impair colonisation ability.

Third: probiotics may inhibit the expression of virulence functions by altering the gene expression program of pathogens. And Lastly: probiotics may create an unfavourable environment for pathogen colonisation by altering the mucus layer, pH, and other factors in the local surroundings [7].

The use of probiotic bacteria is 'generally regarded as safe (GRAS) by the United States Food and Drug Administration (FDA), which is mainly focused on understanding the role of probiotics and their mechanism in GIT [8].

## Probiotics and Immune Response

The use of probiotics for clinical health benefits is a fascinating area of research that the present era has yet to explore. Some of the elite properties of probiotics, such as antipathogenicity, anti-diabetic, anti-obesity, anti-inflammatory, anti-cancer, anti-allergic, and angiogenic activities and their effect on the brain and central nervous system [1].

## The Anti-Pathogenic Activity of Probiotics

Anti-pathogenic activity is regarded as one of the most beneficial effects of probiotics. Unlike classic antibiotics, disturbance or alteration in the composition of the complex population of the gut microbiota is inhibited. Probiotics inhibit pathogens by producing short-chain fatty acids (SCFAs), such as acetic, propionic, butyric, and lactic acids. SCFAs help maintain an appropriate pH in the colonic lumen, which is imperative in the expression of numerous bacterial enzymes and the metabolism of foreign compounds and carcinogens in the gut.

## Urogenital Health Care

It is well-known that there is an association between abnormal vaginal microbial flora and an increased incidence of urinary tract infection (UTI). There are about 50 different species inhabiting the vagina, like Lactobacillus species, Lactobacillus Brevis, Lactobacillus casei, Lactobacillus vaginalis, Lactobacillus delbrueckii, Lactobacillus salivarius, Lactobacillus reuteri, and Lactobacillus rhamnosus, that are regarded as the primary regulators of the vaginal micro-environment. Imbalance in the microbial composition dramatically influences the health of the vaginal microenvironment, potentially leading to a compromised state of bacterial vaginosis (BV) and UTI. These compromised states can be reassured by balancing the number of Lactobacillus sp. *via* probiotics supplementation.

## Antidiabetic Activity

Gram-negative bacteroidetes and the Gram-positive firmicutes are two specific bacterial species that dominate the gut microenvironment. Recent research has proven that obesity is associated with increased Bacteroides over time, concurrent with a reduction in firmicutes. Alterations in the microbiome also increase invasion of opportunistic pathogens, which are resistant to oxidative stress and simultaneously capable of reducing sulfates and inhibiting the growth of butyrate-producing bacteria. Using probiotics and prebiotic interventions, management of type-2 diabetes by modulating gut hormones, such as gastric inhibitory polypeptide and glucagon-like peptide-1, is another effective strategy. Research is focused on generating new prebiotics, such as arabinoxylan and arabinoxylan oligosaccharides, which show promising results in countering related metabolic disorders because both carbohydrates have been linked to adiposity reduction.

## Anti-Obesity Activity

Abnormal or excessive fat (obesity) accumulation that directly impairs health is linked to increased energy availability, sedentariness, and greater ambient temperature control, leading to an imbalance in energy intake and expenditure. Probiotics possess physiological functions that contribute to the health of the host environment regulating microbes. In most instances, thermogenic and lipolytic responses facilitate weight loss by stimulating the sympathetic nervous system.

## Anti-Inflammatory Activity

Crohn's disease (CD) and ulcerative colitis (UC) are among the most chronic inflammatory diseases of the GIT, collectively called inflammatory bowel disease. Crohn's disease can affect any part of the GIT like the mucosa, submucosa, and serosa, and the inflammation can even spread to the whole GIT. Ulcerative colitis characteristically involves the large bowel, specifically the mucosa and submucosa of the colon. Research has shown that an imbalance in the gut microbiota plays an essential pathophysiological role in the positive regulation of IBD. IBD is associated with impaired production of SCFAs, mainly acetate, butyrate, and propionate. Moreover, these SCFAs have been known to play a vital role in maintaining colonic homeostasis.

## Anti-Cancer Activity

In the present decade, intense research on cancer involving genomics, proteomics, and molecular pathology, has enhanced the knowledge about cancer and public awareness. In recent years, natural sources that confer anti-carcinogenic effects, such as probiotics, have received prime focus. These have attracted intense interest from clinical nutritionists, scientists, and industrialists to work collaboratively to bring down the disease and develop an effective drug with minimal or no side effects.

## Effect on Brain and CNS

The colonisation of microbiota in the GIT is well-associated with GIT and gastrointestinal diseases. Moreover, many studies have been devoted to elucidating the influence of gut microbiota on the CNS in recent years. The "microbiota-gut-brain axis" is an interactive, bidirectional communication established by exchanging regulatory signals between the GIT and CNS. The effect of probiotics on the CNS has been mainly studied in clinical trials, where it has been evident that gut microbiota influences human brain development function. In children with autism spectrum disorder, a daily dose of L. Plantarum WCFS1 (4.5 1010 CFU/ day) improved their school records and attitude towards food [1].

## Probiotics in other Fields of Medicine

Traditional applications of probiotics are in gastroenterology.AAD (Antibiotic-associated diarrhoea) is a condition of diarrhoea associated with antibiotic usage and has no other identifiable causes. The incidence of this condition is relatively high and depends upon the population and the used antibiotics. An increased incidence of AAD (25% to 50%) has been described for ampicillin/amoxicillin, cephalosporin, and clindamycin. Seeing the high incidence of this problem associated with antibiotics frequently prescribed in the dental practice is also an essential concern for the dental practitioner. Additionally, there is strong evidence for applying probiotics in treating infectidiarrheahoea in children and adults. The use of, for example, Lactobacillus casei strain GG shortens the duration and reduces the stool frequency. The use of S boulardii in the treatment of a Helicobacter pylori infection. This probiotic can decrease the side effects and enhance the efficacy of the prescribed drug treatment. Results are also shown in the treatment of Clostridium difficile associated diarrhoea, irritable bowel disease, allergic reactions, and acute respiratory infections. Potential future applications include probiotics in rheumatoid arthritis, cancer, ethanol-induced liver diseases, and bacterial vaginosis [9].

## Probiotics in Oral Cavity

### *Probiotics and Dental Caries*

Dental caries is an infectious disease affecting most people. This multifactorial and complex disease process occurs along with the enamel surface and dental biofilm interface. Several methods may alter the carcinogenicity of the biofilms responsible for dental caries. Researchers are developing "probiotic" ways to treat caries causing infection. Probiotic mechanisms selectively remove only the harmful pathogen while leaving the remainder of the oral ecosystem intact. One of the replacement therapy options entails the application of a genetically engineered "effector strain" of mutans streptococci that will replace the cariogenic or "wild strain" to prevent or arrest caries and promote optimal remineralisation of tooth surfaces that have been demineralised but that have not become cavitated. S. mutans strain BCS3-L1 is a genetically modified effector strain designed for use in replacement therapy to prevent dental caries. Recombinant DNA technology was used to delete the gene encoding lactate dehydrogenase in BCS3-L1, making it unable to produce lactic acid. This effector strain was also designed to produce elevated amounts of a novel peptide antibiotic called mutacin 1140. It gives it a substantial selective advantage over most other strains of S. mutans. The extracellular polysaccharides (glucans) promote the adhesion and colonisation of cariogenic organisms and mediate protection against antimicrobial agents and resistance to toxic compounds. These glucans are Synthesis through glucosyltransferase B, glucosyltransferase C, and glycosyltransferase D genes. The introduction of the mutated gtfC gene affects the ability of S. mutans to produce extracellular glucans resulting in a decrease in the extracellular matrix component of mixed oral biofilms from 51 to 33% of the biofilm volume. Several studies suggest that consuming probiotic lactobacilli or bifidobacteria products could reduce the salivary concentration of mutans streptococci [7].

Probiotics can reduce the risk of a high Streptococcus mutans level occurrence in the oral cavity. Lactobacillus rhamnosus and Lactobacillus casei have proven potential to hamper the growth of oral streptococci.

The normal microflora protects the oral cavity from infections; species of bacteria associated with complex microbial floras in the mouth constitute the dental plaque. Dental caries is one of the major diseases caused by human microbial flora. It is postulated that the long-term consumption of milk containing the probiotic Lactobacillus rhamnosus CG strain reduced caries in kindergarten children.

Streptococcus thermophilus and Lactococcus lactis strains are shown to reduce cariogenic bacteria levels. The studies also suggest that consuming products containing probiotic Lactobacilli or Bifidobacteria could reduce the number of mutans Streptococci in saliva. Oral probiotics may help fight tooth decay since acid production from sugar is detrimental to teeth; care needs to be taken not to select strains with high fermentation capacity [6].

## Arginine in Caries Prevention: Prebiotics, Probiotics, and Oral Care Formulations

L-arginine was identified as the main component responsible for the pH-raising effect of saliva. Arginine is found free in saliva in micromolar concentrations and abundant in salivary peptides and proteins. Arginine enters the mouth through dietary components but is also naturally produced by the human body *via* protein turnover and de novo arginine synthesis from citrulline. Among these pathways, arginine degradation, the arginine deiminase system (ADS) is the most widespread anaerobic route for arginine degradation. In supragingival biofilms, arginine is metabolised mainly by the ADS of certain oral bacteria to produce citrulline, ornithine, $CO_2$, ATP, and ammonia. Ammonia production *via* ADS results in cytoplasmic, and environment pH rises and serves as a mechanism used by oral bacteria for Protection against acid killing.

Bioenergetic advantages, including the increase of DPH and synthesis of ATP

They maintain a neutral environmental pH that favours the persistence of ADSpositive (ADS1) bacteria while being competitive against caries pathogens. Salivary levels of free arginine are strongly correlated with caries resistance. Plaque of caries-free individuals has higher pH values than plaque from active caries individuals. This difference has been correlated with elevated ammonia levels in caries-free subjects [5].

## Probiotics and Periodontal Diseases

The probiotic strains reported for periodontal diseases include L. reuteri strains, L. Brevis. Krause *et al*. showed a significantly reduced gingival index and bacterial plaque amount in patients treated with L. reuteri than in a placebo. Most authors have concluded that oral probiotics were associated with improved oral health, including a significantly reduced level of cariogenic and periodontal pathogens and bacterial mixture [9]. Klais *et al*., 2005 studied the effect of Lactobacillus Brevis on chronic periodontitis. It concluded that the improvement in targeted clinical parameters (plaque index, gingival index, bleeding) resulted in a significant reduction in salivary levels of prostaglandins and suppression of periodontal pathogens by oral probiotics [4].

## Probiotics and Halitosis

Halitosis (bad breath) is discomfort rather than a disease. Halitosis occurs due to many reasons, including consumption of foods, metabolic disorders, and respiratory tract infections. It can also be associated with the imbalance of microflora. To be specific, it results from the anaerobic action of bacteria. These can degrade salivary and food proteins to generate amino acids, which are in turn transformed into volatile sulfur compounds, such as hydrogen sulfide and methyl mercaptan, and dimethyl sulfide. Clinical and laboratory studies have proven the potential of preventing halitosis by introducing prebiotics. Marked reduction in the levels of hydrogen sulfide, $CH_3CH$, can be noticed after regular gargling using

*W. cibaria. S. salivarius* strain K12. It produced two lantibiotic bacteriocins, inhibitory compounds to strains of several species of gram-positive bacteria implicated in halitosis. Trials done using chlorhexidine rinse followed by K12 lozenges showed a reduction in halitosis for two weeks [4].

## Probiotics and *Candida albicans*

Candida albicans is a leading cause of infection in the oral cavity. It is widespread in the elderly and immunocompromised patients. Hatakka *et al.* showed a reduced prevalence of *C. Albicans* after taking probiotics in cheese containing *L. rhamnosus* and *Propionibacterium freudenreichii* ssp. Sherman [10].

## Probiotics and aphthous ulcer

A study conducted by a few researchers revealed that there could be a reduction in the recurrence of aphthous ulcers using synbiotics. Even though there are many other treatment modalities for aphthous ulcers, studies on synbiotic bifilar lozenges demonstrated better results. There are no significant side effects for synbiotics. Instead, it is more beneficial for the host [4].

## Probiotics and Orthodontic Treatment

Dental health is affected by fixed orthodontic appliances because they cause the accumulation of microorganisms which leads to the demineralisation of enamel. An ecological environment is created whenever orthodontic bands and brackets are used due to their complex designs, which favour the growth of S. mutans strains. The formation of a white spot occurs due to an imbalance between mineral loss and mineral gain. A clinical study was conducted by Cildir *et al.* in 2009 with probiotics using *Bifidobacterium animalis* subsp. Lactis DN-173010 and noticed that it could reduce the salivary count of mutans streptococci in orthodontic patients who use fixed orthodontic appliances.

## *Adverse effects of Probiotics (Table 2)*

1. Flatulence,
2. Mild abdominal discomfort,
3. Nausea /vomiting
4. Rarely, septicemia

## CONCLUSION

Probiotics are nevertheless an innovative and a different field to be researched in oral microbiology. Probiotic therapy indicates the correlation between diet and health, including oral health. However, this concept is in its early stages.

Although knowledge about the pathogen and host interactions is increasing day by day, this area is still doubtful. There is a great need to find out the role of beneficial bacteria to identify and to conduct proper studies on the uses of probiotics to treat oral health [11].

**Table 2. Precautions and Contraindications.**

| Precautions | Contraindications |
| --- | --- |
| 1) Since probiotics contain live micro-organisms, there is a slight chance that these preparations might cause pathological infection, particularly in critically ill or severely immunocompromised patients.<br>2) Probiotic strains of Lactobacillus have also been reported to cause bacteremia in patients with short-bowel syndrome, due to altered gut integrity.<br>3) Caution is also warranted in patients with central venous catheters since contamination leading to fungemia has been reported. | 1) Lactobacillus preparations are contraindicated in persons with a hypersensitivity to lactose or milk.<br>2) *S. boulardii* is contraindicated in patients with a yeast allergy.<br>3) No contraindications are listed for Bifidobacteria since most species are considered nonpathogenic and non-toxigenic. |

## CONSENT FOR PUBLICATION

Not applicable.

## CONFLICT OF INTEREST

The authors declare no conflict of interest, financial or otherwise.

## ACKNOWLEDGEMENT

Declared none.

## REFERENCES

[1]     Mahasneh S, Mahasneh A. Probiotics: A promising role in dental health. Dent J 2017; 5(4): 26.
[http://dx.doi.org/10.3390/dj5040026] [PMID: 29563432]

[2]     Kerry RG, Patra JK, Gouda S, Park Y, Shin HS, Das G. Benefaction of probiotics for human health: Areview. Yao Wu Shi Pin Fen Xi 2018; 26(3): 927-39.
[PMID: 29976412]

[3]     Pandey KR, Naik SR, Vakil BV. Probiotics, prebiotics and synbiotics- a review. J Food Sci Technol 2015; 52(12): 7577-87.
[http://dx.doi.org/10.1007/s13197-015-1921-1] [PMID: 26604335]

[4]     Jayaraj L, Shenoy P, Chatra L, Veena KM, Prabhu RV, Kumar V. Role of probiotics in dentistry. World. J Pharm Sci 2017; 6(2): 294-301.

[5]     Nascimento MM. Approaches to Modulate Biofilm Ecology. Dent Clin North Am 2019; 63(4): 581-94.
[http://dx.doi.org/10.1016/j.cden.2019.07.002] [PMID: 31470914]

[6]    Acharya S. Probiotics: Current knowledge update. Int J Pedod Rehabil 2016; 1(2): 79-83.
       [http://dx.doi.org/10.4103/2468-8932.196493]

[7]    Tandon V, Arora V, Yadav V, *et al.* Concept of Probiotics in Dentistry. Int J Dent Med Res 2015;
       1(6): 206-9.

[8]    Kumar N, Marotta F, Dhewa T, Mishra V, Kumar V, Bharadwaj A. Management of oral health
       through novel probiotics: A review. Int J Probiotics Prebiotics 2017; 12(3): 1-6.

[9]    Laleman I, Teughels W. Probiotics in the dental practice: a review. Quintessence Int 2015; 46(3): 255-
       64.
       [PMID: 25485319]

[10]   Myneni SR, Brocavich K, Wang H. Biological strategies for the prevention of periodontal disease:
       Probiotics and vaccines. Periodontol 2000 2020; 84(1): 161-75.
       [http://dx.doi.org/10.1111/prd.12343] [PMID: 32844414]

[11]   Agarwal G, Ingle NA, Kaur N, Yadav P, Ingle E, Charania Z. Probiotics, and oral health- a review. J
       Int Oral Health 2015; 7(10): 133-6.

**CHAPTER 15**

# The Setting of a Pediatric Dental Clinic

**Nilima Thosar**[1,*] and **Prachi Goyal**[2]

[1] *Department, of Pediatric and Preventive Dentistry, Sharad Pawar Dental College and Hospital, Datta Meghe Institute of Medical Sciences (Deemed to be University), Wardha-442107, India*

[2] *Department of Pediatric and Preventive Dentistry, MMCDSR, Mullana (Ambala), India*

**Abstract:** Pediatric Dental Clinic should be colourful and pleasantly full of colours and lights. Pediatric patients should like the ambit of the environment. So, the setup of a Pediatric dental clinic should consider the interests and likes of pediatric patients. The clinic should have designated areas for the clinical work of patients. There should be a separate clinical area, waiting area, and play area.

**Keywords:** Dental Clinic Set up, Pediatric Patient.

## INTRODUCTION

Pediatric Dentistry is the speciality concerned with the dental treatment of children. It is rightly said that a "Child's mind is tender and lovely as the petals of a full-blown rose. Beware how you touch it. Meet it with all reverence of your being. Use it with gentle respect and fill it with the honey of love, the perfume of faith, and the tenderness of tolerance."

For the child to like the environment of the Pediatric dental setup, it should be pleasant. Children should not feel bored and restless at any moment. It should be constructed to give the child patient a sense of relaxation and comfort. Dentistry for children is not complex but is different from that for adults. So, the same dental setup also differs accordingly.

Mohammad Karimi, 2018 [1] suggested that dental office setup and environment require knowledge about the science of colour and lighting design; the correct layout is needed.

---

* **Corresponding author Nilima Thosar:** Department,of Pediatric and Preventive Dentistry, Sharad Pawar Dental College and Hospital, Datta Meghe Institute of Medical Sciences (Deemed to be University), Wardha-442107, India; E-mail: drnthosar@rediffmail.com

Satyawan Damle, Ritesh Kalaskar & Dhanashree Sakhare (Eds.)

## Factors to be Considered for Pediatric Dental Set-Up

The design of the Pediatric Dental clinic setup is different as various aspects need to be taken into consideration, such as behaviour management understanding of child psychology as some children have inherent fear and anxiety or it may be related to family/parent/ society related influencing factors causing the fear in the child. Pediatric Dentistry is an age defined as from birth up to adolescent children visiting a dental clinic for their dental problems. A child's first dental visit is an extraordinary task for a Pediatric Dentist who is responsible for creating a positive dental attitude not only in children but also in parents of younger children (Fig. **1**).

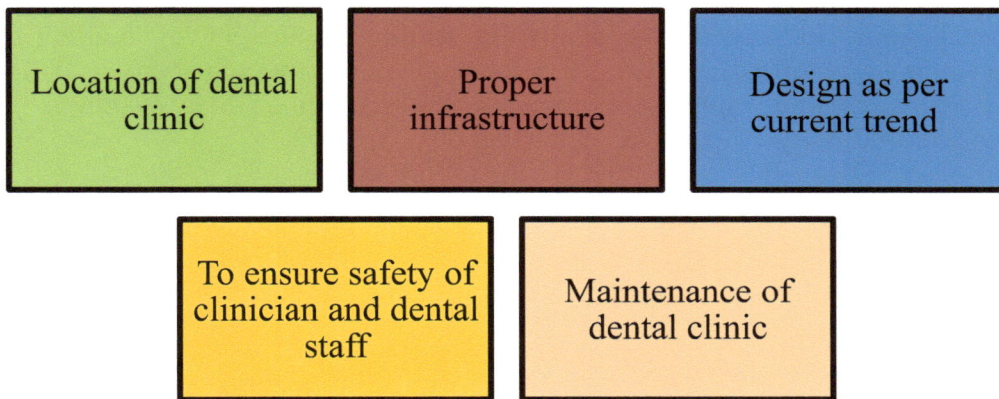

| Location of dental clinic | Proper infrastructure | Design as per current trend |

| To ensure safety of clinician and dental staff | Maintenance of dental clinic |

**Fig. (1).**  Factors to Be Considered for Pediatric Dental Set-Up.

Nowadays, dental practitioners want to develop dental setup designs taking into consideration the following points such as:

Pediatric Dental setup requires knowledge of interior decoration of office, lighting, and proper layout of dental equipment.

Space utilisation for dental setup requires the provision of the following areas [1]:

1. Reception area
2. Waiting area
3. Playroom
4. Dental office set up
5. Audio-visual aids
6. Dentist's private office
7. Examination room
8. Treatment room

9. Radiography room
10. Central Sterilization room
11. Dental laboratory
12. Area for biomedical waste management

## Reception Area

The reception area in the dental clinic is where the child enters first. The receptionist always should address the child with a smile so that child should not feel that they have visited an unknown area. It is the first area that attracts the child. So, this area welcomes the child to the Pediatric Dentistry Department/ Dental clinic. In general, the admission section should convey inviting and welcoming. The office clerk can fill in the required information about the child in various ways like using questionnaires and recording their responses and computerised entry of patients' data (Fig. **2**).

The receptionist should possess communication skills. She can call the patient by their name, preferably by the nickname, so the child feels that the receptionist is their friend who may help develop rapport. The receptionist can engage the child in topics of interest, which can help relieve the child's anxiety.

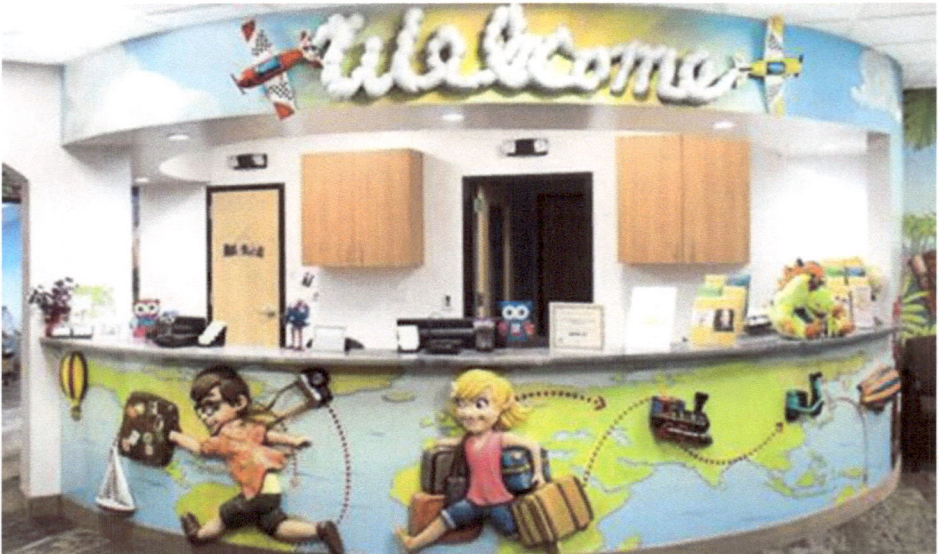

**Fig. (2).** Reception area of a Pediatric dental clinic.

# Waiting Area

Younger children are often accompanied by their parents for dental treatment. Sometimes, children and parents need to wait in the waiting room until their turn comes. Many dental clinics have laptops and phone charging points as it is the need of the hour to remain updated with the latest technology. Colourful chairs can be of help for children to sit quietly. The waiting area should have wall-mounted monitors to sensitise and orient parents about the availability of facilities and various dental procedures for pediatric patients. Children can play cartoon shows of their choice until they are waiting. Mothers should not get bored, so books of their interest such as cookery books and beauty products magazines and books should be kept so that mothers can get engaged until the waiting period. Book cabinets/ shelves/ racks should have separate sections for children's cartoon/comic/educational books and mother's books (Fig. **3**).

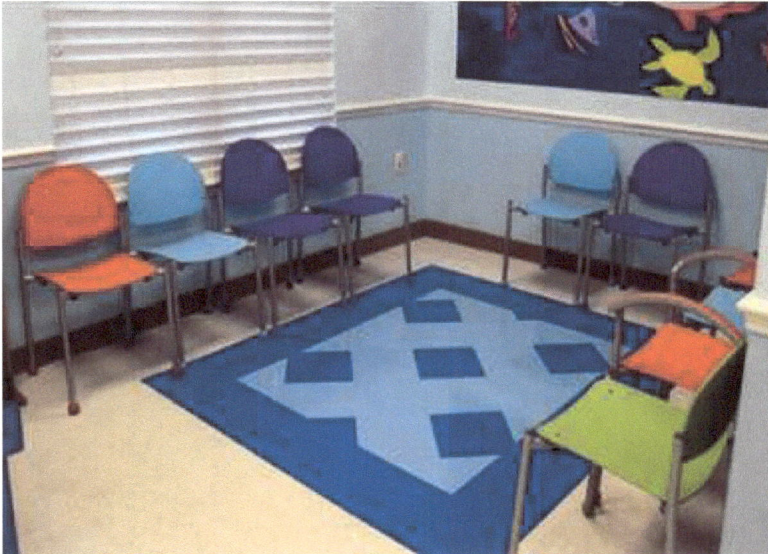

**Fig. (3).** Waiting area in pediatric dental office.

# Playroom

For children to not get bored, the playroom can be made colourful with different toys. Various posters of cartoons can be pasted on the wall. Depending upon the availability of space, creativity-related items or games should be arranged and kept. Children can draw and play together. Cartoon images and characters in the form of posters can be pasted on the walls. Children will be more comfortable with their peers away from their parents with no fears in this environment. Installing DVDs or TVs to play animations is another essential thing that can entertain children. If the waiting room is large enough, considering a playground is an exciting and tempting idea to attract children (Fig. 4).

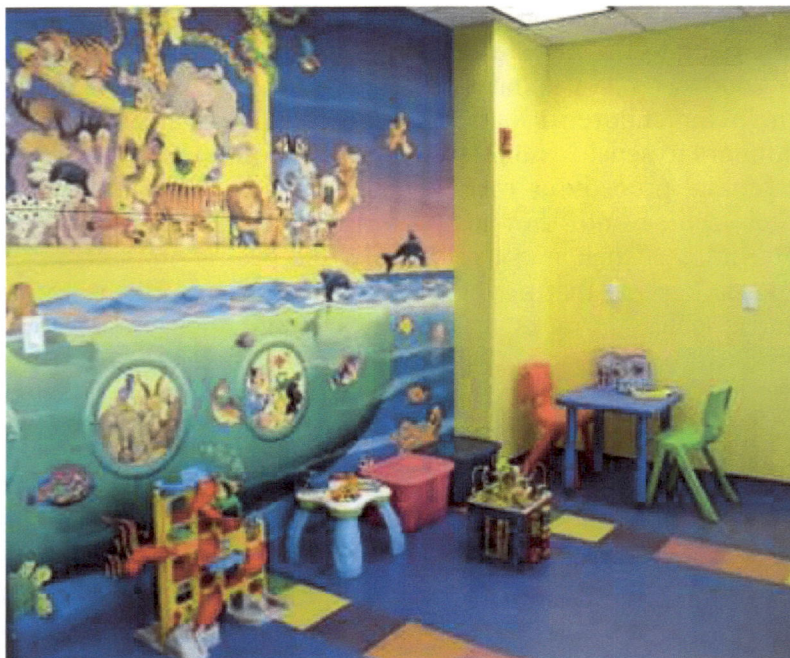

**Fig. (4).** Playroom in Pediatric dental clinic.

## Dental Office Set Up

### *Attire of Clinic Staff*

Some children develop anxiety about dental staff being observed in a white coats. It is in the Dentist's hands to decide the dress code for him and the office staff. The child should be interviewed in a separate consulting room, which will help to develop rapport with the child. At the same time, communication can be established effectively with the child. The dentist should talk about the child's likes/ dislikes, favourite topics, friends, hobbies and skills, and school-related things. The dentist, as well as his staff, should always smile and be pleasant. Finally, the child should be taken to the dental chair.

### *Colours, Smells and Sounds*

The child likes bright colours, so walls or certain areas, curtains, and floors can be made colourful. The child does not like the smell of certain dental materials like eugenol, acrylic monomer, and waxes. Because of the child's uncooperative behaviour, they may not be kept on the tray during initial visits of the child. The noise/ sound of the air-rotor handpiece, an ultrasonic cleaner that can disturb the child, should also be used carefully, and be avoided during the child's 1ˢᵗ dental visit. Otherwise, if the handpiece must be used to mask its sound; light instrumental music can be played, distracting the child (Fig. **5**).

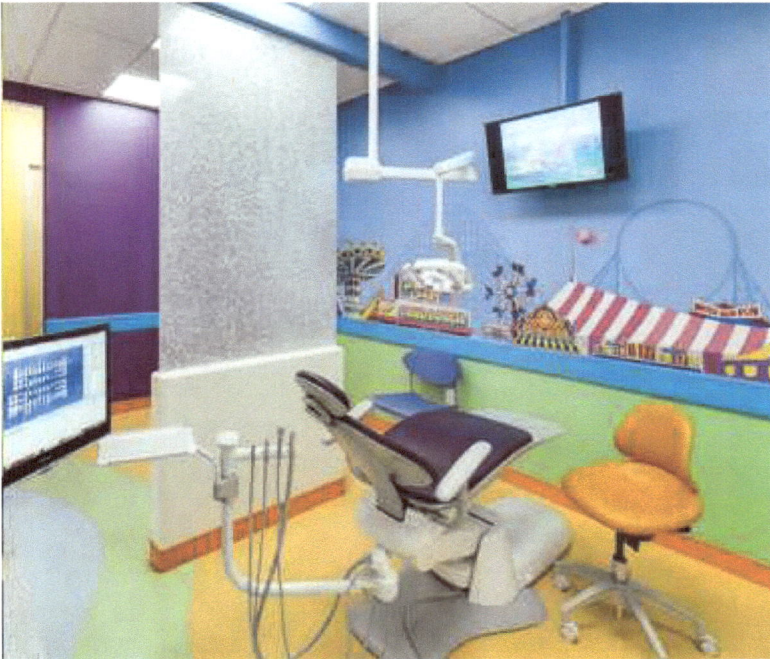

**Fig. (5).** bright colors of the wall and floor.

## *Rewards and Gifts*

- A child should be appreciated for sitting correctly in the dental chair for dental treatment and should be offered gifts like stationery, favourite toy, and educational aid.
- Gifts in sweets/ chocolates/ candies are not to be given as it is cariogenic.
- Reward is compensation for the effort somebody has made. It can be expressed in spoken words like "Thank you." So, providing the gift is also helpful in developing a cheerful outlook in the child about dentistry

## Audio Visual Aids

To prevent anxiety child is encouraged to watch cartoon shows on the dental chair-mounted computer monitor. The monitor can be mounted on the ceiling also.

## Dentist's private office: (Fig. 6)

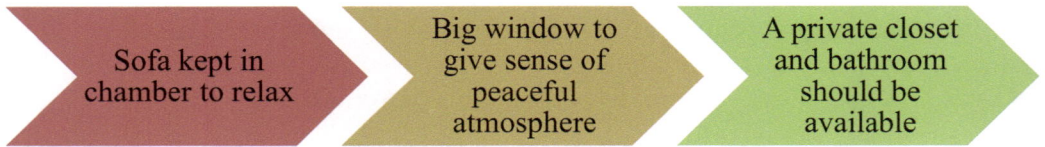

| Sofa kept in chamber to relax | Big window to give sense of peaceful atmosphere | A private closet and bathroom should be available |

Fig. (6).   Dentist's private office.

It should consist of the following setup:

## Examination Room (Figs. 7 - 9)

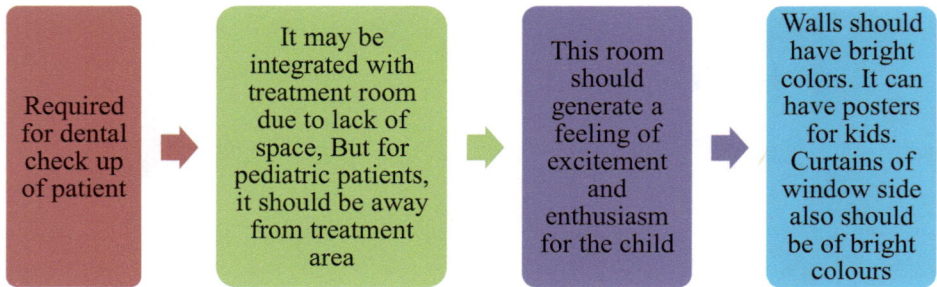

| Required for dental check up of patient | It may be integrated with treatment room due to lack of space, But for pediatric patients, it should be away from treatment area | This room should generate a feeling of excitement and enthusiasm for the child | Walls should have bright colors. It can have posters for kids. Curtains of window side also should be of bright colours |

Fig. (7).   Examination Room.

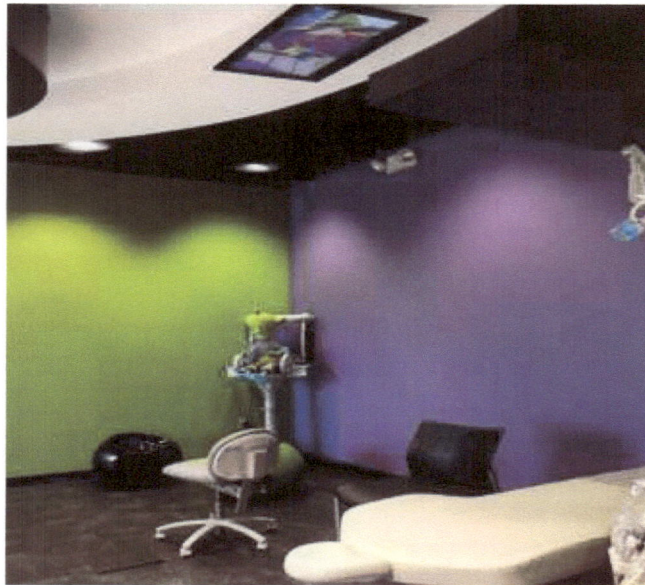

Fig. (8).   Wall mounted monitor.

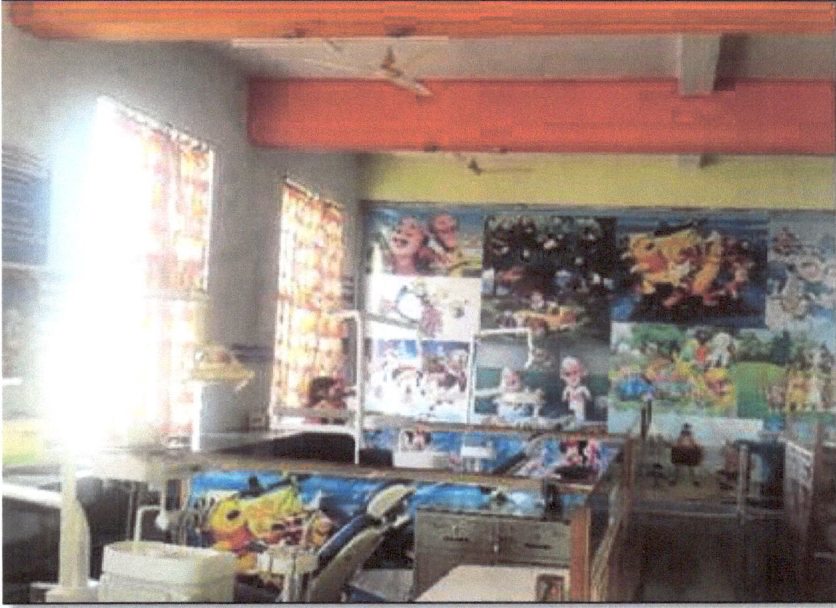

**Fig. (9).** Examination room.

## Treatment room (Fig. 10)

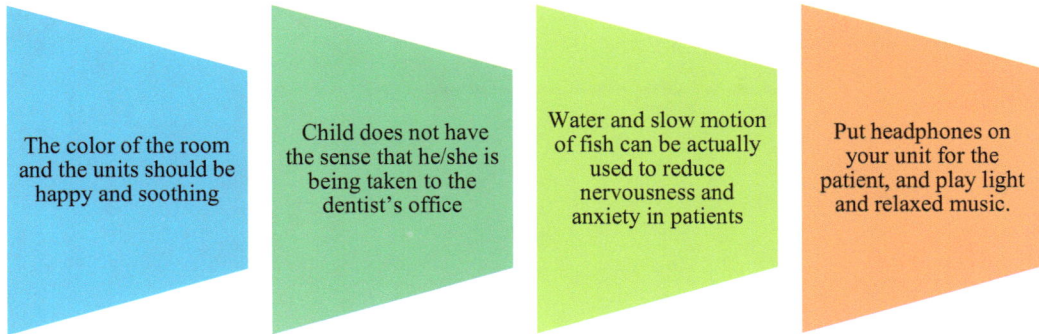

| The color of the room and the units should be happy and soothing | Child does not have the sense that he/she is being taken to the dentist's office | Water and slow motion of fish can be actually used to reduce nervousness and anxiety in patients | Put headphones on your unit for the patient, and play light and relaxed music. |

**Fig. (10).** Treatment room.

## Radiography Room

- X-ray machines should be installed on dental chairs to be easily accessible for shooting on both the right and left sides of the mouth.
- Radiography room door should have a lead coating with 2mm thickness.
- Radiography room should be equipped with radiation protection barriers like lead aprons separately for the operator and child patient, thyroid collars. If the

parent available, then for lead apron be provided to the parent also.
- X-ray viewer should be available. It may be sometimes wall mounted. It ranges from small to large depending upon the use of X-ray.
- There should be a sign of radiographic hazard depicted on the X-ray room door.
- Radiographic room should depict the red and green lamp outside the room. A red light denotes that the X-ray room is not in use, while a green lamp suggests that a Dentist is available in the X-ray room with a child patient and is shooting the X-ray.
- Automatic developer can be installed. But if radiovisiography (RVG) is available, it should be used. For the same, the computerised set-up should be available.
- Record maintenance of patients' X-rays throughout the day can be done for follow-up purposes (Figs. 7 - 12)
- Pediatric considerations for taking radiographs for different age groups children should be well oriented with all staff and X-ray technicians.
- 10. Sterilization Room specifications: The practice of Pediatric dentistry exposes dental health professionals and children to infectious disease agents. The risk is considered to be higher in dental practices than in other health care settings, mainly because there is close and prolonged contact between provider and patient. In addition, most dental procedures generate aerosols that are contaminated with a patient's saliva, blood, other secreta, or tissue particles. To control this risk, the Centres for Disease Control and Prevention (CDC) and other organizations developed recommendations and protocols based on the principle of standard precautions (Fig **13**).

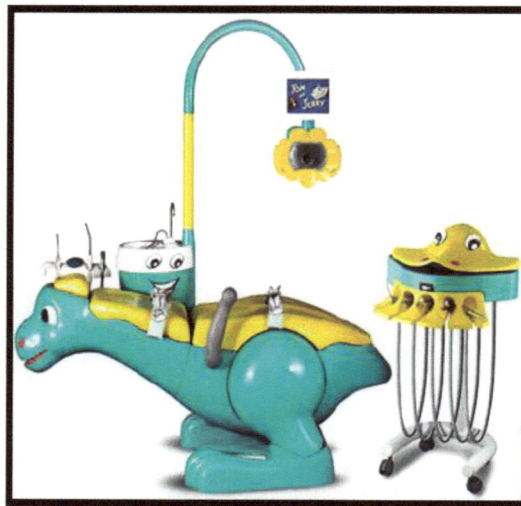

**Fig. (11).** Dental chair specifically designed for Pediatric patients.

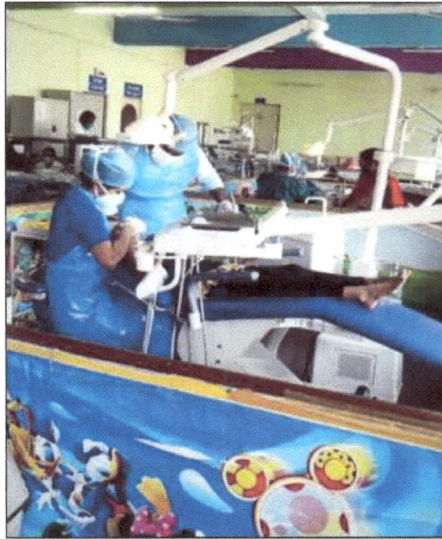

**Fig. (12).** Treatment room.

**Fig. (13).** Sterilization room specifications.

## Dental Laboratory

- Dental Laboratory for Pediatric Clinics should be installed with equipment like a dental lathe machine for finishing and polishing appliances, a model trimmer for trimming the dental casts, plaster dispenser for dispensing the dental plaster and stone.
- Other equipment that can be kept in the laboratory includes hydro solder used to sell space maintainers.
- There should be the installation of mannequins with typodonts for skill training of students for various pre-clinical procedures like cavity preparations, rubber

dam application demonstrations, and tooth preparation for stainless steel crown or strip crown. It is available in a hospital-based laboratory set up in Academic Institute.

## Waste Storage Area (Figs. 14 & 15)

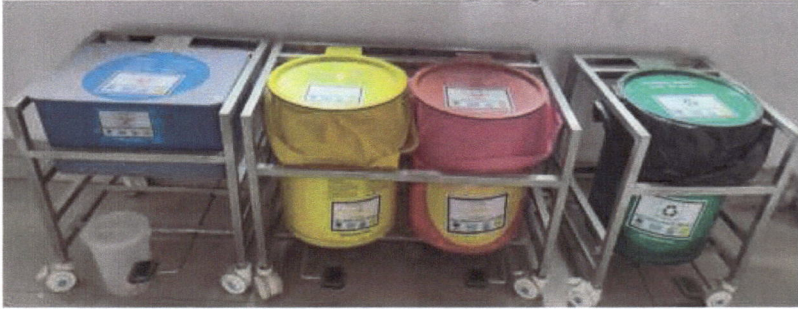

**Fig. (14).** Colour-coded bins for waste disposal.

- The area of waste storage should be in a remote corner.
- The area should be well cordoned by proper fencing and locked.
- The biomedical waste must be stored in rigid/ semi-rigid, leak-proof containers to prevent its spillage and spread of infection through the vectors like flies.
- The Universal symbol of Hazardous "BMW" must be prominently displayed, and warning notice in the vernacular language must be prominently displayed.

## Specifications for Disposal of Waste as Per Colour-coded Bins (Figs. 14 and 15)

**Yellow:** Human and animal anatomical waste, soiled waste like gauze pieces, infected cotton, chemical waste, discarded or expired medicines, discarded linen and beddings contaminated with blood, clinical laboratory waste, microbiology waste, X-ray film developing liquid, discarded formalin, infected secretions, aspirated body fluids, liquid from laboratories and floor washings, cleaning, house-keeping and disinfecting activities etc.

**Red:** Contaminated waste which is recyclable, contaminated tubings, catheters, IV tubes, syringes without needles, gloves

**Blue:** Broken/ discarded and contaminated glass, metallic implants

**White:** It is a white puncture proof container. Needles, syringes with fixed needles, scalpel, blade/ contaminated sharp objects, portion of needle which remains after it is destroyed or burnt

**Fig. (15).** Biohazardous waste management.

## Dental Set Up for Dental Health Care of Special Children [2]

Oral is an integral part of general health and influences the quality of life [3]. The oral health status of disabled children is poor compared to normal children. Such children have higher chances of getting affected with dental diseases like dental caries and periodontal disease. Such poor health is limited manual dexterity due to lack of muscle incoordination and poor neuromuscular skills (Table **1**).

These children also have specific medical problems for which they are being treated. Therefore, it causes a financial burden for the family. The oral health needs of these children are numerous but are not attended to and utilised. This could be because gaining physical access to dental treatment is the biggest challenge. Most dental setups are not accessible to such children. Every dental clinic or dental practitioner designs and furnishes a dental clinic from the perspective of dental treatment of normal children. Since the creation of dental clinics for special children is not kept in mind and is given secondary weightage, such setups are hardly thought of for construction by dental clinicians. Design and Architectural set up in India are not friendly for disabled children. To overcome such a problem Government of India has set guidelines in 2016 [4], which mention the specifications of construction of building with barrier-free set-up to have access to health care needs of such children. As per these guidelines, the following are the requisites for dental clinic set-up (Fig. **16**).

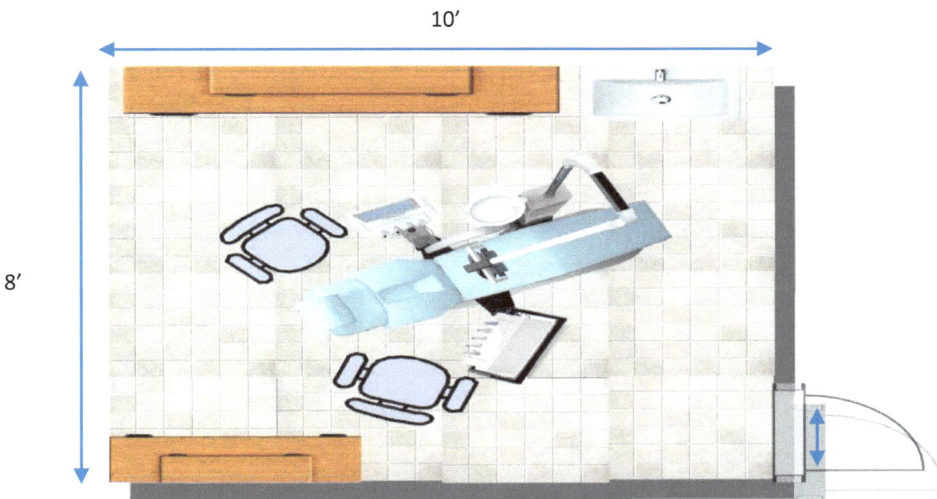

**Fig. (16).** Layout of Dental clinic set up for cerebral palsy patient.

**Table 1. Area specifications for construction of dental clinic for disabled children.**

| Area | Size requirements | Specifications |
|---|---|---|
| **Parking area** | 98 feet distance | To be located near the dental clinic |
| **Walkways** | Length: 60 meters<br>If length is more: rest area with bench/ seat at an interval of 98 feet with a seat height between 17.6 to 19.6 inches.<br>The height of the backrest and hand rest should be 27.54 inch<br>Walkway width: 70.6 inches for 2-way traffic | The surface should be challenging, smooth, and plain levelled for ease of walking and for carrying wheels of exceptional children. |
| **Tactile pavers (guiding and warning blocks)** | - | It is used for visually impaired children.<br>Two types are available: Dot type guiding block type. |
| **Ramp** | Vertical height: 6 inches<br>Width: 47 inches | Handrails should be slip-resistant. |
| **Staircase** | Treads: 12 inches deep<br>Risers: Not more than 6 inches<br>Stair's landing: 48 inches deep and 60 inches in width<br>Grab bars height:30 to 35 inches | It should be with a lift/ ramp<br>It should be grab bars for holding while walking and should be slip-resistant<br>Grab bars should bear a weight of 550 pounds |
| **Lifts** | 48 inches wide by 48 inches deep | The capacity of 13 passengers for easy manoeuvrability of a wheelchair |
| **Door** | Doorway opening: 35 inches<br>For hand-operated door, handle to be kept at the height of 33 inches to 43 inches from the floor. | Sliding or folding door to be used<br>It should not be heavy and should be able to withstand the force of 20N<br>Push-button system to open<br>External doors with warning blocks 30 inches before the entrance<br>For a wheelchair user, the door should have a horizontal handle at the closing face 30 inches from the floor area |
| **Waiting area** | Floor levelling: 35.48 inches<br>If greater: to be designed as a ramp | For corridor flooring, complex patterns to be avoided<br>Carpet to be adequately secured with a firm cushion<br>Exposed edges to be trimmed |
| **Lighting** | - | White (High-pressure sodium) |
| **Operatory room** | - | Tap: Hand or electronically operated |
| **Signs** | - | Direction signs at reception, doorways, toilet, drinking water area |

*(Table 1) cont.....*

| Area | Size requirements | Specifications |
|------|-------------------|----------------|
| **Restrooms** | Internal dimensions: 86 by 86 inches | Unisex accessible toilet facility<br>Western closet with grabrails<br>Toilet paper dispenser 2 to 8 inches height above the top of the closet |

## Dental Setup for the Cerebral Palsy Patient (Fig. 16)

These children should be given special consideration, and proper arrangements should accompany their needs. These are:

1. Apprehension: Several of these children are not accepting to meet outsiders.
2. Difficulty of communication: Communication needs to be modified if there is any visual, or audio, or if the patient cannot understand the dentist.
3. Low intelligence: The child's cooperation is hampered in these cases.
4. Poor concentration: This may be a characteristic aspect of the cerebral dysfunction, inconsequential things disturbing the attention.
5. Convulsions: A child with a history of these conditions should be treated with special care.
6. Posture: Ataxic patients must be treated with the dental chair tilted well behind to give steadiness and backing.
7. Ability to cooperate: Self-assurance and relaxation can solve the problem.

## Infection Prevention and Control in Dental Practice Adopted by The General Assembly of the United States of America

This policy statement provides basic principles of infection prevention and control.

## Policy Statement [5]

Members of the oral health team are obliged to keep their knowledge and skills up to date about diagnosis and management of infectious diseases that may be transmitted in the clinical setting, adhere to standard precautions, and where necessary transmission-based precautions as set forth by the relevant authorities and to act appropriately to protect their patients and themselves against infections.

## FDI Urges Oral Health Professionals

1. To protect themselves by physically wearing surgical masks, gloves, and protective eyewear.
2. To be appropriately vaccinated against infectious diseases according to current guidelines issued by relevant authorities from time to time.

3. Immediately initiate appropriate post-exposure prophylaxis for occupational exposure to blood-borne pathogens, including HBV, HCV, and HIV6.
4. To be aware of signs and symptoms indicative of blood-borne and other infectious diseases and undergo the necessary diagnostic tests when the infection is suspected.
5. To comply with medical advice and relevant regulations regarding continuing clinical practice if an infection is diagnosed.

## CONCLUSION

The dental needs are not limited to a specific age group. All individuals, young or old, may require the service of a dental surgeon either for preventive, maintenance, or treatment, so dental surgeons are trained to deal with patients of all ages. A child, a compact human being, may undergo the same problems as any adult patient may have. Still, it is essential to recognise that children have different needs, and this is what Pediatric dentists keep in mind when deciding to open a Pediatric dental office. A child's body is a lot different from that of an adult. The anatomy and physiology of a child's oral cavity may have some similarities to that of an adult, but there are also distinct differences that require special attention. When the decision is taken to start Dental Clinic exclusively for children, it must have an amalgamation of different criteria which need to suit a child patient. Pediatric dentistry is a specialised field in Dentistry because children are a special breed of patients requiring a more specialised treatment approach. When choosing a Pediatric dental office, the art and skill of handling children should need to be mastered, appealing much to their interests, temperament, and oral health requirements. Apart from what is apparent, however, when we choose a pediatric dental clinic to be set up, one must follow all the necessary criteria, including space, decorum, and ambience.

## CONSENT FOR PUBLICATION

Not applicable.

## CONFLICT OF INTEREST

The authors declare no conflict of interest, financial or otherwise.

## ACKNOWLEDGEMENT

Declared none.

# REFERENCES

[1]     Karimi M. A standard pediatric dental clinic. Mod App Dent Oral Health 2018; 3(1): 219-22.

[2]     Lakshmi K, Madan Kumar P, Das D. Design considerations for dental health care for patients with special needs. J Access Des All 2018; 8(1): 80-101.

[3]     Mehta A, Gupta R, Mansoob S, Mansoori S. Assessment of the oral health status of children with special needs in Delhi, India. South Braz Dent J RSBO 2015; 12(3): 244-251.

[4]     Government Of India Ministry Of Urban Development (2016). Harmonised Guidelines And Space Standards For Barrier Free Environment For Persons With Disability And Elderly Persons. Retrieved from: http://cpwd.gov.in/publication/harmonisedguidelinesdreleasedon23rdmarch 2016.pdf

[5]     Rachael E. Infection prevention and control in dental practice: Adopted by the General Assembly: September 2019, San Francisco, United States of America Original version adopted by the General Assembly: September 2009, Singapore, Singapore. Int Dent J 2020; 70(1): 17-8.

**CHAPTER 16**

# Child Abuse and Neglect

**Vishwas Chaugule[1,*], Vishwas Patil[2] and Bhagyashree Shetty[3]**

[1] *Ex Professor, Department of Paediatric and Preventive Dentistry, Sinhgad Dental College and Hospital, Pune, India*

[2] *Ex Professor, Department of Paediatric and Preventive Dentistry, Dr. D.Y. Patil Dental College and Hospital, Pimpri, Pune, India*

[3] *Junior Research Officer, Pune, India*

**Abstract:** Child abuse and neglect are synonymous with the current term "Child maltreatment", a multifactorial problem affecting the health and well-being of large numbers of children worldwide. "Child Abuse and Neglect" has been discussed from public health and a professional perspective, focusing on global problems. It narrates the consequences of being exposed to this form of brutality on the minds and bodies of the child, their detection and measures being taken to prevent these types of violence. Also, the extent of the problems, the risk factors, the consequences of child abuse, and what is being done to avoid child abuse and neglect have also been discussed.

**Keywords:** Child Abuse, Dental Neglect, Emotional Abuse, Physical Abuse.

## INTRODUCTION

Child abuse is a state of emotional, physical, economic, and sexual maltreatment meted out of a person below the age of eighteen and is a globally prevalent phenomenon. The growing complexities of life and the dramatic changes brought about by socioeconomic transition have played a leading role in increasing the vulnerability of children to various and new forms of abuse. It has severe physical and psycho-social consequences that adversely affect a child's health and overall well-being.

One of the significant problems in understanding the scope of the subject of "Child Abuse and Neglect" is that it is tough to get a response from children on such a sensitive issue because of their inability to understand the different dimensions of child abuse and to talk about their experiences.

---

* **Corresponding Author Vishwas Chaugule:** Department of Paediatric and Preventive Dentistry, Sinhgad Dental College and Hospital, Pune, India; E-mail: vbchaugule@gmail.com

**Satyawan Damle, Ritesh Kalaskar & Dhanashree Sakhare (Eds.)**

As health guardians, the medical and dental fraternity should plan and concentrate their efforts on addressing child abuse and neglect. "Be human and stop child abuse" should be a motto to change children's prospects of safety and well-being.

## Definitions

The term "Child abuse" may have different interpretations in the unfamiliar cultural milieu and socioeconomic situations. A universal definition of child abuse in the global context does not exist and needs to be defined.

## Child Abuse

WHO, in 1999, defined child abuse as a violation of the fundamental human rights of a child. It includes all forms of physical, emotional ill-treatment, sexual harm, neglect, negligent treatment, commercial or other exploitation, and the likelihood of harming the child's health, survival, or dignity in a relationship of responsibility, trust, or power [1].

## Child Maltreatment

WHO, in 2006, defined child maltreatment as all forms of physical and emotional ill-treatment, sexual abuse, neglect, negligent treatment or commercial or exploitation, resulting in actual or potential harm to the child's health, survival, development, or dignity in the context of a relationship of responsibility trust or power [2].

## Types of Abuse

### *Physical Abuse*

The WHO (2006) defines child physical abuse as the intentional use of physical force against a child that results in or has a high likelihood of harming the child's health, survival, development, or dignity. This includes hitting, beating, kicking, shaking, biting, strangling, scalding, burning, poisoning, and suffocating. Much physical violence against children in the home is inflicted with the object of punishment [2].

### *Warning Signs of Physical Abuse*

The child may:

- Have frequent injuries or unexplained bruises, wounds, or cuts. Their injuries may have patterns such as marks from a hand or belt (Fig. **1**).

- Be constantly watchful and "on alert," as if waiting for something terrible to happen.
- Shy away from touch, flinch at sudden movements, or appear to be afraid to go home.

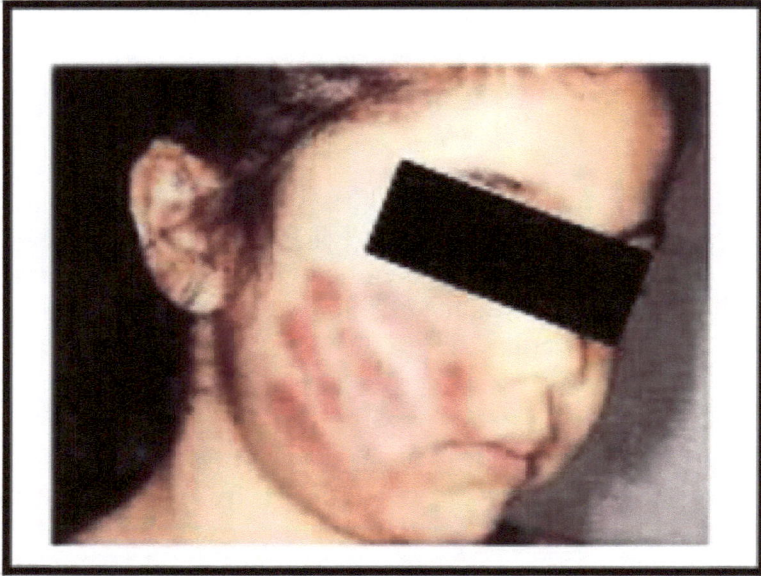

**Fig. (1).** Physical abuse.

### *Emotional Abuse*

Emotional and psychological abuse involves both isolated incidents and a pattern of failure over time of a parent or caregiver to provide a developmentally proper and supportive environment. Acts in this category may have a high probability of damaging the child's physical or mental health or mental, spiritual, moral, or social development. Abuse of this type includes the restriction of movement; patterns of belittling, blaming, threatening, frightening, discriminating against or ridiculing; and other non-physical forms of rejection or cruel treatment [2].

### *Warning Signs of Emotional Abuse*

The child may:

- Be excessively withdrawn, fearful, or anxious about doing something wrong.

- Show extreme behaviour (extremely compliant, demanding, passive, aggressive).
- Not seem to be attached to the parent or caregiver.
- Act either inappropriately adult (taking care of other children) or inappropriately infantile (thumb-sucking, throwing tantrums).

## Child Sexual Abuse

The WHO 2006 defines child sexual abuse as the involvement of the child in sexual activity that they do not fully understand and cannot give informed consent to, or which the child is not developmentally prepared or else that violates the laws or social taboos of society. Children can be sexually abused by both adults and other children in a position of responsibility, trust or power over the victim [2].

### Incidence and Prevalence

The reports of WHO in 2020 provide global data on the problem of child abuse and neglect. According to those reports, a billion children aged between 2-17 years have experienced physical, sexual, or emotional violence or neglect in the past year (Fig **2**). It estimated 40150 homicide deaths in children under 18 years due to child maltreatment. $1/3^{rd}$ of students aged 11-15 years worldwide have been bullied by their peers. Emotional violence affects 1 in 4 children worldwide, while 3 in every four children aged 2-4 years regularly suffer from physical punishment and psychological violence at the hands of parents or caregivers. Around 120 million girls under 20 years have suffered from sexual contact [2].

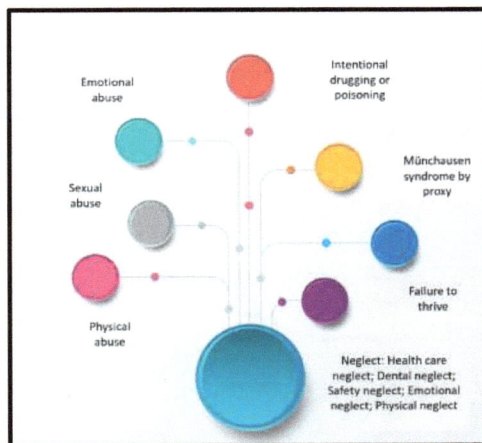

**Fig. (2).** Types of child abuse.

## Global Perspectives of Child Abuse and Neglect

Child Abuse and Neglect (CAN) is in plenty in many countries worldwide. Sadly, much of the world's response to CAN has been linked to funding levels. Although the proportion of developing countries establishing formal child abuse policies and response systems is growing, wide discrepancies remain in service availability. No universal standards exist for the best children. This is because child-rearing beliefs and behaviours differ across cultures. Many international communities have focused only on children's societal/ extra familial abuses. It has been related to child labour, beggary, prostitution, intrafamilial abuses, etc.

- International barriers to preventive efforts
- Limited resources
- Widespread support for corporal punishment
- Use of physical discipline
- Lack of effective systems to investigate abuse reports
- Protecting children on international levels

Prevention and proper response to violence against children remain an ongoing and worldwide concern and challenge. The world report on violence against children noted that documentation of the size of violence against children clearly showed that this is a very substantial and severe problem. This report highlights the importance of equipping parents and caregivers of children with the knowledge and skills to parent without violence. Abuse of children and adolescents is a complex international problem that defies simple analysis and easy answers. There may be hope for an emerging global agreement on the significant behaviour of child abuse and neglect. Some differences will continue to exist between definitions embraced in various parts of the world. This would be true in developing versus developed countries [3].

There is a select group of strategies based on the best available evidence to help countries and communities intensify their focus on the prevention programs and services with the most significant potential to reduce violence against children. INSPIRE is an evidence-based resource for everyone committed to preventing and responding to violence against children and adolescents -from the government to grassroots and civil society to the private sector. The "INSPIRE" strategies are based on the best available evidence-based recommendations to help countries focus on the prevention programs and services with the most significant potential to reduce violence against children.

I - For implementation and enforcement of laws

N – For norms and value

S- For a safe environment

P - For parents and caregivers

I - For income and economic strengthening

R - For response and support services

E - For education and life skills [4]

## Medical Recognition of the Condition

However, the current concerns about the wrongful diagnosis of child abuse centre on a trio of quite different clinical situations whose defining characteristic might be described as one of uncertainty or ambiguity.

- Sudden Infant Death Syndrome SIDS is the most typical cause of unexpected death in childhood, where primary aetiology, despite much research, has proved elusive.
- Childhood Injuries Children are by nature accident-prone, but sometimes the severity of their injuries might seem disproportionate to the explanation provided
- Medically Unexplained Symptoms All doctors have patients whose signs and symptoms are difficult to explain.

## MUNCHAUSEN SSYNDROME BY PROXY (MSP)

(Factitious Disorder Imposed on Self / Medical Child Abuse / Caregiver - Fabricated Illness in a Child)

It is a mental health disorder where one falsifies, exaggerates, or induces physical, emotional, or cognitive conditions. People with factitious disorders act this way because of an inner need to be seen as ill or injured, not to achieve a concrete benefit, such as getting medications or financial gains.

Munchausen syndrome is named after Baron von Munchausen, an 18th-century German officer who was known for embellishing the stories of life and experiences. Most symptoms in people with this disorder are related to physical illness symptoms such as chest pain, stomach problems or fever -rather than those of a mental disorder. Some signs are self-imposed, while others are exaggerated.

The term was coined by Roy Meadow in 1977. The exact cause of MSP is not known, but researchers are looking at the roles of biological and psychological factors in its development. Some theories suggest that a history of child abuse and neglect as a child or the early loss of a parent may be the factors in its development. It is a relatively rare behavioural disorder. It affects a primary caretaker, often the mother.

## Symptoms of MSP

- Parent / Caregiver – usually a mother.
- Very friendly and cooperative with the healthcare provider.
- Appears overly concerned about the child.

## Signs of MSP

- The child has a history of many hospitalisations, often with a strange set of symptoms.
- Worsening the child's symptoms is generally reported by the parent and is not witnessed by the hospital staff.
- The child's reported conditions and symptoms do not agree with the test results.
- There may be more than one unusual illness or death of children in the family.
- The child's condition improves in the hospital, but symptoms recur upon the child's return.
- Blood in lab samples may not match the child's blood.
- There may be signs of chemicals in the child's blood, stool, or urine.

## Diagnosis of MSP

- Diagnosing MSP is difficult because of the dishonesty that is involved.
- Doctors must rule out any possible physical illness as the cause of the child's symptoms before diagnosing MSP.
- A thorough review of the child's medical history, family history and parent's medical history, and parents' medical history may provide clues to suggest MSP.
- Remember, it is the adult, not the child, diagnosed with MSP.

## How to Manage or Treat MSP?

- Ensure the safety and protection of any actual or potential victims first. This may require that the child be placed in the care of another.
- MSP management team must have a social worker, foster care organisation, law enforcement and doctors.

# SHAKEN BABY SYNDROME

(Abusive head trauma, shaken impact syndrome; Whiplash shake syndrome)

It is a severe brain injury to a child's brain resulting from forcefully shaking an infant or toddler. In this, a child's brain cells are destroyed and are prevented from getting enough oxygen. The shaken baby syndrome is a form of child abuse that can permanently damage /death (Fig. **3).**

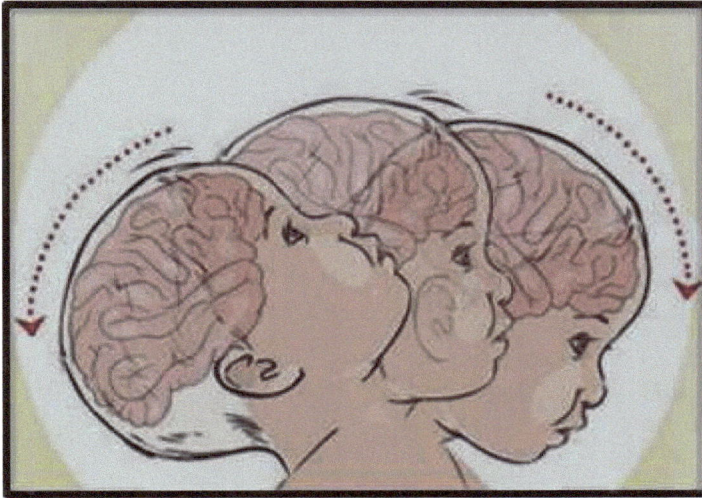

**Fig. (3).**  Shaken Baby Syndrome.

## *Causes*

- It occurs when a parent or a caregiver severely shakes a baby or a toddler due to frustration or anger, often because the child will not stop crying.
- It is usually not caused by bouncing a child on your knee, minor falls, or even rough play.
- The baby's brain is very fragile. So, when shaken vigorously, it results in a back-and-forth position in the skull. This causes bruising, swelling, and bleeding.

## Signs

- Physical injury to the child's outer body.
- Pale or bluish skin
- Bruised face
- Bleeding in the eyes
- Damaged spinal cord
- Fractures of ribs, skull, legs, and other bones.

## Symptoms

- Excessive fussiness/ irritability seen in a child
- Difficulty in staying awake.
- Breathing problems.
- Poor eating
- Vomiting
- Seizures
- Paralysis
- Coma

## Risk Factors

- Unrealistic expectations of babies
- Young/single parenthood
- Stress
- Domestic violence
- Alcohol and substance abuse
- Unstable family
- Depression
- A history of mistreatment as a child

## Complications

- Irreversible brain damage
- Death
- Lifelong medical care
- Partial or total blindness
- Developmental delays, learning problems or behaviour issues
- Intellectual disability
- Seizure disorder
- Cerebral palsy

## Prevention

- New parent education classes to help parents understand the dangers of violent shaking
- Tips to soothe a crying baby.
- Stress management.
- Seek counsellor's help [5].

## BATTERED CHILD SYNDROME

Henry Kempe, in 1962 described 'battered child syndrome. The battered-child syndrome is a clinical condition in young children who have received severe physical abuse and may be a frequent cause of permanent injury or death. The syndrome should be considered in any child showing evidence of fracture of any bone, subdural hematoma, failure to thrive, soft tissue swellings or skin bruising, in any child who dies suddenly, or where the degree and type of injury are at variance with the history given about the occurrence of the trauma. Psychiatric factors are essential in the disorder's pathogenesis, but knowledge of these factors is limited. Health care professionals have a duty and responsibility to the child to require a complete evaluation of the problem and to guarantee that no expected repetition of trauma will be allowed to occur. It is now known by the term 'non-accidental injuries.

## THE ABUSED CHILD AND THE ABUSER

Research has linked specific characteristics of the caregiver and features of the family environment. Factors related to the caregiver's psychological and behavioural characteristics or aspects of the family environment may compromise parenting and lead to child maltreatment.

**Abused or neglected children**: Some everyday observations are found among the abused or neglected children-

1. New-born to 3 years (new-borns because of their crying and wakefulness; toddlers because of preverbal frustration, feeding times with bottles, spoons, and toilet training).

2. Youngest in a large family

3. Physical or mental disabilities

4. Unwanted child

5. Purposefully evoking negative responses from parent

6. Lying, disrespect, disobedience, low performance in school

**Abuser characteristics:** Research and clinical experience help in finding specific abuser characteristics. These may help the dentist intercede before abuse occurs and eliminate or confirm suspicions when found.

1. Parents or caregivers have low self-esteem and may feel unloved, unwanted, and frustrated that their needs are not met.

2. Severe psychotic tendencies where the abuser is often a recidivist who repeats and escalates the amount and severity of abuse.

3. A lack of trust and tension often characterises relationships with others.

4. Perceive the child as a burden, different or wrong.

5. Poor parenting skills, lack of knowledge in child development and child-rearing practices.

6. The parent's reaction is either lack of control or fear of losing control.

7. Manifesting their childhood deficits and using the same coping methods as did their parents.

8. Unaware of the child's problems and give absurd contradictory explanations.

Fortunately, most abusive parents or caregivers can be rehabilitated; only 10% are considered mentally ill.

## Child Neglect

It is an act of omission or commission that denies a child's basic needs. Neglect can be physical, educational, emotional, or psychological.

Neglect is defined as "a type of maltreatment that refers to the failure by the caregiver to provide needed, age-appropriate care although financially able to do so." Poverty is mistaken for neglect — but they are not the same. Low-income families do not have the means to provide adequate care — neglectful parents and caregivers do (Fig. **4**).

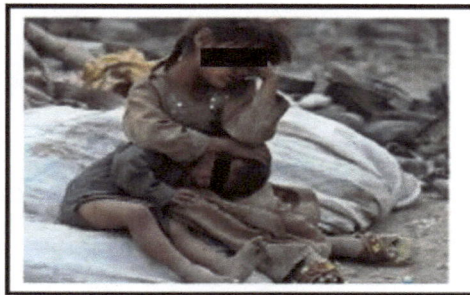

**Fig. (4).** Socially deprived neglected children.

## Dental Neglect

Dental caries, periodontal diseases, and other oral conditions, if left untreated, can lead to pain, infection, and loss of function (Figs **5a, 5b, 5c, 5d**). These undesirable outcomes can adversely affect learning, communication, nutrition, and other activities necessary for average growth and development.

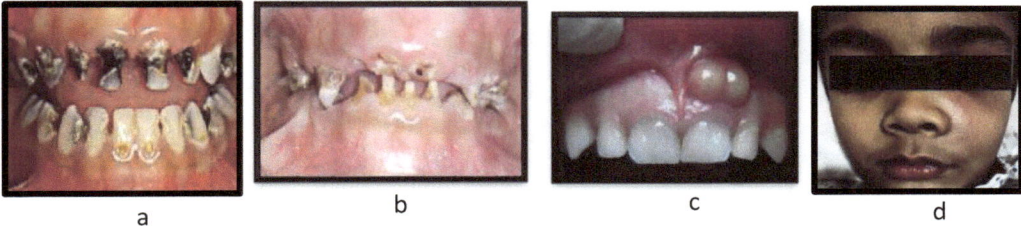

**Fig. (5 a, b, c, d).** Severe early childhood caries and facial swelling due to Dental Neglect.

The American Academy of Pediatric Dentistry defines it as the "willful failure of parent or guardian, despite adequate access to care, to seek and follow through with treatment necessary to ensure a level of oral health essential for adequate function and freedom from pain and infection." This definition was developed by the Child Abuse Subcommittee of the Clinical Affairs Committee and adopted in 1983. This is the sixth reaffirmation of the 1992 version [6].

Several factors are considered necessary for the diagnosis of neglect:

- A child is harmed or at risk for harm because of a lack of dental health care.
- The recommended dental care offers a significant net benefit to the child.
- The anticipated benefit of the dental treatment is significantly more significant than its morbidity so that parents would choose treatment over non-treatment.
- Access to health care is available but not used; and
- The parent understands the dental advice given.

Failure to look for or obtain proper dental care may result from family isolation, lack of finances, transportation difficulty, parental ignorance, or lack of perceived value of oral health. The point at which to consider a parent negligent and begin intervention occurs after the parent has been appropriately alerted by a health care provider about the nature and extent of the child's condition, the specific treatment needed, and the mechanism of accessing that treatment. Because many families face challenges accessing dental care or insurance for their children, the health care provider, including the dental provider, will evaluate whether dental services are readily available and accessible to the child when considering whether negligence has occurred. A child's social, emotional, and medical ability to undergo treatment also should be considered when finding dental neglect.

To the best of their ability, the health care provider should be sure that the caregiver understands the explanation of the disease and its implications. When barriers to the needed care exist, try to aid the family in finding financial aid, transportation, or public transportation facilities for needed services. The risks and benefits of dental treatment should be explained. Parents should be told that good analgesic and anaesthetic procedures will be used to ensure the child's comfort during dental procedures. If the parent does not obtain therapy despite these efforts, the case should be reported to the appropriate child protective services agency.

### Difference Between Neglect and Abuse

People often interchange the terms nursing home abuse and nursing home neglect, but the concepts are not the same. Although it is helpful to distinguish between the different subtypes of child abuse and neglect to understand and find them more thoroughly, it can also be slightly misleading. It is deceptive if it creates the impression that there are always strong lines of distinction between the different abuse subtypes or that abuse subtypes usually occur in isolation. There is a growing body of evidence to suggest many children who are abused or neglected are subjected to multiple forms of abuse and neglect (Table 1).

## THE ROLE OF PAEDIATRIC DENTIST IN IDENTIFICATION AND PREVENTION OF CHILD ABUSE AND NEGLECT

Child abuse, a reprehensible act, pervades all strata of society. Dentists are more likely to meet such cases in their daily practice. However, such cases go unnoticed or unreported due to inadequate knowledge. Practitioners keep themselves from reporting topics for several reasons that set up a vicious circle that traps the victim, leading to grave long-term consequences.

Dental practitioners and auxiliaries come in regular contact with children and their caregivers and thus have an opportunity to assess not just their dental health but also their family milieu. A dentist's onus in preventing child abuse and neglect was taken in 1970. The ADA appended the required recognition and reporting of perioral signs of child abuse to its Principles of Conduct and Code of ethics. Dentists are at an advantage in finding child abuse as most characteristic signs can be visualised in the craniofacial and oral regions. The identification and reporting of abuse become not just a moral but legal responsibility as well. Not just this, it is seen that perpetrators keep changing hospitals and clinicians to avoid suspicion; however, they visit the same dentist repeatedly.

**Table 1. Difference between child abuse and child neglect.**

| Child Abuse | Child Neglect |
|---|---|
| • Abuse is the intentional infliction of harm on someone, whether physical, emotional, or sexual harm.<br>• Abuse is the misuse of power, person, and trust<br>• Abusing is harming someone or something<br>• Physical abuse is when a person hits; slams, pulls hair, hurts using weaponry, murder, bites, or burns.<br>• Emotional abuse is inadequate emotional and physical care, isolation, withholding of care and love. | • Neglect refers to the failure to supply the necessary care for an individual, resulting in injury or illness.<br>• Neglect is the deliberate act of forgetting and not caring.<br>• Neglect is not preventing harmful action.<br>• Physical neglect is a failure or delays to supply healthcare, abandonment, and expulsion.<br>• Psychological neglect is also different from psychological abuse, as neglecting a person means delaying or refusing to provide physiological care to a person and allowing abusive behaviours. |

## Detecting Child Abuse in the Operatory

The characteristic features may lead the physician to diagnose child abuse and neglect. It is thus regarded as a diagnosis rather than an identification. It is the task of professionals from multidisciplinary backgrounds working together to supply care and evaluation in the child's best interests since it involves many grey areas and disagreements in defining the "abusive" nature. The dentist who suspects child abuse or neglect needs to do a thorough dental and general physical examination.

A responsible dental team follows 4 Rs when it comes to child abuse -

1. Recognize

2. Record

3. Report

4. Refer

## Diagnosis of Child Abuse

The following symptoms should alert the dentist of abuse:

1. Incomplete history or inadequate explanations of injuries should raise a concern about maltreatment.

2. Delay in seeking treatment

3. History of multiple injuries

4. An adult other than the parent(s) seeking treatment

5. Injuries attributed to a sibling

6. Children show violent behaviour,

7. Withdrawal from touch

8. Oblivious of the environment or watchful

9. Unusual sexual behaviour or knowledge

10. Wearing unique clothing for the season.

When suspicion of child abuse is present, a thorough examination is needed. The dentist should begin with reviewing the child's lips and go ahead in a systemic order to other parts of the oral cavity and the body.

**1.** Lips: lacerations or scars from trauma, burns from heated implements, or rope marks on the corners of the mouth from a gag being placed over the mouth **(Fig. 6)**

2. Palate: any unexplained petechiae or bruises that may be indicative of forced oral sex (fellatio), particularly at the junction of the complex and soft palate

3. The floor of the mouth: Contusions

4. Teeth: fractured or nonvital teeth that appear to be non-accidental trauma and any teeth missing or displaced for which there is no obvious explanation

5. Edentulous patients: bruises on edentulous ridges or severe lacerations.

6. Labial frenum: lacerated from forced feeding or blunt trauma from an instrument or hand.

7. Tongue: scars or abnormal mobility from repeated trauma or damage from forcibly biting down.

8. Oral mucosa burns from caustic substances or scalding liquids in the mouth. This will appear as a white slough from the necrotic epithelium. In addition, the child may salivate excessively, drool, and may have difficulty swallowing.

9. Radiographs: exhibit healed or recent fractures

10. Venereal warts, HIV-associated lesions, or any sexually transmitted diseases.

11. Injuries, bruises, and handcuff marks on the overlying soft tissues that are not directly supported by bone, such as the cheeks (below the zygoma), lips, neck, inner thighs, and inner aspect of the upper arm, should be viewed with suspicion, as they are more likely to result from abuse **(Fig. 7).**

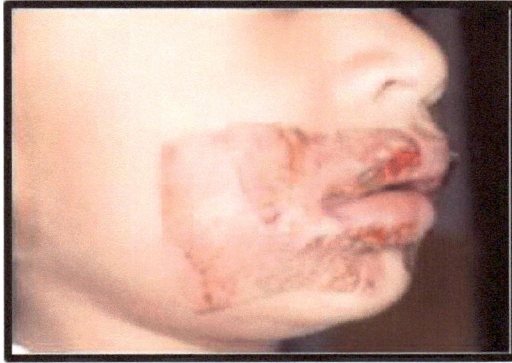

**Fig. (6).** Iron burn on cheek and lips -a sign of child abuse.

Bite marks: Acute or healed bite marks are indicative of child abuse. A dentist can help health care providers detect and evaluate bite marks related to physical and sexual abuse. Bite marks are suspected when ecchymoses, abrasions or lacerations are in elliptical, horseshoe-shaped, or oval patterns. It is usually seen because of positive pressure from the closing of teeth or with disruption of small vessels or negative pressure caused by suction and tongue thrusting. An inter-canine distance measuring more than 3 CMS is suspicious for an adult human bite (a linear distance between the pivotal points of the cuspid tips) (Fig. **8**) [7].

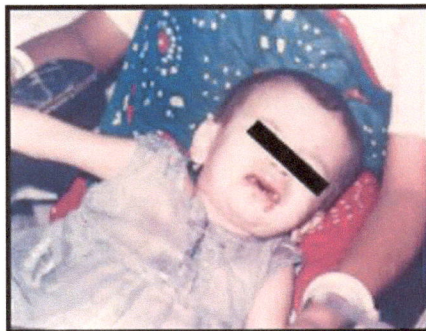

**Fig. (7).** Child with a severe wound on lips and peri-oral structure.

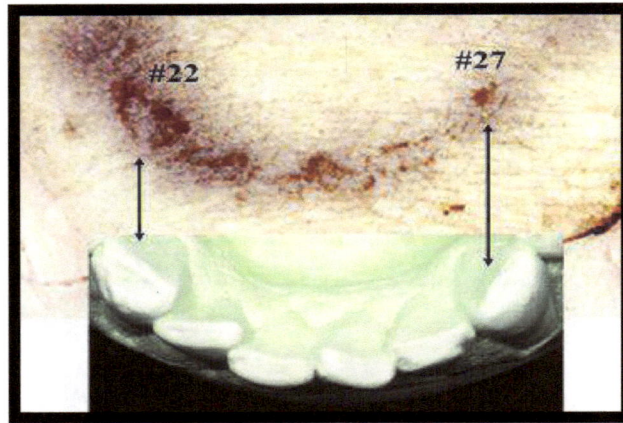

**Fig. (8).**  Recording adult bite marks on child's body.

## Recording and Documentation of Child Abuse

Conducting and documenting the interviews with the child and parents forms the first critical step in recognising and reporting child abuse. A dentist should begin with an overall assessment of the child as soon as they walk into the treatment room.

- An interview should be done in the presence of a witness, and if possible, the child and parent should be interviewed separately.
- Questions should be open-ended and nonthreatening that require a descriptive answer. While dealing with the parent, they should be informed about the reason for the interview.
- The dentist needs a goal to discuss concerns about the child's injury or lesion, reassure the parent of support, and should not try to prove abuse or neglect.
- The dentist should decide if the parent's story conflicts with the child's story or if their explanation makes any sense before reporting the case to the proper authorities.
- In cases of severe abuse where the dentist suspects the parents may abscond with the child, it is recommended to notify the proper authorities before informing the parents of suspicions of abuse. However, the ideal situation is that the oral healthcare professional should try to gain as much information as possible as well as the confidence of the parent before making any report.

## Why Report?

A report of child abuse should have the following information if it is known:

- Name and address of the child and parents, age.

- Child's present condition.
- Nature and extent of the injury and proof of earlier injuries. (Size, shape, colour, location, number, photographs, and radiographs)
- Child's behaviour alone and with parents.
- Document all interviews with the child and parents.
- Sign and date the report and get a witness to sign for the injuries and interview [8].

## The AAPD Recommendations for Dentists are as Follows

1. Health care providers (including dental providers) must report concerning injuries for abuse or neglect to child protective services by local or state legal requirements. Abusive injuries often involve the face and oral cavity and, thus, may be first met by dental providers.

2. Similarly, sexual abuse may involve the mouth, even without overt signs. Thus, healthcare providers (including dental providers) should know how to collect history from eliciting this information and manage laboratory tests to support forensic investigations appropriately. The general provider is encouraged to become aware of and consult with proper specialists in their area for specialised forensic interviews and specimen collection.

3. Bite marks on human skin are challenging to interpret because of the distortion presented and the time elapsed between the injury and the analysis. Ideally, a forensic odontologist should evaluate the pattern, size, contour, and colour of the bite mark when one is available.

4. Health care providers (including dental providers) are encouraged to ask their patients about bullying and advocate for anti-bullying prevention programs in schools and other community settings.

5. Health care providers (including dental providers) should be aware of the risk factors for human trafficking, find these in their patients (both girls and boys), safely connect the patients to resources, and advocate for anti-trafficking efforts.

6. If parents do not obtain therapy after barriers to care have been addressed, the case should be reported to the appropriate child protective services agency concerning dental neglect.

7. Providers are encouraged to collaborate with colleagues (including psychological and educational resources) to supply support to families if any of maltreatment has occurred [6].

## Why do Dentists Flinch from Reporting Abuse?

- Fear of legal entanglement
- Fear of losing patients
- Apathy for the gravity of the crime
- Wary of being accosted by the family
- Lack of faith in child protection services
- Improper education and training on the subject.

Dentists should know that they are mandated to report suspected cases of child maltreatment, with immunity granted to voluntary reporters acting in good faith [5].

## How to Help an Abused Child? (Fig. 9)

- Avoid denial and remain calm.
- Do not interrogate
- Reassure the child that they did nothing wrong.
- Safety comes first.

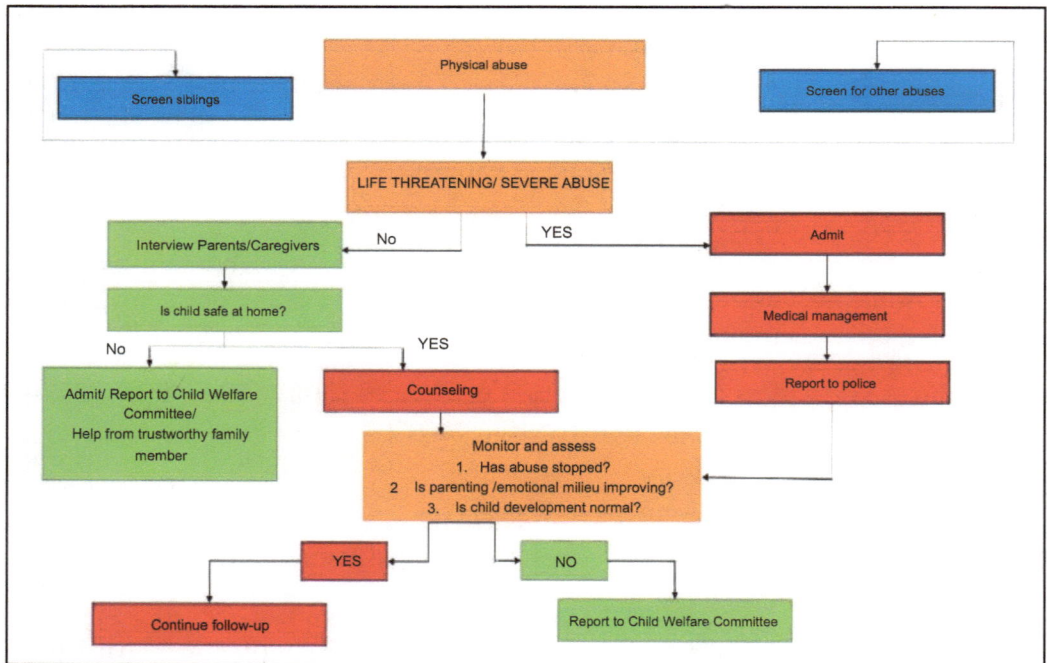

**Fig. (9).** Flowchart showing the role of dentists in the identification of child abuse.